FIGHTING FOR NEW YORK

NICHOLAS FREUDENBERG

FIGHTING FOR NEW YORK

Activism for Health and Social Justice Since the 1960s

Columbia University Press / *New York*

Columbia University Press
Publishers Since 1893
New York Chichester, West Sussex
cup.columbia.edu

Library of Congress Cataloging-in-Publication Data
Names: Freudenberg, Nicholas author
Title: Fighting for New York : activism for health and social justice since the 1960s / Nicholas Freudenberg.
Description: New York : Columbia University Press, 2026. | Includes bibliographical references and index.
Identifiers: LCCN 2025052211 (print) | LCCN 2025052212 (ebook) | ISBN 9780231221412 hardback | ISBN 9780231221405 trade paperback | ISBN 9780231565639 ebook | ISBN 9780231563710 pdf
Subjects: LCSH: Social movements—New York (State)—New York—History—20th century | Social movements—New York (State)—New York—History—21st century | Public health—New York (State)—New York | Social justice—New York (State)—New York | Housing policy—New York (State)—New York
Classification: LCC HN80.N49 F74 2026 (print) | LCC HN80.N49 (ebook)
LC record available at https://lccn.loc.gov/2025052211
LC ebook record available at https://lccn.loc.gov/2025052212
Printed and bound by CPI Group (UK) Ltd, Croydon, CR0 4YY

Cover design: Tim Jones

GPSR Authorized Representative: Easy Access System Europe, Mustamäe tee 50, 10621 Tallinn, Estonia, gpsr.requests@easproject.com

CONTENTS

PREFACE

In the last sixty years, New York City has experienced recurrent health crises—the AIDS epidemic in the 1980s, spikes in homicide and other violence, and repeated surges in the addiction to crack cocaine, heroin, and fentanyl. By the end of 2025, the COVID-19 pandemic had caused almost 47,000 deaths, 209,000 hospitalizations, and approximately 3.4 million cases in New York City over five years, as well as exacerbating the city's persistent problems of hunger and food insecurity, housing instability, and economic hardship.

Below these headline-grabbing crises, in my sixty years living in New York I have also watched other health disasters emerge or endure: a rise in type 2 diabetes, especially among younger people and people of color, deaths and injuries of construction workers and food delivery workers, a widening gap in Black and white maternal mortality, and increasing rates of anxiety, depression, and traumatic stress.

In my roles as health researcher, health practitioner, and health activist, I have also had the privilege over the years to observe, study, and participate in multiple initiatives to tackle these front-page and back-page health crises. I worked at Harlem Hospital to improve school health programs, helped to organize community education and screening programs to prevent childhood lead poisoning in Washington Heights and the South Bronx, then joined a lawsuit against the city government for failing to enforce the health and housing laws designed to prevent lead poisoning. I spent more than a decade at the Rikers Island Detention Center helping to develop and evaluate reentry programs to assist people leaving jail to find the housing, jobs, and health care that would reduce their risk of HIV, tuberculosis, drug addiction, and reincarceration. For several years, I led the CUNY Urban Food Policy Institute, an organization that helped community groups and advocates to take on food insecurity, diet-related disease, and food worker hazards in neighborhoods around New York.

From these experiences, I learned two key lessons. First, New York City is blessed with people, communities, and institutions committed to improving the health of our residents. For more than a century, the city health department, the public hospital system, thousands of health professionals, and the staffs of hundreds of community health and social service agencies have strived to make the people of New York City healthier, improve their living conditions, and reduce the wide racial/ethnic, class, gender, and other gaps across the city's populations. Together, these people have made New York City a cradle of public health innovation.

However, I also observed that these efforts were not enough to prevent the health crises the city experienced, to deploy effectively existing scientific knowledge and evidence to improve health, or to close the persistent gaps between the city's well-off and less well-off residents. In just the one year from 2019 to 2020, life expectancy—the average number of years a person can expect to live from the time of birth—dropped from 82.6 years in 2019 to 78 years in 2020, the biggest and fastest drop in lifespan in a century, primarily due to the COVID-19 pandemic. These decreases in life expectancy hit some populations harder than others. The largest decreases were among Black and Latiné New Yorkers, for whom the COVID-19 pandemic worsened existing health inequities. (I use "Latiné" to describe people of all genders who are of Latin American origin or descent.) Even before the pandemic, between 2015 and 2021, drug overdose deaths almost tripled and pregnancy-associated deaths among Black people rose almost 6 percent.

As a longtime student, teacher, and researcher of public health practice and history, I recognize the critical roles that health activists, social movements, and other reformers have played in calling attention to public health problems, introducing new ideas for solutions, and mobilizing communities to demand action from business and government leaders. I have learned that many of the advances in public health in New York City, the United States, and other parts of the world have come from activists' success in challenging the political and economic status quo that so often produced health crises or maintained enduring problems.

These insights raised some questions for me, and I wrote this book to find answers. First, why has New York City, long one of the wealthiest cities in the world, had such a hard time overcoming its most serious health problems, especially given its earlier history as a leader in urban health innovation? Second, what have health activists and social movements in New York City accomplished in the last sixty years? What specific improvements have they made in promoting health or advancing social justice, and where have they failed to achieve these goals? Finally, as the world faces new political, environmental, and social threats to well-being, what lessons can an assessment of sixty years of health activism in New York City provide for those seeking to improve health in New York and other cities in the decades to come?

New York City has long been home to a heterogeneous mix of activists, social movements, and rabble-rousers. Over the years, these collections of people have campaigned for changes in policies, institutions, and ideas that have made New York a healthier city. They helped to create the largest urban public hospital system in the nation, legal protections for tenants, the right to shelter for the unhoused, recognition of labor unions' right to organize and protect workers' health and safety, protection from police violence, prevention and treatment services for people with AIDS or mental illness, drug users, and other vulnerable groups, easier access to abortion and other sexual and reproductive health services, legal protections for the rights of gay and lesbian people, and more.

In *Fighting for New York: Activism for Health and Social Justice Since the 1960s*, I explore the roles activists have played in protecting the health of the people of New York City. I analyze the successes and failures of their campaigns and seek to extract lessons that can guide future activism that enables New York and other cities around the world to better prevent or mitigate new and recurring threats to health. Another goal of this book is to document how health activists have changed New York City over the years—and how New York City's changing politics and economy have in turn transformed the practice of health activism.

As a public health researcher, practitioner, and activist who has explored health activism for many years, I want to document and celebrate the successes of generations of activists. Of equal importance, I want to understand when, how, and why activists have failed to achieve their most ambitious goals and missed opportunities for making the city a healthier, more just place to live.

In the book, I identify possible causes for these shortcomings. Internal factors include the fact that many activist campaigns are siloed, few activists systematically study their own or their predecessors successes and failures, and few take a step back from the intensity of their campaigns to reconsider whether the goals, strategies, tactics, and allies they choose will best help them achieve their vision of a healthier city. External obstacles include the growing power of business elites over the last six decades, the increasing concentration of wealth, and the rise of an ideology that promotes market solutions to all health and social problems. I explore some of the ways activists have encountered and overcome these obstacles in New York City and suggest approaches that can make health activism more effective in the coming decades.

WHY NEW YORK CITY?

For more than 150 years, New York City has been the epicenter of multiple health crises as well as an incubator of public health innovation. Its large and diverse population, its robust history of activism and social movements, and its role as a model for the best and worst of urban policy and planning make it ideal for examining the impact of specific activist campaigns and the cumulative effect of health social movements. I also chose New York City because I have lived here for more than sixty years, giving me the benefits of a long-term insider's perspective.

While the book is focused on New York City, its content and lessons are relevant to activists working on health problems in urban and nonurban areas in the United States and abroad. By examining several decades of varied activist experiences in one of the world's largest, most diverse cities, *Fighting for New York* can extract lessons with relevance to activists, health professionals, and policymakers in the United States and around the world. As I show, community mobilizations, social movements, public policies, and new ideas on health that start in New York do not stay in New York.

WHY START IN THE MID-1960S?

The book begins with activism that started in the 1960s and moved into the 1970s, a decade that marked transitions in the New York, national, and international political economies and concurrently in the goals and tactical and strategic repertoires of activist movements. In response to the Great Depression, World War II, and growing concerns about the social impact of unrestrained market economies, between the 1930s and the 1970s, new movements in labor, civil rights, women's rights, antimilitarism, decolonization, and the environment emerged to challenge the status quo and to pose a sometimes inchoate but often powerful alterative to business as usual.

These movements continued to flourish in the 1970s, but they also encountered backlash from both ordinary citizens and the powerful economic and political interests they threatened. "Backlash" describes the negative reaction of significant sectors of a population to a social or political development. On the national level, business leaders created new organizations to challenge the spate of new federal regulations to protect the environment, workers, and consumers. In New York City, the 1975 fiscal crisis triggered new austerity policies to limit the city's commitments to the health, education, housing security, and the welfare of its residents, approaches to public policy that soon spread to the federal government.

In 1980, the election of President Ronald Reagan further consolidated this national shift to the right. In the following years, this swing forced activists to act more defensively and to seek new ways to influence and interact with government, business, and civil society. The labor, housing, and women's movements in New York and nationally, for example, looked more to defend earlier victories rather than win new rights.

And in 2016 and 2024, Donald Trump again amplified this shift, bringing to the White House the perspectives of both New York's wealthiest and most powerful residents and the partisans who had long opposed the advances of the New Deal and the civil rights, labor, women's, gay rights, and environmental movements. The election of Zohran Mamdani, a young activist democratic socialist, as New York City mayor in 2025, demonstrated another shift. Once again the city is a crucible where activists and their opponents clash to realize their competing visions for the city and the nation.

By focusing on this post-1960s era, I hope to provide enough perspective to generalize beyond a single issue, community, or election cycle. At the same time, the geographic boundary of one city allows this work to stay grounded in the specific transitions in politics, economy, and activist trajectories that have characterized New York City for the past sixty years. Readers from other places can decide how these changes played out in their own settings.

WHO IS THIS BOOK FOR?

I wrote this book for activists—past, present, and future—who are determined to bring about improvements in the well-being of people and communities. By carefully describing and comparing activism across multiple problems, I hope to engage readers who have had experience in taking on one issue—housing, health care, labor, environmental justice, or sexual and reproductive health and justice—so that they can learn from those working on other issues. By including insights and lessons derived from three or four generations of activists who have worked on various health problems, I hope to spark intergenerational, intersectoral, interdisciplinary, and intersectional conversations that can yield new insights to guide health activism in the future.

Another intended audience for *Fighting for New York* is undergraduate and graduate students in public health, medicine, nursing, other health professions, and in social sciences such as sociology, anthropology, urban studies, and political science. Today students from varied disciplines are interested in the potential and limitations of activism and social movements. The world our children and grandchildren live in and the health problems they encounter will depend on what the current generation of young people accomplish. By offering lessons extracted from the intense microcosm of health activism in New York City, I hope these students will be better prepared to define their own roles in local, national, and global health activism.

PLAN OF THE BOOK

To better enable readers to pull together the many compelling stories from health activism across the range of health problems, communities, and time periods covered in *Fighting for New York*, I have organized each chapter to answer a question that activists grapple with in planning and implementing their campaigns. Chapter 1 provides a framework for investigating activism and defines some of the book's concepts and ideas: activism, social movements, advocacy, and social determinants of health. It describes why, in my view, the mobilization of communities to improve housing, policing, working conditions, and food access can be considered health activism.

In each chapter, I profile one or a series of campaigns working on a single issue. These nine profiles in the book's chapters tell the stories of specific campaigns, organizations, and leaders, introducing readers to the accomplishments and limitations of many of the city's most important health activist battles. Together these stories constitute a tapestry that illustrates the deeper narrative of communities and populations mobilizing to make New York a healthier, more just city.

The first chapter profiles the Young Lords Party, a militant Puerto Rican group that integrated 1960s- and 1970s-style activism to take on several of New York City's major health and social problems. Its goal was to transform neighborhoods that undermined health and self-respect to create places where Puerto Ricans in New York City could win dignity and respect while pursuing education, health care, improved sanitation, and public safety without discrimination. The Young Lords showed that a militant group addressing a range of international, national, and local issues could center its organizing on improving the well-being and living conditions of specific New York City populations. Its demise in the mid-1970s illustrates the difficulty of sustaining activist groups over time.

In chapter 2, I explore how changes in New York City politics and the economy have influenced activism. The profile describes Make the Road New York, a group that has organized immigrant New Yorkers, low-wage workers, and others to improve living conditions related to work, housing, and health care since 2007. I examine how Make the Road crafted a plan that took advantage of the opportunities presented by the city's changing political economy and compare its successes and limitations to those of the Young Lords Party.

The subsequent chapters follow approximately the sequence of questions that activists seek to answer over the course of their campaigns. I chose this structure so that readers would encounter the questions and decisions that activists face as their campaigns unfold. In practice, I recognize, activists will sometimes jump from one stage to another or go back to a previous phase based on a victory, defeat, or changing conditions.

In chapter 3, I ask how organizers and activists have defined the problems they seek to fix. I also examine how they have used the frame of health to describe these threats to well-being and mobilized communities in New York City to confront them. The profile describes Housing Justice for All, a statewide housing group that has fought multiple battles to expand rent control, prevent evictions, limit the power of landlords and developers, and defend the interests of the many New Yorkers who struggle to find and keep affordable housing.

Chapter 4 asks how activists have decided to fix the problems they have identified. By analyzing the causes of these problems and the feasibility and importance of various solutions, they can choose a path that matches their analysis, their resources, and the specific windows of opportunity for mobilization and action. In the profile, I describe three campaigns of the AIDS Coalition to Unleash Power (ACT UP) to tackle problems their members had identified: inadequate treatment for AIDS, the greed of pharmaceutical companies, and the role of the Catholic Church in opposing public policies to prevent and treat AIDS.

After activists have decided what to fix, they need to map the constellation of potential supporters and opponents of their proposed solution, the topic of chapter 5. With this information, campaign organizers can decide which individuals and groups to engage and how to recruit them. A profile of WE ACT for Environmental Justice, a Harlem-based group that started its work to advance environmental justice in Upper Manhattan and then expanded to consider New York City and the nation, shows how this group mapped supporters and began to engage them in activist campaigns. The chapter also explores how stratification systems based on race/ethnicity, gender, age, or sexual or gender identities can undermine efforts to engage supporters and some of the ways activists have overcome these pervasive forces.

Once activists have defined the problem, identified a solution, mapped partners and opponents, and engaged a core group of supporters, they face the challenge of what to do to achieve their specific goals. They must choose the mix of strategies, tactics, and alliances they will use to advance their cause.

Chapter 6 examines how activist health campaigns in New York City have made these choices and how they have worked through the obstacles that arise as they translate their plans into action, then modify the plan based on the results of their activities. To illustrate this process, I profile the Lunch for Learning campaign, a successful effort to convince New York City schools to provide free lunch to all children enrolled in New York City public schools. To provide a context for this campaign, I also briefly describe earlier efforts to improve the food served in New York City schools by the Young Lords, the Black Panthers, United Bronx Parents, and other groups.

In chapter 7, I examine how activists have forged relationships with the external actors who support or oppose their campaigns. By identifying the kinds of interactions with allies and opponents that tend to advance or block campaign victories, this chapter provides evidence to inform future activism. I profile the campaign to close the Rikers Island Detention Center, New York City's jail complex, examining its interactions with supportive and opposing city and state government and elected officials, nonprofit groups, the media, foundations, and the union representing correctional officers.

Most campaigns also connect with other local, national, and global social movements. These relationships can provide new ideas, opportunities for expanded impact, and resources, as well as complications or conflicts. Chapter 8 profiles Fight for $15, a successful campaign to raise the hourly pay of fast-food and other low-wage workers in New York City. Fight for $15 worked with a national union, the Service Employees International Union, that organizes low-wage workers in multiple sectors across the country, as well as with the locally based New York Communities for Change, a city-based community organizing support center, and many local groups of fast-food workers in New York and around the country.

Activists need to assess their campaigns to decide their next moves. Chapter 9 describes some of the formal and informal ways that New York City groups have evaluated their successes and failures in achieving their policy goals. To determine their accomplishments and plan their next steps, activists consider various outcomes. These include changes in policy or institutional practices, in the capacity and power of activist organizations and movements, and in the public acceptance of their ideas and vision.

To illustrate these processes, I examine how sexual and reproductive justice activists have assessed their success and limitations since 1970, when New York State first made abortion legal, through the efforts to respond to the Supreme Court's 2022 *Dobbs* decision to overturn *Roe v. Wade*. The profile charts how New York City groups like the Committee to End Sterilization Abuse, the Committee for Abortion Rights and Against Sterilization Abuse, Black and feminist activists working to reduce Black maternal mortality, and others have modified their goals and strategies based on their analysis of their accomplishments. Exploring how these appraisals and the changes they led to altered the quest to advance sexual and reproductive justice in New York City and beyond can inform evaluation strategies that contribute to greater success.

Finally, chapter 10 considers the cross-cutting lessons from the previous case profiles and my other investigations of the experiences of health activists in New York. I seek to highlight their insights in ways that health activists can incorporate into their future practice. By proposing several strategies for strengthening health activism in New York City based on the bodies of evidence I consider in this book, I hope to provide practical guidance for current and future activists.

The 2024 election of Donald Trump and the subsequent transformation of federal policies and programs to benefit the wealthy and stigmatize or punish the poor, immigrants, women, LGBTQI people, and opponents of US foreign and military policies reprised many previous setbacks for activists seeking healthier, more just communities. I assess the insights gained from comparing the backlash and defeats across the past sixty years and suggest cross-cutting lessons for the coming decades. The book ends with the call for a New York City people's movement for health, an alliance among the various social movement organizations, activist campaigns, community leaders, and supportive public officials that can, over time, define and enact a shared agenda for a healthier and more just city.

MY SOURCES

Fighting for New York relies on a variety of sources. These include academic and scientific articles, the reports of governments and advocacy groups, archival records of activist organizations and their leaders, and media accounts of campaigns and activism. Where possible, first-person accounts, interviews with activists undertaken at the time of the campaigns, and contemporary news stories are used to describe key events and their interpretation by participants.

I also rely on several bodies of scholarship: historical accounts of activism in New York and other cities, social science research on urban health, social movements, health movements, and activism, public health literatures on the social and commercial determinants of health and health governance, and emerging work on human rights and health, urban health, and the right to the city. The reference notes for each chapter provide interested readers with these sources.

I also base the book on my own experiences. I have observed, planned, evaluated, or participated in dozens of health activist campaigns and written more than twenty peer-reviewed articles and five books focusing on health activism in New York City or elsewhere. During this time, I have learned from, listened to, counseled, sponsored research, and supervised dissertation projects for hundreds of students who were themselves health activists in New York City or who worked as health professionals interacting with activists. I acknowledge the potential subjectivity of this perspective, but I trust that critical analysis by my readers and my own immersion in the wider academic and activist literature will counteract any lacunae in my judgments.

This book is not a comprehensive historical record of health activism in New York City since the 1960s. Others have documented parts of this history, and I have relied on many of these accounts for this work. Inevitably, I have left out some crucial activist campaigns and movements. Nor is this book a scholarly analysis of social movements for health, also a subject considered by others. Rather, my aspiration is to provide evidence that can inform the next stage of activism in ways that lead to new accomplishments in advancing health, health equity, and social justice in New York and beyond.

1

FRAMEWORKS FOR INVESTIGATING ACTIVISM FOR HEALTH AND SOCIAL JUSTICE IN NEW YORK CITY

Imagine a New York City without the activists and movements that have fought to improve living conditions and health over the last sixty years. Imagine a city where public housing had been destroyed or left to crumble, as in other US cities, without rent control or restrictions on evictions by landlords, and without public shelters for homeless people, however inadequate those shelters are. A city with wage laws stuck at the federal minimum wage, set at $7.25 an hour in 2009 and not raised since, a city without guaranteed sick pay or fair job scheduling laws, and with unionization rates as low as the nation, rather than double that. Police would continue to stop, frisk, jail, and occasionally shoot people without public oversight. Imagine a city without the nation's largest public hospital system, where immigrants would have no subsidized health care and where access to sexual and reproductive health services might be as restricted as in Florida or Texas. Its schools would continue to charge some children for school lunch and breakfast, ensuring that some would go hungry. In short, it would be a different city, a less healthy, less just, more polluted, and less safe place to live, a harsher environment for New York's poor, working-, and middle-class residents.

Then envision a city whose activists and movements had achieved their most ambitious health goals. It would be a city where universal health care was available to all residents, forcing no one to forgo needed physical or mental health care. It would be a city that had eliminated homelessness by building ample affordable and public housing. It would be a city where all people—regardless of race/ethnicity, disability, gender, sexual orientation, or identity—would be protected from discrimination and violence; and have equal access to healthy food, clean air, and other pillars of health. It would be a city where more than a million residents were no longer hungry, nor worried about having enough food. It would be a city where the 25 percent of New Yorkers now living in poverty would have the resources they need to protect their health. This city would show the world that affluence can be used to benefit all people, not just the wealthiest. It would be a city that could anticipate, prevent, or mitigate health and environmental crises, not just await them with dread. This New York, too, would be quite different from the current reality, a New York that had made steady progress toward becoming a healthy, safe, and equitable home for all its inhabitants, where all residents had powerful voices in shaping their well-being.

Fighting for New York analyzes the successes that activists and movements in New York City have achieved to avoid the first, dystopian vision and the obstacles that prevented them from realizing the more utopian goals of the second vision. My aspiration is to provide evidence and insights that activists can use in the coming years to make New York a healthier and more equitable place to live, work, and play. More broadly, the lessons from health and social justice activism in New York City can also inform, guide, and inspire those seeking healthier cities and communities elsewhere.

Yes, New York City is unique, but its energy, diversity, and multiple problems make it an appropriate testing ground for new approaches to urban activism that can then be applied elsewhere. The dissemination to other cities and states of the early successes of New York activist movements in making abortion legal, raising the minimum wage to $15 an hour, banning discrimination against pregnant workers, and making free lunch universal in the city's public schools testifies to the contributions these activist campaigns bring beyond city limits. Conversely, New York City has long been a magnet for activists from around the world; their experience and wisdom have assisted the city's social movements to achieve success. This reciprocal impact further highlights the value of activists from inside and outside the city learning from each other.

* * *

Throughout the nineteenth and twentieth centuries, health activism was a force for health in New York City and the nation. Alliances between health professionals and social movements helped to confront the epidemics of cholera, smallpox, and yellow fever that plagued New York in the nineteenth century, improve working conditions, housing, and access to safer and healthier food in the first part of the twentieth century, and bring health care, education, and clean water and air to urban residents in the second part of the twentieth century. A rich body of historical and public health scholarship documents and analyzes the improvements in housing, diet, and longevity and the reductions in infectious diseases, premature deaths, and infant mortality that public health reformers, municipal government, and social movements achieved in this period.[1]

In the last century, social movements have organized and mobilized people in New York City, the United States, and around the world to take on powerful actors who have contributed to inequality, poverty, injustice, and violence. In New York City, the labor, civil rights, environmental and climate, women's, and antiwar and peace movements have shaped the living conditions, rights, and the practice of democracy in the city and beyond. Here, too, scholars from many disciplines have examined the accomplishments, limitations, and characteristics of these social movements.[2]

These previous explorations of the role of activism in advancing health and social justice inform my investigation of health activism in New York City since the mid-1960s. To extract useful lessons from recent campaigns, I apply several concepts from current scholarship to the accounts of more recent health activism. These include "social determinants of health," "health equity," and "intersectionality," defined below. These definitions explain how I use these terms and give readers the opportunity to explore recent relevant scholarship.

A framework that synthesizes these concepts and applies them to the study of health activism asks several questions, questions I seek to answer in this book. First, how have health activists in New York City tackled the "social determinants of health"? The World Health Organization (WHO) defines these as "critical influences on health," the "non-medical factors that influence health outcomes." They include "the conditions in which people are born, grow, work, live, and age, and the wider set of forces and systems shaping the conditions of daily life." These forces and systems incorporate "economic policies and systems, development agendas, social norms, social policies, and political systems,"[3] and, according to WHO, account for between 30 and 55 percent of deaths and illnesses around the world.

By examining how activist campaigns to improve housing, diet, environmental quality, policing, and working conditions have shaped the well-being of New Yorkers, I expand the definition of health beyond health care and medicine. In the last sixty years, activists have also made promoting "health equity" a more central focus of public health practice. "Health equity" is defined as a state where "everyone has a fair and just opportunity to be as healthy as possible. Achieving this requires removing obstacles to health—such as poverty and discrimination and their consequences, which include powerlessness and lack of access to good jobs with fair pay; quality education, housing, and health care; and safe environments."[4] Analyzing to what extent these initiatives have narrowed racial/ethnic, class, and gender gaps in the health of New Yorkers provides a metric for assessing the impact of activism.

Second, I ask how the relationships among health campaigns, activist organizations, and social movements influence the outcomes of activism. I define health campaigns as coordinated, time-limited series of actions that activists carry out to achieve specific policy goals.[5] Activist organizations are structured groups created by their members to support or oppose given goals and recruit and educate new members to bring about desired policy or institutional change.[6] Finally, social movements bring together campaigns, activists, and organizations to achieve more lasting changes in the environments, policies, and beliefs that shape social justice and patterns of health and disease in communities, nations, and across the world.[7] In each chapter, profiles of activist campaigns in New York illustrate how the elaborate dances of campaigns, organizations, and movements shape the outcomes of health activism.

New York City is home to what Mayor David Dinkins called the "gorgeous mosaic," a diverse population of all races, ethnicities, and classes that have sometimes acted together to improve the city for all. It is also a city characterized by high levels of wealth inequality, racial segregation, and discrimination against people of color, LGBTQI people, immigrants, women, and others. To what extent have health campaigns and health activism in New York City succeeded in engaging participants across these categories?

Black feminist scholars have used the term "intersectionality," defined as "the ways that multiple forms of inequality or disadvantage sometimes compound themselves and create obstacles that often are not understood among conventional ways of thinking,"[8] as a lens through which to examine activism. What strategies have worked to bring people together across these boundaries? When have the structures and systems of inequality undermined activist campaigns? By exploring these questions across health problems, communities, and time, I hope to find guidance that can assist activists to bring groups together to dismantle racism, sexism, and other forces that have so often harmed health and activist success.

Effective activism depends not so much on abstract theories or manifestos as on thoughtful, grounded analysis of what strategies and tactics work in the real world at a particular time and place. In each chapter, profiles of an activist organization highlight their contributions to our understanding of what constitutes successful activism. In the late 1960s and early 1970s, the New York City branch of the Young Lords Party mobilized Puerto Ricans and other disenfranchised New Yorkers to improve living conditions and well-being, illustrating an approach to activism rooted in the national social movements of the 1960s. In this chapter's profile, I examine how these roots both facilitated and limited the Young Lords' capacity to influence policy, win power, and improve health—the interrelated goals of New York's health activists across the years.

Third, I ask how health activism intersects with and differs from other forms of social justice activism. Barbara Klugman, a reproductive rights scholar and evaluator in South Africa, has written that social justice activism seeks to increase fairness in the distribution of resources, end discrimination and foster values that recognize all people as equal, and promote the participation of people in deciding the polices that affect their lives.[9] The political theorist Nancy Fraser has argued that advancing social justice requires both more equitable distribution of resources and the recognition of social differences and identities.[10] As the following profile of the Young Lords and subsequent profiles of other New York City activist organizations show, every group working to improve well-being grapples with finding the right balance between redistributing the necessities for health and recognizing the distinct needs and aspirations of different population groups. By exploring the complex interactions among activist campaigns for better health and those for more social justice, I hope to identify ways that these strands of activism can amplify their cumulative impact.

PROFILE: THE YOUNG LORDS PARTY IN NEW YORK

In the late 1960s and early 1970s, the New York chapter of the Young Lords Party fought to increase the power and voice of Puerto Rican New Yorkers and to improve their living conditions. The Young Lords, which started as a street gang in Chicago in 1968, worked on many issues—education, sanitation, policing, protesting the US war in Vietnam, and advocating for the independence of Puerto Rico. While the group confronted local, national, and international problems, health was at the center of many of their appeals to Puerto Ricans and others to join their movement. The organization campaigned to improve public hospitals, make abortion safe as well as legal, prevent lead poisoning and tuberculosis, clean up dirty streets, and reduce police violence.

It was the social circumstances of Puerto Ricans in New York that created the opportunities for the Young Lords to organize. In 1966, almost half (47 percent) of Puerto Ricans in New York were unemployed, underemployed, or out of the workforce. Two-thirds of all Puerto Rican families earned less than $6,000 a year—twice the proportion for the city as a whole. Nationally, only 25 percent of Puerto Rican men aged eighteen to thirty-four and 52 percent of women had four years of high school or more, compared with more than 70 percent of the total labor force within the same age range.[11]

By organizing Puerto Ricans and others in East Harlem, the South Bronx, and other low-income neighborhoods, the Young Lords engaged community residents in political action to improve their living conditions and reduce the daily burdens that poverty and racism imposed. A deeper understanding of how this group organized campaigns that integrated health and other issues provides a starting point for analyzing subsequent health activism in New York.

Before expanding to New York, the Lords evolved from a street gang into a multiracial alliance that brought residents of the Windy City together to fight for improved living conditions and civil rights.[12] In New York, the Young Lords based their analysis of the problems facing the city's Puerto Rican community in the late 1960s and early 1970s on two sources.

First, their organizing was grounded in their understanding of the daily experiences of Puerto Ricans living in New York City. By recognizing the obstacles that Puerto Ricans—including Young Lords members and leaders—faced in finding education, employment, housing, health care, protection from police and community violence, and respect, the Young Lords hoped to mobilize action to change these circumstances. The group recognized that for many Puerto Rican New Yorkers, poverty and disrespectful treatment by landlords, employers, health-care institutions, schools, and the police were continuing insults and sources of distress.

Second, the Lords' political analysis was shaped by other activist movements of the 1960s, particularly the Black Panthers, an important influence on the Lords in Chicago and New York and on the late 1960s activist left in general, as documented by several activists and scholars.[13] Other influences included movements for civil rights, labor, the struggle for Puerto Rican independence, the fight against the war in Vietnam, and for women's rights. Notably, several women served as leaders of the Young Lords and insisted the organization address the issues facing Puerto Rican women (see figure 1.1). These mobilizations created a political environment that supported and reinforced the more radical ideology of the Young Lords, especially in comparison to the activism of, for example, the 1950s or the 1980s. The problems the Young Lords defined emerged from this cauldron of life experience and prior activism.

The Young Lords also acknowledged the many approaches to mobilizing communities for action. Civil unrest—called "urban riots" by some—had hit more than 500 American cities between 1962 and 1973. These disturbances led to 125 deaths, as many as 7,000 injuries, 45,000 arrests, and property damage of about $1 billion in today's dollars.[14] Johanna Fernández, a historian of the Young Lords, observed that activist responses to police violence in New York City in 1964 and 1968 persuaded these radicals that they needed to "address material impoverishment and psychological trauma produced by northern racism. They felt compelled to set aside the moderate solutions to the urban crisis adopted by an older generation of Puerto Rican reformers."[15] By seeking to connect the grievances and actions of people who took to the streets with more traditional activist campaigns, the Young Lords hoped to create a more powerful force than either approach offered by itself.

The Young Lords' personal experiences and those of their families and neighbors growing up Puerto Rican in New York, or coming to the city from the island, gave them an emotional and intellectual understanding of the problems their community faced. It also gave them personal ties and lifetime connections with those they hoped to mobilize, a powerful asset for any organizer.

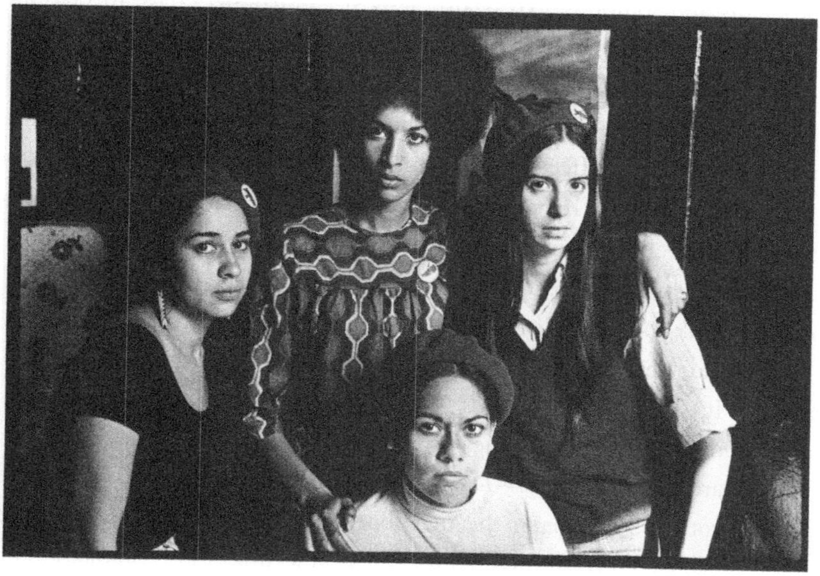

FIGURE 1.1 Women activists from the Young Lords Party. From the left: Iris Morales, Denise Oliver, Nydia Mercado, and Lulu Carreras. Describing the Lords at the time, Morales later wrote, "The struggles of the Women's Caucus [in 1969 and 1970] successfully moved the Young Lords Party to adopt feminist principles as central to its political agenda. Women advanced into leadership and developed campaigns centered on issues of reproductive justice and raised awareness about the institutional oppression of women."

Quote: Iris Morales, *Through the Eyes of Rebel Women: The Yong Lords, 1969–1976* (Red Sugarcane Press, 2016), 110.

Source: Michael Abramson, 1970. From Young Lords Party and Michael Abramson, *Palante: Voices and Photographs of the Young Lords, 1969–1971* (Haymarket Books, 2011).

In this profile, I describe three campaigns of the Young Lords—the Garbage Offensive, their work to prevent childhood lead poisoning, and their takeover of Lincoln Hospital in the Bronx. These campaigns show how the Young Lords identified the causes and consequences of the hardships and threats their constituents faced, how they came to define the problems they sought to fix, and what role health played in framing problems and solutions. All health activist campaigners have to take on these tasks to decide how to proceed.

For more than a century, community residents in New York's low-income neighborhoods and public health reformers had advocated for stronger and more effective city sanitation services.[16] The Young Lord's first campaign, the Garbage Offensive, applied this tradition, giving it a 1960s spin. Felipe Luciano, the chairman of the Young Lords in 1969, recalled, "So we're on 110th Street and we actually asked the people, 'What do you think you need? Is it housing? Is it police brutality?' And they said, 'Muchacho, déjate de todo eso—LA BASURA!" [Listen kid, fuggedaboutit! It's THE GARBAGE!] And I thought, my God, all this romance, all this ideology, to pick up the garbage?"[17]

A March 1969 *New York Daily News* report described the "horror" of tons of rotting garbage in the neighborhood's forty-square-block zone, where uncollected trash lingered for weeks at a time.[18] The first action of the Young Lords was to sweep neighborhood streets with brooms they had taken from a local sanitation depot. When the Sanitation Department failed to pick up this garbage, the Young Lords dumped it in the middle of the street, adding old mattresses, armchairs, sofas, and sinks found in empty lots, blocking drivers passing through East Harlem.

As Hiram Maristany, a member of the Young Lords, later told a reporter, "We were using the instrument of our protest, which was garbage, to protest even more. Meanwhile, the traffic is backing up. Now, it's O.K. to inconvenience Puerto Ricans and people with no power, but you start to inconvenience people with power. All the rich white folks were trying to get out of town. It created so much hell!"[19] As Fernández concluded, "Street sweeping had turned into an act of civil disobedience."[20]

The Garbage Offensive illustrates the Young Lords' radical communications strategies.[21] In the year after the Vietcong had launched the Tet Offensive against the US military in South Vietnam, the choice of the word "offensive" demonstrated the group's commitment to opposing the war in Vietnam and admiring resistance to established power. Media images of people throwing garbage in the streets after the Sanitation Department failed to make promised pickups showed the power of action.

In the weeks after the protest, mayoral candidates addressed the issue of inadequate sanitation, a topic not previously on their political agenda.

As Fernández wrote, the garbage offensive expanded the Young Lords' impact through the "simultaneous deployment of civil disobedience, political muckraking, and the symbolism and vocabulary of the era's defining decolonization struggles."[22] It also opened new channels of communication. The Garbage Offensive, explained Pablo Guzman, a Young Lords leader who later became a television reporter, allowed the group to "rap with the people of East Harlem about the revolutionary changes going on in society at large and then to connect these changes with the need to make revolutionary changes in the immediate society around them. Right now."[23]

Lead poisoning resulted from exposure to peeling leaded paint, a consequence of landlords' failure to maintain their buildings and the presence of lead in the air from leaded gasoline. At high levels, it causes brain damage, learning problems, or even death. In the 1960s, lead poisoning was the most common harmful environmental exposure facing low-income urban children.[24]

To prevent lead poisoning, the Young Lords Party launched its "Lead Offensive" in 1969 by conducting door-to-door lead testing with health professionals from Metropolitan Hospital. The group organized a sit-in at the Department of Health, successfully demanding the release of two hundred lead-testing kits that they claimed were not being used at Metropolitan Hospital.[25]

Its members tested over sixty children in a day and held a press conference to release their findings to expose government inaction. The announcement that one-third of the children tested positive for lead pressured the Department of Health to act to either disprove these findings or to expand treatment and prevention programs to address the issue. A later report by the city Health Department physicians responsible for community health programs in East Harlem, Central Harlem, and the Bronx credited the Young Lords—and crusading journalist Jack Newfield—with having pressured the city government to deal with childhood lead poisoning.[26] By defining the problem as one of government inaction and indifferent public officials, they sparked the anger that mobilized community residents to act on this and other concerns.

A party member explained the broader context of this campaign as follows: "When we began testing the children of El Barrio for lead poisoning, we did it out of necessity. Before any of us were Young Lords, we experienced what our children are going through today: getting bit by rats, sleeping with bed bugs, but most of all eating lead paint. Many of our children die every year of lead poisoning, while the landlord is only concerned if we pay the rent for the rathole that is killing our children."[27] In the next two decades, many New York City housing and health activists mobilized their communities to force the government to act more forcefully to prevent lead poisoning. The Young Lords' campaigns of testing children and then pushing for a government response served as a model for these later mobilizations.[28] As a result of these and other actions, between 1970 and 1998, the number of cases of lead poisoning in New York City fell by 60 percent and the number of children with the highest blood lead levels (55 micrograms per deciliter or more) declined by almost 99 percent.[29]

The Young Lords' brief occupation of Lincoln Hospital provides a third example of their health campaigns. In the 1960s, Lincoln Hospital in the South Bronx, a part of the New York City public hospital system, was a symbol of underfunded, understaffed health care, decaying facilities, and low quality of care. It was known in the community as the Butcher Shop. Building on several community initiatives to improve care at Lincoln, the Young Lords partnered with other organizations and launched their own campaign. In 1970, the Young Lords and the Health Revolutionary Union Movement (HRUM) created the Think Lincoln Committee (TLC). HRUM, whose members were health-care workers at Lincoln and other city hospitals, believed that patients and workers acting together could achieve more reforms than either group was capable of making on their own. TLC opposed budget cuts proposed by the newly formed Health and Hospital Corporation, the body created to run the city's public hospitals. TLC members educated community residents and hospital staff about the impact of the cuts, especially at Lincoln, where the steepest cuts were proposed.[30]

In response to the many complaints they heard in their conversations, the Young Lords created a patient and worker complaint table in Lincoln's emergency room that was open from 9:00 a.m. to 9:00 p.m. on weekdays and for twenty-four hours on weekends. In the initiative's first month, party members documented two thousand complaints, evidence they brought to hospital administrators, community residents, and elected officials—a compelling example of community research that serves organizing. Although hospital leaders were wary about the Lords' visible presence, a report prepared by Lincoln's chief administrator, Antero Lancot, concluded that "the watchdog activities of persons strongly committed to good, humanized and personalized health care, created immediate, visible, positive changes."[31]

In July 1970, frustrated by the lack of progress in resolving the problems they had identified, the Young Lords decided it was time for direct action. More than 150 members of the Young Lords, HRUM, and TLC put on long white lab coats and occupied the nurses' residence at Lincoln Hospital, a site they chose so as not to disrupt patient care. They set up clinics to screen for anemia, lead poisoning, and tuberculosis, a day-care center for the children of patients and workers, and a classroom for political and health education.[32] Hundreds of community residents visited the hospital, but by the end of the day, as police surrounded the building, the Young Lords decided not to battle the police. Again donning their white coats, they exited without being detected.

Several months later, thirty activists from the Young Lords and their partners again occupied Lincoln, this time demanding the creation of improved services for drug users. With the South Bronx's high rates of heroin addiction and the lack of sufficient or effective treatment programs, the Lords demanded a drug program that would "serve the community effectively and be run by the community." In the aftermath of this occupation, Lincoln won a new grant from the city's Addiction Services Agency and the hospital created "the People's Drug Program," staffed by Young Lords members and volunteers. The program added acupuncture and political education to the methadone treatment the clinic already offered.[33] For several years, the Lincoln clinic served as a model for community-oriented drug programs.[34]

By 1976, a new, more modern Lincoln Hospital had opened, and a citywide movement of community residents, activists, and health-care workers had emerged to defend public hospitals against growing calls for cuts in public funding. Over the years, this movement, originally sparked by the austerity measure imposed during the city's 1975 fiscal crisis, has experienced successes and failures in protecting the city's public hospitals. But through to the present, its activists have served as a catalyst for improvements in health care in New York City. By combining and aligning activism to improve health care with activism to improve broader living conditions, the Young Lords created a model that continues to inspire health activists in New York and beyond.

In their campaigns at Lincoln, the Young Lords encountered a frequent dilemma for activists. On the one hand, they immersed themselves in the mundane and daily work of improving health care, one patient and one complaint at a time—critical but frustrating work. On the other hand, many Young Lords members believed only fundamental changes would truly improve the care at Lincoln and other hospitals. As Carlito Rivera, a Young Lords member, wrote about the work at Lincoln in *Palante*, the party's newspaper, "The only way we can stop all this is not by electing someone into office, because we have tried that and it does not work. It is not done by going to college and getting doctor degrees, because that leads to an intellectual trip that takes us away from our people . . . and that we also tried. The only way to make this racist government serve us right is by knocking it down and building a new one of our own."[35] Finding an effective balance between these sometimes contradictory goals tested the Young Lords and subsequent activists for a healthier New York.

Through their campaigns, the Young Lords developed several themes that have long motivated health activists in New York City. First, they believed that when public agencies failed to protect public health, they must be held accountable. Iris Morales, a leader of the group, explained that the Young Lords "exposed what the government could and should do, and what it was not doing. Our grassroots organizing was a combination of revolution and reform. . . . [We] were determined to improve poor people's lives. After all, the richest nation on the planet had the resources to provide food,

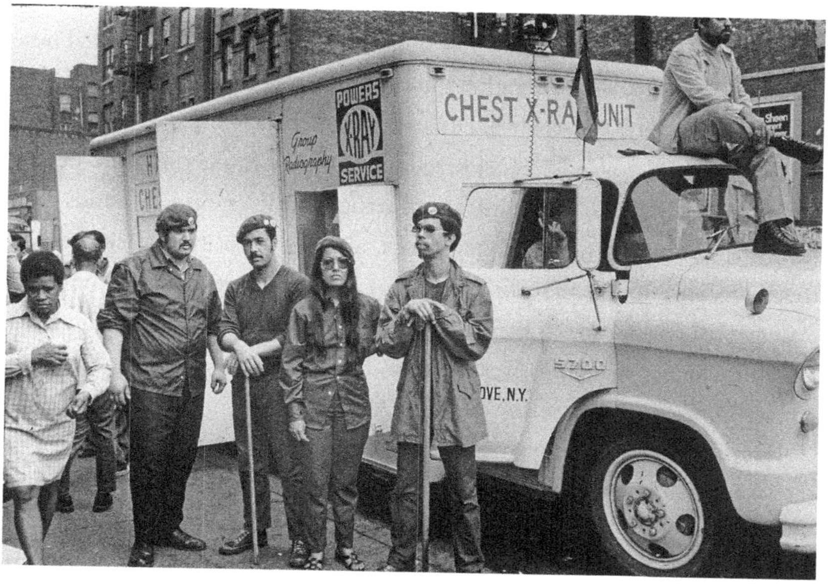

FIGURE 1.2 Members of the Young Lords stand watch by the TB testing truck they "liberated" from the Health Department while doctors administer X-rays to members in the community, 1970.

Source: Meyer Liebowitz / Getty Images.

clothing, housing, and health care for everyone. It was unconscionable to have so few with so much, and so many with so little."[36] Their seizure and use of city testing equipment for tuberculosis (see figure 1.2) and lead poisoning illustrated their commitment to holding government accountable.

Second, the Lords showed the potential for allying with other movements and groups working for related goals. In the same neighborhoods where the Lords organized, the New York City Black Panthers were offering free breakfast programs and calling out police violence. The alliance between these two groups provided a visible manifestation of Blacks and Latinés working together to achieve common goals. Parents were organizing to improve and desegregate New York City's largely segregated public schools. Many of the early founders of the Young Lords were themselves activists in campaigns for Puerto Rican independence, civil rights, women's rights, or against the war in Vietnam, making them familiar with a repertoire of tactics and strategies that other movements had used. These relationships, experiences, and networks constituted the assets the Young Lords used to mobilize their neighbors.

The Young Lords also recognized another key asset: the pride people felt as Puerto Ricans. Their history of struggle, the emotional bonds they felt with family, friends, and neighbors, and the aspirations that had led them to come to New York constituted powerful antidotes to the daily experiences of disrespect. By tapping into these emotions, the group reinforced the belief that by acting together, Puerto Ricans could create stronger communities for themselves.

From other social movements and their own experiences as activists, the Young Lords acknowledged the power of a broad vision of a better society. Through their community meetings, their bilingual newspaper *Palante*, the posters and flyers they distributed, and their demonstrations and media coverage, the Young Lords put forth a vision of communities where residents controlled their health centers, schools, and police precincts and used this power to shape the policies and practices of these institutions, and where professionals and politicians recognized the dignity of all community residents and treated them with respect.

The Young Lords identified as Puerto Ricans. But through their support for other anticolonial struggles as well as Puerto Rican independence, their opposition to the war in Vietnam, and their alliances with the Black Panthers, health-care workers organizations, and others, the Young Lords envisioned a movement that was both local and global, antiracist, and nationalist. The organization was determined to bring about transformative changes by immersing itself in people's daily lives and the issues and people they cared about most.

Although the Young Lords did not define themselves as a health organization, personal and community well-being was central to their vision and practice. The group recognized that ensuring access to health care was a priority in their communities. Their Ten Point Health Program, which emerged from and shaped their health campaigns, called for "total self-determination of all health services in East Harlem" by creating a governing board for health facilities made up of both community residents and staff.[37] The program also called for "free publicly supported health care for prevention and treatment," an end to all fees for health services, and "door-to-door" preventive health services emphasizing environment and sanitation control, nutrition, drug addiction, and maternal, child, and senior citizen services. The program also demanded "education programs to expose health problems—sanitation, rates, poor housing, malnutrition, police brutality, pollution, and other forms of oppression."[38]

As Fernández observed, these "quiet and deliberate medical campaigns were a vital part of the young organization. Involving many hours of face-to-face organizing, they represent the kind of immersive work that truly characterized a typical day in the life of a Young Lord."[39]

Almost fifty years before Senator Bernie Sanders proposed Medicare for All,[40] and almost forty years before WHO's Commission on Social Determinants of Health called for concerted action to close the socioeconomic gaps in health caused by social influences on health like sanitation, housing, work, and health care,[41] the Young Lords sought to realize in a few New York City communities the vision implicit in these two later influential proposals.

In 1948, WHO had defined health as "a state of complete physical, mental, and social well-being and not merely the absence of disease or infirmity,"[42] an aspiration the Young Lords sought to turn into practice. The Young Lords expressed their plan with the revolutionary rhetoric of the period. "Any community, union, or workers organization must support all the points" of their ten-point health program and "work and fight for them or be shown as what they are—enemies of the poor people of East Harlem," they wrote.[43] This rhetoric no doubt offended some Puerto Ricans, but it also attracted young people, those living in extreme poverty, and those inspired by the visible local, national, and international social movements. In short, it appealed to just those constituencies most ready to heed the Young Lords' calls to action.

Long before the concept of "social determinants of health" became standard public health terminology, the Young Lords took on housing, police violence, and education as threats to the well-being of their communities. In 1970, with the Met Council on Housing, a citywide housing group, the Black Panther Party, and I Wor Kuen, a radical Asian American collective in the city's Chinatown, the Young Lords staged the People's Court Housing Crimes Trial, where landlords and city government were charged with exposing tenants to "slum conditions, evictions, demolition of sound homes, soaring rents, criminal negligence and racism."[44] The Young Lords opposed police violence with boisterous demonstrations that framed abusive policing as both a social justice and a health issue. These and other actions illustrate the group's many campaigns to tackle social influences on health and to name and shame the perpetrators they believed were responsible for these conditions.

According to the historian Johanna Fernández, the Young Lords won support because they confronted the everyday issues of life: "Is my neighborhood clean? Do I have access to a hospital that will save my child in an emergency? Lead poisoning disfigured the lives and learning possibilities of children and is a problem people cared about. These issues had been discussed and debated in New York City and other cities for some time, but no organization had mounted a political education campaign around it and a strategy to force the city to respond."[45]

The Young Lords' experiences also reveal the difficulty of maintaining high levels of activism and of translating radical ideas into sustainable policies and institutional practices. By 1975, police repression, discord within the group over strategies, and a shift in its attention to the political conflicts in Puerto Rico led to the demise of the Young Lords organization in New York City. As I will show, such internal conflicts have contributed to the demise of other activist organizations in New York.

Like other movements of the 1960s, the militancy, rhetoric, and passion of the Young Lords did not always fit the changing political economy of the 1970s. The growing emphasis on austerity, the rise of conservative movements, and the increasing belief on both the left and the right that government was the problem, not merely an institution in need of reform, as well as forceful police repression, undermined the appeal of the Yong Lords and similar radical groups.

The Young Lords in New York City lasted less than ten years. The group's swift rise and fall illustrates both the potential for capturing widespread support from activists and community residents and the obstacles to building militant and sustainable activist movements that can improve living conditions of poor and working-class communities in New York City and elsewhere. As the movements of the 1960s lost strength and visibility, the Young Lords Party was unable to forge new messages, campaigns, or practices that might have enabled it to grow and change, or to sustain the support it had mobilized in its earlier years.

Despite the demise of the organization, however, through the ideas it promoted and its activities in Puerto Rican communities in New York City, the Young Lords Party left a legacy of ideas and activism that continues to influence activist leaders and movements in the city and elsewhere. I explore three such ideas that have shaped health activism since the 1960s, concepts that predate the Young Lords, but which the group turned into practical strategies for change.

HEALTH ACTIVISM AND THE SOCIAL DETERMINANTS OF HEALTH

Growing public health evidence shows that social determinants of health—the living conditions that shape access to housing, food, clean air, work, and other fundamental causes of well-being—play a critical role in shaping patterns of health and disease. The history of public health shows that social movements and citizen action have played transformative roles in sparking reforms that led to health improvements. The sanitary movement in England in the 1830s and 1840s,[46] the labor movement in the United States in the 1930s and 1940s,[47] the AIDS movement around the world in the 1980s and 1990s,[48] women's health movements,[49] and the environmental and climate justice movements today[50]—each of these illustrate that popular mobilizations are capable of convincing or forcing reluctant governments and businesses to act to counter threats to health.

Over the last sixty years, as the case profiles will show, activists in New York City have focused on modifying several key social determinants, including housing, working conditions, health care, environmental exposures, and policing, in order to improve health. In its era, the Young Lords wrote the playbook on how to do this in attention-grabbing, effective, and practical ways.

Activists are not alone in taking on the deeper determinants of health. Municipal and state health departments, government agencies with the mandate to protect public health, have also contributed to expanding the scope of public health to address social determinants. Over the years, health professionals working for New York City have played key roles in public health advances such as providing free milk to infants and children, improving school health programs, strengthening public hospitals, and winning new policies to reduce tobacco use by changing the practices of the tobacco industry.[51]

While public health agencies and activist campaigns share the goals of improving health, they differ in some important ways. Health departments seek to create systems, structures, and practices that coordinate municipal, business, and community-based efforts to improve health, sometimes requiring compromises with powerful actors who may also undermine health. And while most public health officials are fully committed to improving public health, they must answer to elected officials who are subject to political and economic forces that may require them to choose other priorities, such as promoting economic development, obtaining campaign contributions, or winning elections.

Social movements, however, may seek to oppose or disrupt influences that harm health. This might include dismantling structures, systems, and practices that reinforce or exacerbate racism, sexism, or homophobia, perpetuate the inequitable distribution of the necessities of life, or undermine democracy and community voice. These differing roles can lead to conflicts between movements and governments. The case profiles analyze these conflicts. The Young Lords, for example, seized unused testing equipment from the Department of Health and occupied city hospitals to pressure these city agencies to change their practices. They also created new structures to bring community voices into the governance of hospitals, schools, and sanitation services.

Since the 1970s, new ideologies have emerged in New York and nationally that disparage the role of government in protecting health. Instead, these neoliberal proponents of market solutions to social problems emphasize the role of individual responsibility in protecting health.[52] In New York City, the fiscal crisis of 1975 enabled those favoring this ideology to test their policies of austerity, privatization, and deregulation, experiments that later moved to the national stage in the 1980s.

In the last two decades, partly in response to the rise of neoliberalism, scholars from several disciplines have recognized new fundamental influences on health, further expanding the social determinants of health perspective. Political determinants of health describe how the structure of relationships among societal actors, the distribution of resources, and the administration of power operate to advance health equity or exacerbate health inequities.[53] Commercial determinants of health are defined as "the systems, practices, and pathways used by commercial actors" such as corporations, banks, financial institutions, and trade associations to influence health and equity.[54]

The intertwined influences of social, political, and commercial determinants of health constitute the powerful forces that shape health and health equity. Social epidemiologists label these forces the "cause of the causes"—making them suitable targets for health activists.[55]

A central premise of *Fighting for New York* is that effective collective action can be a powerful strategy for improving health and equity. By putting pressure on governments, businesses, or charitable organizations, activists can help to overcome the limitations of these other actors. They can convince these decision-makers to take up problems they would otherwise ignore. They can give those with power the backbone to pursue solutions they would prefer to avoid. They can introduce new ideas that promise realistic and effective alternatives to the unhealthy or unjust status quo. Moreover, by using unconventional or disruptive strategies, activists may be able to change the rules of the game from those that favor supporters of the status quo to ones that level the playing field.

In New York City, activist campaigns have acted on social determinants of health by organizing to increase the supply and access to safe, affordable housing and healthy food. They have taken on political determinants by supporting or opposing candidates for mayor and the city council, advocating for legislation promoting well-being, and mobilizing communities and populations to pressure government officials, politicians, and voters to advance their campaign goals. Activists have challenged commercial actors by seeking to close polluting facilities, limit the power of landlords to raise rents or evict tenants, or force medical institutions and drug companies to act in the interest of their patients rather than to increase their revenues in ways that harm patients.

Why do I believe that health activism can play an important role in overcoming the current public health crises facing New York and other cities? First, the experience of the last several decades shows that in New York City and elsewhere, the business-as-usual approach to improving health has not prevented massive harm from the AIDS epidemic, cycles of heroin, crack, and fentanyl addiction, the COVID-19 pandemic, rising inequality, persistent racial and gender inequities in health, or shortened lifespans, premature deaths, and preventable illnesses.[56] The professional mandate to pursue ethical practices requires New York (and other cities) to consider alternatives. Moreover, the new threats to health and democracy posed by the Trump administration and the Make America Great Again movement highlight the urgency of creating alternatives to the deteriorating status quo.

Second, the cumulative successes—albeit sometimes transitory—of groups like the Young Lords and others in mobilizing ordinary people to take collective action to improve their health provides an alternative to the limited impact of health departments and health-care organizations in the Sisyphean task of changing the health behavior of one individual at a time. The capacity of social movements to activate people over time also provides a powerful asset for a public health community that often lacks the resources to achieve its goals.

Finally, a historical perspective shows that the most impressive improvements in the health of populations result from the synergistic impact of health professionals, reform movements, and activists together tackling the most important influences on health.[57] Together this evidence compels those seeking to improve public health today and in the future to consider appropriate roles for health activists.

Three key concepts inform my definition of activism: Activists challenge those in power, they seek to spark policy or social change, and they work to bring meaningful benefits to communities or populations with higher burdens of disease. The profiles of New York City activist campaigns will examine how health social movements approached these ideas.

Campaigns such as Lunch for Learning's win in making school lunches free for all public school students in New York,[58] or the Committee to End Sterilization Abuse's successful advocacy for new rules to protect women from sterilization abuse in the city's public hospitals,[59] launched coordinated activities carried out over time with the goal of changing *specific* policies, programs, practices, or ideas that widened health inequities. By considering these campaigns as an appropriate subject of study—a useful unit of analysis, in the language of researchers—activists and scholars can define the characteristics of more and less successful campaigns.[60]

Such definitions build on previous work on activism. Using a community organizing strategy, Saul Alinsky, a community activist and political theorist, created the Industrial Areas Foundation in Chicago to assist poor communities to demand action from landlords, politicians, bankers, and business leaders. His books *Rules for Radicals*, first published in 1971, and *Reveille for Radicals*, which appeared in 1989, continue to influence activist thinking and action.[61]

Alinsky identified the tasks of organizers as identifying problems that require community action, stirring up dissatisfaction and discontent in the community to mobilize residents to act, and then encouraging residents and communities to develop and harness the necessary power to effectively challenge and change existing conditions. Organizers support this by creating broad coalitions and training community members to conduct campaigns on issues and problems that let them win.[62]

Alinsky and his followers were influential in New York City organizations such as ACORN (Association of Community Organizations for

Reform Now), New York City Communities for Change, a sponsor of the Fight for $15 campaign to increase the wages of fast-food workers in New York City, and Make the Road New York, whose campaigns to protect the well-being of immigrant New Yorkers are profiled in the next chapter.[63]

While activists and scholars debate the similarities and differences between activism and organizing,[64] in my view all those seeking to mobilize people and build power to promote health need to be able to identify the specific solutions to the problem they have identified in a particular time and place. This requires developing strategies that adapt to changing contexts rather than following one playbook or another. Most campaigns depend on the work of both organizers and activists.

Defining features of social movements are grievances, demands, and a repertoire of tactics, strategies, and messages. A rich literature on social movements and health informs my assessment of the contributions of these movements to health activism in New York City.[65] Some of the campaigns I describe are closely affiliated with these broader social movements, others less so. The assessment of these connections can yield insights into the variable impact of social movements on activism and on improving health and justice in New York City.

Health and social justice movements pose "collective challenges to medical policy, public health policy and politics, belief systems, research and practice," which can include "an array of formal and informal organizations, supporters, networks of cooperation and media."[66] In New York City, several established movements have supported, sometimes amplified, health activist campaigns in recent decades. In the 1980s and after, the labor movement shifted from "business unionism," an approach used in the 1950s and 1960s that emphasized collective bargaining achieved through top-down hierarchies, to "social movement unionism" that made organizing low-wage workers and advancing social justice priorities. In the last few decades, the labor movement in New York has supported campaigns to improve working conditions and workplace safety, housing, and health care.[67]

The racial justice movements played important roles, long before as well as after Black Lives Matter emerged in the wake of recent fatal shootings (Trayvon Martin in Florida in 2012, the police killing of Eric Garner in New York City in 2014, the police murders of George Floyd in Minneapolis and Breonna Taylor in Louisville in 2020, and too many others).[68] Beginning in the late 1960s, movements promoting racial justice, including the Black Panther Party and the Young Lords in New York City, provided political support to activist campaigns in housing, labor, health care, environmental justice, women's health, and policing and incarceration.[69]

Other national social movements that nurtured and augmented health activism in New York City included movements for women's rights and health,[70] gay and lesbian rights,[71] environmental justice,[72] immigrant rights,[73] disability rights,[74] and, in the last two decades, climate justice.[75] These national movements, as subsequent profiles show, offered New York City health activists new ideas, local and national leaders, an expanded repertoire of strategies and tactics, the possibility of extending local victories to other places, and the vision of multiple coordinated and aligned popular mobilizations that pursued a varied but partially shared political agenda.

My explorations of health activism in New York City map the pathways and interactions between activist campaigns, activist organizations, and social movements.

Activism, supported by social movements, can lead to improvements in health via overlapping but distinct routes. Activism in New York City has improved living conditions, promoted justice and freedom, and increased access to quality health care. In New York City, activists primarily focused on living conditions have campaigned for better, more affordable housing, safer and better-paid work, and access to healthy, affordable food. Those emphasizing justice organize to ensure that all people and communities have the rights, freedoms, and public safeguards to pursue their health and autonomy. The city's movements for sexual and reproductive justice and health, environmental justice, and just policing and incarceration reform illustrate this pathway.

Finally, New York City activists who target health care pursue inclusion and access to health care and mental health services through movements for public and universal health care, improved prevention, and care for people with or at risk of AIDS or drug use, and for the rights to care and dignity for people with mental illnesses or other disabilities.

Together, the movements and campaigns pursuing these three sometimes intersecting pathways constitute several streams of activism that have been visible in New York City since the mid-1960s. Table 1.1 shows nine such streams, which together constitute a powerful force for improving the health of all populations and reducing current health inequities. Throughout the book, I provide evidence that shows some of the ways that this activism has contributed to a healthier and more just city.

It is also true that across these pathways and within their constituent streams of activism, the health campaigns in New York City in this period have at times been siloed, in conflict, duplicative, or ineffective. These shortcomings have diminished activists' capacity to achieve their goals. In the case profiles, I describe these obstacles and suggest alternative routes to shared goals. In the last chapter, I propose strategies for creating a more unified health movement in New York City.

THE CONTRIBUTIONS OF NEW YORK'S HEALTH ACTIVIST CAMPAIGNS

Fighting for New York focuses on several streams of activism that played out in New York City from the late 1960s and early 1970s to the mid-2020s. These currents of activism, shown in table 1.1, focus on distinct health problems and population, but they also share common goals such as improving well-being, reducing inequalities, fighting racism, and promoting social justice. I selected these nine areas because they take on the major underlying causes of health and disease in New York City in this period, are well documented, and are relevant to activists and health professionals in other places around the world. Other streams not adequately considered here—transportation,[76] education,[77] and protection from violence,[78] for

TABLE 1.1 Selected Streams of Health Activism in New York City, 1965–2025

STREAM	ACTIVIST GOALS	EXAMPLES OF CAMPAIGNS
Housing	Provide safe, affordable housing for all; end homelessness	Expand and extend rent control; pass Good Cause Eviction law; expand and fully fund public housing
Work	Ensure safe working conditions; adequate pay and benefits; and the right to organize for all New York City workers	Fight for a $15 minimum wage; city pregnancy discrimination act; and Carlos' Law to increase fines and penalties for construction company practices that cause deaths of workers
Food	Make access to heathy, affordable food and adequate nutrition for all New Yorkers a right; end hunger and food insecurity	Lunch for Learning to provide free lunches to all schoolchildren; mobilize against SNAP (food stamp) budget cuts; advocate for policies and funding that make reducing food-system injustice a priority for city government.
Sexual and reproductive health and justice	Ensure that all New Yorkers have full access to sexual and reproductive health care; the right to have or not have children; and the support they need to raise healthy children	End sterilization abuse in public hospitals; ensure abortion and other reproductive services are available and affordable for all residents; close Black-white maternal mortality gap
Environmental and climate justice	End inequitable exposures to toxic environments; reduce carbon emissions and inequitable exposure to adverse effects of climate change; ensure residents have voice in making decisions about their neighborhoods and city	Close diesel bus terminals in Upper Manhattan; pass zoning rules that protect Black and Latiné communities from disproportionate exposure to pollution; close Sunset Park power plant

(*continued*)

TABLE 1.1 (*continued*)

STREAM	ACTIVIST GOALS	EXAMPLES OF CAMPAIGNS
AIDS and drug use	Make prevention of AIDS and problem drug use policy priorities; ensure access to comprehensive services; end discrimination against people with AIDS or drug users	Fund housing and food programs for people with AIDS; make condoms available to high school students; distribute free clean needles to drug users
Health care	Make quality health care available and accessible to all; make prevention and primary care priorities; ensure patients and health-care workers have a voice in shaping systems; end practices, policies, and attitudes that perpetuate racism, sexism, and other forms of domination in health care	Pass universal health care law; prevent closure of Sydenham and Gouverneur Hospitals; stop funding cuts to public hospitals
Mental health and disabilities	Make quality mental health care available and accessible to all; make prevention a priority; eliminate discrimination and stigma against those with mental health or other disabilities	Reduce or end arrests of people with mental illness; pass laws to require public agencies and employers to meet needs of people with mental health or other disabilities; close Willowbrook State School; create humane, community-based alternatives
Policing and incarceration	End violent and abusive policing practices and those that reflect or perpetuate racism and other forms of domination; ensure community oversight of police; reduce or end reliance on incarceration as a public safety strategy	End stop-and-frisk policy; decriminalize marijuana; close Rikers Island Detention Center

example—warrant documentation and analysis by other scholars and activists.

Since the late 1960s, health activist campaigns and organizations in New York City working across these nine intersecting streams have made several major cross-cutting contributions, summarized here, and examined more fully in subsequent chapters.

First, activists and their campaigns have introduced Big New Ideas that have led to changes in policy, government practices, and public beliefs. Examples include the rights of all communities to avoid disproportionate exposure to pollutants, of gays and lesbians to be protected from discrimination, of all children to get free lunches in city schools, and of men and women to receive the services and support that enable them to choose whether and when to have children and fully support the children they choose to have. These ideas that activists offered the public and policymakers have provided a vision and an alternative to business as usual. On their own, these ideas may have been seen as utopian, but as they circulated, they disrupted conventional thinking, opened space for new alliances and coalitions, and revealed practical paths for transitional changes, thus shaping New York's public and political discourses on health and social justice. These ideas have made New York City an incubator of public health innovation.

By serving as enduring and persistent advocates for public health, activist movements counteract the wavering support, limited attention spans, or term limits of the elected officials who may also champion these policies. In this way, they have helped to keep the public spotlight on their new ideas.

Second, these movements have shown that framing a problem as a health concern can be a compelling call to action, a useful platform for collaborating with other constituencies, and an approach that puts powerful opponents on the defensive. Protecting the health of one's family and community has motivated environmental justice, health care, food, and women's health activist campaigns. Lunch for Learning, the campaign that brought free lunches to all New York City public schoolchildren in 2017, enlisted students, parents and parent-teacher associations, unions of school lunch staff, teachers and their union, school principals and their professional association, pediatricians and their organizations, faith-based groups, city council members, and others, all under the banner of promoting the well-being and educational success of New York City's children, a story I tell in chapter 6.

In this and other campaigns, special interest groups or austerity-minded officials who opposed the measure found it hard to say, "We do not want healthier children, families, or communities," or "We are ok with the wide racial/ethnic, class, and gender gaps in health that characterize New York." By challenging the ideas and proposals their opponents advocate, activists can help to set the stage for success. They can also shift the discussion from a narrow focus on individual responsibility for health to a greater emphasis on public and collective responsibility.

Third, health movements have made important contributions by stopping harmful practices or policies. During the economic dislocation caused by the COVID-19 pandemic, housing activists in 2020 won passage of one of the nation's strongest anti-eviction laws, which put a two-year moratorium on landlords evicting tenants who could not pay rent because they had experienced pandemic-related hardships.

Sometimes even defeat can protect against future losses. In the late 1970s, activist campaigns to keep two public hospitals open—Sydenham Hospital in Harlem and Gouverneur Hospital on the Lower East Side of Manhattan—failed, in contrast to the successful efforts of the Young Lords and their allies to support rebuilding Lincoln Hospital. However, the community mobilization and public support these activists had generated contributed to the subsequent defeat of Mayor Koch, who had closed these hospitals, by the more progressive David Dinkins and helped persuade subsequent legislators and mayors that cuts to public hospitals incur the wrath of voters, who want accessible and affordable health care in their own neighborhoods.[79]

Fourth, health activist campaigns have expanded democracy and civic engagement. The 1960s national civil rights, women's, antiwar, and antipoverty movements believed that promoting more democratic processes would contribute to a more equitable society.[80] Following their lead, in the

1970s and beyond, health activists in New York helped to create and serve on community advisory boards for public hospitals, community districts, and other public bodies, and used these forums to win support for their health goals. Over the decades, members of activist groups testified in support of more equitable health policies and programs at legislative hearings, supported candidates who ran for office, and elected labor, housing, and health-care activists to the city council, state legislature, and Congress. They built an infrastructure for democracy that may serve as a useful model and asset in future activist campaigns to counter recent efforts by President Trump to undermine democracy and dismantle the public benefits that activists have won in the past.

Over the decades, the efforts of successful activist campaigns sometimes helped to win majority support in legislative bodies, and to convince mayors and governors that they would lose more votes, political support, or campaign contributions if they opposed these policy initiatives than if they were to support them. A related accomplishment is that these activities helped to prepare a new cadre of leaders and activists for subsequent rounds of health activism and strengthened the capacity of activist organizations to gain power, influence policy, and deepen their connections to their constituents.

As a result of these achievements, activists have contributed to specific and meaningful improvements in the well-being and equity of people living and working in New York City, the fifth accomplishment. A few indicators suggest the cumulative and synergistic impact of these contributions. In New York City, infant mortality (the number of deaths of babies under one year per one thousand live births), a commonly used measure of the public health status of a community or population, fell from 21.6 in 1970 to 4.2 in 2019, a fivefold reduction.[81] Mortality rates (deaths of people of all ages per one thousand residents), another commonly used measure of overall health, fell from 11.2 in 1970 to 6.3 in 2019, an almost twofold reduction.[82]

These dramatic reductions in key indicators of health reflect real improvements in population health. Throughout *Fighting for New York*, I explore what is and is not known about the impact of specific activist campaigns and what steps can be taken to fill these gaps in knowledge. But the fact that evidence is lacking because of insufficient previous study of activism need not lead to inaction. In my view, failing to consider the past and future role of activism in confronting the ongoing political, economic, environmental, and social risks to health that the people of New York and other cities face constitutes public health malpractice.

A VISION FOR A HEALTHIER, MORE JUST CITY

In *Fighting for New York*, I identify the problem framing, tactics, and strategies that activists can use to continue to achieve, amplify, and scale the victories they have won in the last sixty years. I also examine the systemic obstacles and the unsuccessful approaches that have prevented health activists in New York City from realizing their most ambitious goals.

Theoretical frameworks, scholarly analyses, and activist manifestos may be necessary, but they do not suffice to guide the decisions that activists make about what to do tomorrow or next year. Those choices are forged in their daily practice, their interactions with their constituents and powerful actors, and changes in politics and the economy.

All activists, however, are motivated and inspired by a vision of another city, another world, where today's problems are fewer and smaller and the potential for achieving higher levels of well-being and social justice are greater. By charting the changing characteristics of the sometimes explicit, and often implicit, visions that have motivated health activists in New York City over the years, I hope to contribute to the creation of a vision that can lead to more effective action for health in the decades to come.

2

HOW NEW YORK CITY'S POLITICS AND ECONOMY SHAPE ACTIVISM

The success of activists depends on their skills in engaging and mobilizing core supporters, forming alliances with other constituencies, and choosing the right strategies and tactics to pursue their goals. But to achieve changes in policy that lead to improvements in health, activists must understand how the political and economic context in which they carry out these tasks affects the daily lives of the people and institutions they seek to organize. With such insights, organizers of activist campaigns can identify new ways to engage people, connect their political aspirations to the problems they are experiencing, and choose strategies that fit the times. Without such a grounding, activism can become empty gestures unlikely to have an impact.

Since the late 1960s, New York City has experienced profound changes in the people who live in the city, the economy that supports the region, and the politics that determine who decides what about the city's direction. These fluctuations in turn shape patterns of health and disease and the opportunities and constraints faced by activists. I begin this chapter with an overview of the changes in New York's people, economy, and politics over the last sixty years and consider the implications of these transformations for activism.

To show how these changes affected one activist organization, the chapter ends with a profile of Make the Road New York (MRNY), an organization founded in 2007 and still active in 2026. In the first decades of the twenty-first century, MRNY organized the many Latiné, Caribbean, and Asian immigrants who had recently come to Brooklyn and Queens, New York City's most diverse boroughs. They joined with labor groups to organize car-wash workers and later fast-food workers to win better pay and safe working conditions. They helped more than eleven thousand people to enroll in health insurance under the Affordable Care Act. By comparing MRNY to the Young Lords, I illustrate some of the ways that changing times leads to changing activism, but also the consistencies over time among people and groups dedicated to improving health and promoting social justice.

CHANGES IN PEOPLE

In 1970, 7.9 million people lived in New York City, of whom 37 percent were Black or Latiné, and less than 15 percent lived below the federal poverty line, then defined as making less than $4,000 a year.[1] Fifty years later, in 2020, almost a million more people lived in New York City. Blacks and Latinés now constituted 48 percent of the population. The proportion of foreign-born New Yorkers doubled, from 18.2 percent in 1970 to 36 percent in 2020. And using an expanded definition of poverty that considered the rising costs of housing, food, and other necessities, the Robin Hood Foundation and Columbia University's Center on Poverty and Social Policy reported that in 2023, the city's poverty rate hit 25 percent—two million people, one in four New Yorkers—nearly double the 2023 national poverty rate of 13 percent calculated using the same definition.[2]

Throughout the last sixty years, New York City had the highest population density of any big city in the United States. In 2020, the density was

29,091 people per square mile, compared to the US average population density of 94 people per square mile, or Los Angeles with 8,304.[3] Population density is relevant to this discussion for two reasons. On the one hand, dense populations, especially of low-income people, have higher rates of infectious diseases, mental health conditions, and a variety of other health problems.[4] For better-off populations, density is less harmful.

On the other hand, social movements thrive in high-density areas, perhaps because activists find it easier to organize and mobilize in packed populations, where likely supporters are easier to find and engage, social networks are denser, and, especially in New York City, media can amplify activists' messages. For activists, New York City's density and diversity have made it easier to find and mobilize the critical mass of people necessary to jump-start political action.

Three major global and national trends served as drivers of New York City's population changes in this period: (1) increased migration to New York City from other countries and other parts of the United States; (2) the departure of many middle-class and white New Yorkers for the suburbs; and (3) beginning in the 1970s and 1980s, gentrification brought wealthier residents to some city neighborhoods and concentrated the poor in others.

From New York's earliest days, changing patterns of immigration have brought new residents into the city. The Great Migration, the movement of Black Americans from the South to the North to escape segregation and seek greater opportunities, brought two waves of new residents to New York, the first from 1916 to 1940, and the second from 1941 to 1970.[5] Between 1940 and 1970, the number of Blacks living in New York City almost quadrupled and their proportion of the population more than tripled.[6] In her book *The Warmth of Other Suns*, Isabel Wilkerson describes the profound impact of this migration on the people who moved and the communities in which they settled.[7] In the 1960s and 1970s, many of New York City's leading Black activists came from families who were part of this wave—just one example of its impact on social mobilization.

Who lives in and leaves New York molds the city's politics, but politics also shapes who comes to the city. From the late 1920s to the early 1970s, most New Yorkers had been born in America, due to the 1924 federal immigration quotas that shut what New York poet and activist Emma Lazarus called the "golden door" that "glows world-wide welcome." In a recurring trope in US history, the law was motivated by nativist fears of losing the country's white dominance.[8]

By the 1950s, more than 80 percent of New Yorkers were native-born. In 1965, the Immigration and Nationality Act, signed by President Lyndon Johnson, dropped some of the earlier ethnic restrictions. The law made it easier for immigrants from Asia and Africa and those joining family members already here to come to New York, leading to a surge of migration that brought new people, new opportunities for economic growth—and new problems to the city.

New York City was also the destination of choice for people from other parts of the world, often pushed from their countries of origin by poverty, conflict, and stark inequalities. Since 1965, millions of Chinese, Dominican, Jamaican, and Mexican immigrants have come to New York City,[9] transforming the city's neighborhoods, cultures, diets, and eventually its politics. Some came to escape poverty and seek new opportunities, others to join family members who had already settled in the city. Some migrants brought a history of activism from their previous residences, adding to the repertoire of ideas and strategies available to the city's social movements.

Across the city, ethnic enclaves emerged: Puerto Ricans in East Harlem and the South Bronx, Dominicans in Washington Heights, Haitians in Flatbush, Brooklyn, and Chinese in Corona, Flushing, and Elmhurst in Queens. These new ethnic communities, adding to or replacing earlier European enclaves, became important sites for organizing and activism for the Young Lords, MRNY, and other groups.

In the last two decades, fluctuations in US immigration policy brought new migrant groups to New York—Venezuelans, Haitians, people from West African nations, Russia, Uzbekistan, India, and Peru. Especially in the first and second Trump administrations, new policies and politics also deterred immigrants from coming to the United States and made the city's immigrants targets for federal law enforcement agencies.[10]

In 2021, Governors Greg Abbott in Texas and Ron DeSantis in Florida began busing recent immigrants from Central America and elsewhere from their states to New York and other cities on the East and West Coasts. By June 2024, more than 45,000 migrants had been bused from Texas to New York City, with their tickets paid for by Texas. "I took the border to them," Mr. Abbott told a cheering crowd at the 2024 Republican National Convention. "Those buses will continue to roll until we finally secure our border."[11]

By the end of 2023, more than 175,000 migrants had come to New York City, overwhelming the city's shelter system, emergency food programs, and other social services—and aggravating conflicts among politicians and voters who favored and opposed immigration restrictions and within neighborhoods struggling to cope with their new residents.[12] These new populations provided opponents of immigration with new targets for restrictive policies, an illustration of how changes in populations can be used to trigger changes in politics and the landscape for activism on immigration.

In the second half of the twentieth century, many white working- and middle-class people moved from New York and other cities around the country to the rapidly growing suburbs, the second population shift of this era. Between 1970 and 1980, New York City lost 10 percent of its population, mostly to surrounding suburbs on Long Island and north of the city.[13] Their departure reduced the city's tax revenues and made many neighborhoods more segregated.

By 1990, New York City had 3.6 million fewer white residents than in 1950 and more than 3 million additional residents who were Black, Latiné, or Asian, a historic change with profound implications for the political landscape of the city.[14] In 2024, two-thirds of the city's population were people of color, making New York a "majority minority" city, a place that had to realign its housing, work, health-care, and education policies to more closely match the needs of its people.[15] This process, playing out across the United States, has sparked a fierce backlash and created new cohorts of Black and immigrant political leaders. These two trends set the stage for the immigration activism that will shape New York City's politics in the coming years.

The third and final population trend is gentrification, simply defined as "the production of urban space for more affluent users."[16] Gentrification moves people, but it results from moving money and investing in housing and other development in some neighborhoods and disinvesting in others. In New York City, gentrification has pulled wealthy people into some neighborhoods in Manhattan and Brooklyn and displaced lower-income residents into lower-cost neighborhoods in Queens and the Bronx, concentrating poverty in some neighborhoods and disrupting the social networks that sustain health.

Urban planning scholars point out the costs of gentrification for low-income New Yorkers: higher housing prices, more segregated schools and hospitals, and policing that targets people of color.[17] But they also note benefits: better access to healthy food, improvements in some local schools that now also serve wealthier New Yorkers, and retail outlets that provide a wider range of choices.[18] In the last few decades, housing, health-care, policing, and education activists have fought to minimize the harms, maximize the benefits, and claim a voice in shaping the pace of gentrification.[19]

Cea Weaver, a leader at Housing Justice for All, an activist coalition profiled in chapter 3, explained how organizers can best understand the connections between gentrification and politics. "Gentrification is happening because people at the top want to make money by extracting it from already divested communities so following the money is the most important thing. . . . That's how you are going to find the best strategy to fight gentrification."[20]

CHANGES IN THE ECONOMY

Changes in who lives and works in New York City modify who is at risk for poor health and what issues are likely to activate residents to work to improve their well-being. As the overview of demographic changes in

New York City showed, these population shifts are inextricably linked to economic changes in the city and the nation since the 1960s.

These economic changes constitute the second profound transformation that has shaped the city's health and the landscape for activism. Three interrelated economic shifts have served as drivers: increasing wealth and income inequality, reductions in the availability and affordability of housing, and the dynamic collapse and growth of job markets. Mapping these trends helps activists to understand emerging threats and to identify the paths leading to more effective strategies for improving health.

No economic development has more fundamentally altered New York City than the rise of wealth and income inequality. From the mid-1940s to the late 1970s the share of total income going to the wealthiest 1 percent in the United States and in New York City stayed remarkably steady—about 10 percent of all income. A post–World War II economic boom, federal policies that supported working people, more equitable income tax rates, and a vigorous labor movement contributed to this stability.

By 1990, however, the share of income going to the top 1 percent in New York City rose to almost 20 percent, reaching a peak of 44 percent in 2007, almost twice the also skyrocketing national share of 23.5 percent going to the 1 percent.[21] Since 2014, income inequality has continued to widen in New York City, although not as rapidly as in earlier decades.[22] Between 2019 and 2023, New York City's high-wage workers gained 18.2 percent in real wages while low-wage workers saw their wages increase by only 6 percent.[23]

Wealth inequality describes the unequal distribution of assets among individuals, groups, or organizations, making it a more durable measure of inequity than annual income. New York City is also a national leader in wealth inequality, and wealth gaps reflect and widen racial/ethnic gaps. According to a 2025 report by the Robin Hood Foundation, the median value of all assets for white New York City residents was $320,000, for Asian New Yorkers $43,100, for Black residents $2,800, and for Latiné residents $0, meaning debts and assets balanced each other out.[24] Differences in home ownership rates were the largest contributor to wealth gaps, followed by differences in employment and income.

How does wealth inequality lead to health differences and changing opportunities for activism? In New York City and around the world, household wealth and income are the most powerful and consistent predictors of differences in longevity, premature death, and preventable illness.[25] During the COVID-19 pandemic, to give just one example, people living in the poorest New York City neighborhoods died from coronavirus infection at more than double the rate of more affluent neighborhoods, according to New York City Health Department data.[26] In zip codes where at least 30 percent of people live in poverty, the death rate from COVID-19 in 2020 was 232 for every 100,000 people—compared to 100 in low-poverty neighborhoods.[27] The excess burden of COVID-19 deaths resulted from the cumulative impact of income-associated risks, including less access to health care, more dangerous working conditions, less ability to isolate, and more crowded housing.

During the pandemic, 1.1 million New Yorkers worked outside the home during the time when most businesses were shut. These workers in food, health care, emergency services, and other sectors came to be known as "essential workers." Almost three-quarters (72 percent) were people of color, 46 percent had been born outside the United States, and 46 percent identified as female. While the media, public officials, and the public celebrated the dedication of these workers, they contracted COVID-19 at higher rates, worked in unsafe conditions, often lacked job benefits, and were usually paid low wages.[28] They illustrate some of the ways that in the context of high rates of economic inequality, disasters have disparately harmed vulnerable New Yorkers.

While the political mobilization generated by COVID-19 was less evident and enduring than the activism the AIDS epidemic had triggered forty years earlier, it was low-wage workers in health care and food service who demanded better workplace protections, residents of low-income neighborhoods in the Bronx who organized mutual aid support, and tenants at risk of eviction who mobilized to demand changes in city policies that contributed to the disparate impact of COVID-19 by class and race.[29] Once again, a health crisis precipitated a wave of activism.

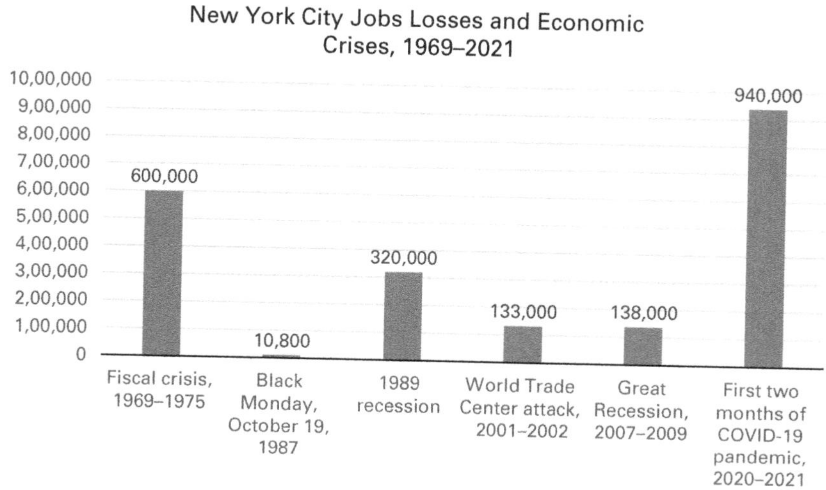

FIGURE 2.1 Contractions of the New York City Labor Market, 1969–2021.

Sources: See notes 33–37 in this chapter.

New York City's prominent role in the national and international economies has long attracted capital and wealthy individuals from around the world, but it has also made the city vulnerable to the shocks of global economic expansions and contractions. Key metrics of these changes are jobs lost and jobs gained, and the resulting impact on income distribution in the city.

Between 1970 and 2025, New York City experienced economic contractions in 1975, 1987, 1989, 2001, 2007, and 2020, often connected to national recessions. These downturns contributed to staggering job losses, a total of more than 2 million jobs lost across these six economic crises, as shown in figure 2.1. Two years after the start of the COVID-19 pandemic in New York City in March 2020, the worst short-term shock to employment in the city, the New York City economy still had 200,000 fewer jobs than before the pandemic.[30]

These recurrent yet unpredictable recession-related job losses have triggered a cascade of health-damaging consequences for the people of New York City.[31] Families of workers who lost their jobs could no longer afford housing, food, health care, and other necessities of life. Lost government revenues (and austerity-minded politicians) led to cuts in social benefits and safety net programs, further increasing misery. In each crisis, unemployment rates were higher for Blacks and Latinés than for whites, further widening the gap in health.

Young people were especially hard hit by spikes in unemployment. Teen unemployment in the city soared from about 10 percent in 1969 to more than 30 percent in 1976.[32] In the immediate aftermath of the 2007–2009 Great Recession, the unemployment rate among the city's eighteen- to twenty-nine-year-old labor force—18 percent—more than doubled in one year, making it 8 percentage points above the overall city rate.[33] As young people lost opportunities for legal jobs, the illegal economy suddenly had an eager workforce of thousands of young people looking for pay, leading to an expansion of the drug, gun, and sex trades, with resulting increases in addiction, violence, and infectious diseases.[34]

Recoveries followed recessions, but by the second decade of the twenty-first century, these cycles had transformed New York's job base. Between 1970 and 2014, the number of private-sector jobs in manufacturing in New York City fell by almost 12 percent, a loss of 864,174 jobs that reduced the proportion of city private-sector jobs in manufacturing from 21.5 percent to 2.8 percent. This precipitous decline hit hardest working-class families and the neighborhoods where they were concentrated.[35] It also reduced the membership and power of the labor unions that had been progressive forces in New York City for more than a century, depriving activist movements of the political impact of their most influential partner.

With the shrinking of the city's industrial and manufacturing economy, which had supported New Yorkers moving into the middle class for the last century, the number of low-wage jobs in services, construction, finance, and food blossomed. A new precarious workforce emerged, characterized by low wages, low job security, few benefits, and unsafe working conditions. In 2022, low-wage workers held 24 percent of the city's jobs, accounting for 64 percent of the job growth between 2020 and 2022.[36] Between 2013 and 2022, this growing low-wage group lost income while middle- and high-income workers gained.[37]

Triggered by changes in the global, national, and New York City economies, new patterns of employment have modified the incomes, working conditions, and workplace exposures of millions of New Yorkers. These alterations have created new threats to health, widened socioeconomic and racial/ethnic inequities in health—and sparked bouts of activism to modify these emerging threats.

For activists, mapping the pathways by which economic changes such as fiscal crises and recessions influence people's working and living conditions, as well as their freedoms and rights, can suggest new directions for political mobilization and organizing as well as identify emerging threats to the success of their campaigns.

The fate of the welfare rights movement illustrates how economic changes can derail a movement. This movement erupted in New York and other cities around the country in the 1960s to protect and expand the rights and public benefits created in the New Deal. Inspired by the African American civil rights movement, the welfare rights movement organized recipients of welfare to demand a voice in welfare policy and the right to be treated with respect.[38] Unlike some movements, which accepted outsiders as leaders, welfare activists insisted that people on welfare had to lead the movement. While organizing welfare recipients continued into the 1970s, the fiscal crisis led New York and other cities and states to cut rather than expand benefits. A strategy that had seemed to fit the times no longer achieved successes, leading to the slowdown of this approach.

In the past half century, a cascade of changes at the global, national, and municipal levels have transformed New York's political economy, making any simple explanation of cause and effect difficult. However, two changes stand out as they profoundly altered the well-being of millions of New Yorkers and served as catalysts for forceful activism in this period.

The first is the rise of low-wage precarious labor in New York's workforce, and the second is the rising role of global and corporate capital and investment in the city's housing market. Together these trends accelerated the transfer of wealth from working- and middle-class residents to business owners, investors, and big landlords.

Changes in housing and neighborhood development also transformed the city and the health of its people. For the last sixty years, New York City neighborhoods have experienced dynamic processes of disinvestment, abandonment, reinvestment, and gentrification. Changes in the city's population, investors' ongoing quest for new sources of profit from the city's real estate, the consolidation of the city's development and real estate industries, and the decreasing availability of land for new developments served as economic drivers of these changes.

As middle-class people left the city for the suburbs during and after World War II, it became less profitable for small- and medium-sized landlords to operate buildings in the neighborhoods where lower-income people of color were replacing departing middle-income whites, trends accelerated by zoning laws and real estate practices that perpetuated racial segregation.[39]

In the 1970s, high fuel costs and rising inflation further challenged landlords. Landlords cut back on maintenance, failed to pay property taxes, and, eventually, some abandoned their buildings, triggering a cycle of disinvestment. Local stores went out of business, visitors avoided the areas, and city agencies moved their offices to more populated areas. As a result, the better-off moved out, leaving many neighborhoods more segregated by race/ethnicity and income than they had been.

In 1976, a city housing official told *The New York Times* that he estimated about 36,000 buildings a year had been abandoned since 1970—a staggering loss of housing.[40] Empty lots and vacant buildings proliferated in the city's poorest neighborhoods. In the South Bronx, where abandonment rates were highest, neighborhoods that had been cut in two by the Cross Bronx Expressway, championed by Robert Moses, were especially hard hit. After the highway was built, property values in the South Bronx plummeted. Subsequent disinvestment, arson, and cutbacks in city services combined to destroy about 80 percent of the housing stock and displace about 250,000 residents.[41]

As public health researchers Deborah and Rodrick Wallace have shown, these declines in living conditions and public safety contributed to the rise of tuberculosis, drug addiction, HIV infection, maternal mortality, and other health problems.[42] These trends also sparked new activism around housing, health care, public safety, sanitation, and other city services, creating organizations and movements that helped to ignite the city's subsequent rounds of health activism.

By the 1980s, some groups found that these disinvested neighborhoods offered new opportunities. People returning to the cities from the suburbs, artists looking for affordable housing and studios, college graduates settling in the city, and others began to buy the inexpensive properties in these neighborhoods, fix them up, and move in—early harbingers of gentrification. Gentrification pushed poor people from mixed neighborhoods to ones that concentrated poor people of color. But it also changed the mix of housing available in many neighborhoods.

For activists, a key challenge posed by these trends is how to make New York City safe for those populations displaced or harmed by gentrification. In the 2020s, as the historian Mark Naison has observed, "it is more likely that the Bronx will receive refugees from gentrification in other boroughs than to be gentrified itself."[43]

By the 1990s, the capital needed to restore the larger or more damaged buildings was often beyond the reach of the early gentrifiers. The pursuit of more profitable rates of return by the city's real estate industry led to a new interest in redevelopment. The growing financialization of the city's economy supported this trend in two ways. First, banks and real estate investors in New York and around the world decided that property was a promising avenue for the pursuit of higher returns on investment, especially in New York, where the city's existing built footprint and its geographic limits ensured that values could only go up. As the city's real estate industry became increasingly consolidated, it provided most of the capital needed for housing development, especially as the federal, state, and city governments lost interest in financing new housing.[44] The real estate industry's absorption of capital is a defining characteristic of the city's current financialized, real estate–driven economy. It also illustrates how market actors have become such a dominant political force, requiring activists to take on these commercial powers in addition to their efforts to influence government actors.

Over the next few decades, the financial and real estate industries pursued several overlapping ventures: building new middle- and high-income housing in poor and wealthier neighborhoods, investing in deteriorated real estate in poor neighborhoods with the hope of reselling as property values increased, and buying up occupied buildings and driving out the tenants with poor maintenance and harassment to flip the building as neighborhoods gentrified. Each of these strategies made housing less affordable, worsened housing segregation, drove out working-class and low-income residents, and concentrated poor people in under-resourced neighborhoods.[45]

* * *

As the city's economy improved, in the 1990s the city allocated more than $5 billion in public money to encourage housing development and revitalize neighborhoods.[46] This reduced vacant land and housing and improved housing conditions, but it also increased housing demand, rents, and property values. Other factors helped to reconstitute the city's housing market by driving up prices. Almost a million immigrants migrated to the city and financial and business services, now pillars of the city's economy, further accelerated employment and income growth.[47]

Again, these new investments contributed to gentrification. A 2017 study by researchers at University of California, Berkeley, New York University, and several community organizations found that New York City had 314 "super gentrified" areas in Manhattan, Brooklyn, and Queens with extremely high concentrations of wealthy residents.[48] In many of these neighborhoods, city-subsidized projects like the Barclays Center, the sports stadium in Brooklyn, became focal points for gentrification—and protest.[49] "The Plaza at the Barclays Center will quickly become one of Brooklyn's great public spaces," said Bruce Ratner, the president of Forest City, the developer for the center. "I knew, way back when, that the plaza at Barclays would come in handy as a central spot for protest in Brooklyn," Daniel Goldstein, a cofounder of Develop Don't Destroy Brooklyn, wrote on Facebook. "One silver lining."

By the 2020s, the New York City Economic Development Corporation, a nonprofit organization sponsored by the city's government and business organizations, proclaimed that "real estate is in New York City's blood. Its properties, valued at a combined $1.3 trillion, are a testament to the premium that people and businesses all across the globe place on being able to live and work in our city."[50] By portraying the real estate industry as a beneficent force advancing the economic well-being of all New Yorkers, city government and the business community obscured the industry's role in determining the housing choices of New Yorkers and limiting the supply of affordable housing.

For housing and other activists, these changes in the city's housing markets presented new opportunities and new threats. On the one hand, more New Yorkers than ever were experiencing housing anxiety, the fear that they could not pay the next mortgage payment or rent increase, afford to move, or avoid eviction. This experience created a receptive audience for housing organizers. On the other hand, the consolidation of the real estate and development industries and their growing control of capital and therefore political influence made this sector a more formidable opponent for housing activists.

In the Progressive era in the first decades of the twentieth century, housing activists had won new laws making tenements safer, and after the Great Depression they had supported the construction of the city's public housing system.[51] From the 1970s to the present, however, New York City's housing movement has fought mostly defensive battles against an alliance of landlords, real estate developers, and wealthy investors from around the world. Both its victories and defeats were shaped by this increasingly unlevel playing field.

In sum, by the mid-2020s, these post-pandemic changes in the city's economy led to another bout of widening inequality and growing poverty, a trend that had slowed in previous decades. Everywhere, income and wealth inequality are the most fundamental determinants of health inequities.[52] By accepting these gaps as normal, perhaps inevitable, New York City business and political leaders implicitly guaranteed that the inequities in health between better-off and poor New Yorkers would continue to widen. For activists, challenging the belief that inequality was now as inevitable as the outsize role of billionaires in city politics became a key priority. Economic changes opened windows of opportunity for political changes, the third major post-1960s transformation of the city's landscape. New York's growing housing-affordability crisis defined the issues for Zohran Mamdani's successful 2025 election campaign for mayor of New York City and for the next period of activism.

CHANGES IN POLITICS

Compared to activists organizing in the late 1960s and early 1970s, those working in the aftermath of the 1975 fiscal crisis, when Rudy Giuliani was mayor, or when Donald Trump became president in 2017 and again 2025, faced a very different political landscape. The stories of how organizers of health campaigns in New York City assessed these changing circumstances and made decisions about what to do and not do show how the changing context shapes the opportunities and obstacles that activists encounter. It also shows how their actions in turn affect the city's political and economic dynamics.

The political scientist Julia Lynch has observed that "political and economic structures shape the allocations of social determinants of health."[53] These structures determine who has the power to distribute resources like food, housing, jobs, and health care; to what extent the law differentially protects the 1 percent versus the 99 percent; and in what ways the practices of public agencies promote or undermine health. The profile of the Young Lords and the following profile of Make the Road New York illustrate some of the ways that activists have assessed and responded to the city's changing political context.

Since 1965, New York City has had 9 mayors, 3 Republicans and 6 Democrats; New York State has had 9 governors, 3 Republicans and 6 Democrats; and the United States has had 11 presidents, 6 Republicans and 5 Democrats. Each of these elected leaders assembled and was supported by a coalition that helped them win office and achieve (or fail to achieve) their policy goals. In each electoral cycle, mayors, governors, and presidents cooperated and clashed in ways that shaped the choices open to activists in New York City. For those who did not live through these regime changes, mapping the shifting alliances and their respective priorities helps to illuminate the political choices that activists made in these different periods.

To plan their goals, strategies, and allies, activists must sort out what changes are possible within existing city, state, and federal political alignments. Even more challenging, they need access to the political intelligence that alerts them to conflicts within Democratic and Republican political coalitions, disputes that can facilitate or block desired policy changes.

Longer-term changes in public finance and governance also shape the political dynamics of setting policies and allocating resources for health. After World War II, the role of the federal government in funding municipal services, including health, increased greatly. Later, the New York State government also expanded such assistance. From 1965 to 1973, 55 percent of the public revenue growth in the city came from state and federal aid and only 37 percent from local revenues.[54] The remaining 8 percent came from borrowing—debt. For activists, these numbers emphasized the important role of the federal and state governments in determining what benefits the city offered.

Over the next three years, the proportion of new revenues that came from the federal and state governments plummeted to 8 percent and borrowing skyrocketed to 70 percent, the short-term cause of the city's 1975 fiscal crisis.[55] As tax revenues declined, for a time, borrowing became the path to maintain public services and avoid cuts in safety net programs. For elected officials and activists, these dramatic shifts, reinforced by the rightward shift of national politics under Presidents Nixon and Ford, changed the calculus of what was and was not politically feasible.

Two examples of changing political alignments at the city level illustrate the potential for activists to take advantage of such opportunities. In 1979, community and health activists in Harlem and other Black and

Puerto Rican neighborhoods opposed Mayor Ed Koch's plan to close Sydenham and other public hospitals to save money. Then as now, public hospitals in New York City provide more affordable and accessible health care than the private hospitals and medical centers run by the city's medical schools.

Although their campaign to keep Sydenham Hospital open failed, activists mounted several large demonstrations, won media coverage, and earned strong support from multiracial progressive legislators. Koch's turn toward austerity politics opened the door for activists to win new supporters for preserving the public hospital system. Koch's proposals to close several other public hospitals were defeated.

The battle to keep Sydenham open had political consequences as well. After shutting Sydenham in 1980, despite a campaign promise to keep it open, Ed Koch lost his 1982 primary race for New York State governor to Mario Cuomo, the more progressive Democratic candidate. A few years later, Koch lost both the primary and the general election for mayor to David Dinkins. While several factors contributed to Koch's losses, Ebun Adelona, an activist leader of the fight to keep Sydenham open, observed, "I'm proud of how we came together as a community and supported one thing. And then when we lost that hospital, [we] turned around and elected another mayor, a Black mayor, the first Black mayor in New York City."[56]

And while Dinkins experienced the same pressures to cut budgets as Koch did, his support for public hospitals enabled the system to stay relatively intact, a legacy that continues to benefit low-income, Black, Latiné, and immigrant New Yorkers. Strong support for public funding of hospitals from the labor movement also limited the scope of austerity-inspired cuts. In 1992, for example, when President George H. W. Bush proposed additional reductions in funding for Medicaid, an alliance of New York City health-care worker unions demonstrated against these cuts (see figure 2.2).

Another example of the interactions between activists and mayoral politics comes from the campaigns to end the stop-and-frisk policies of Mayor Michael Bloomberg. This police practice had allowed officers with the New York City Police Department (NYPD) to stop, interrogate, and

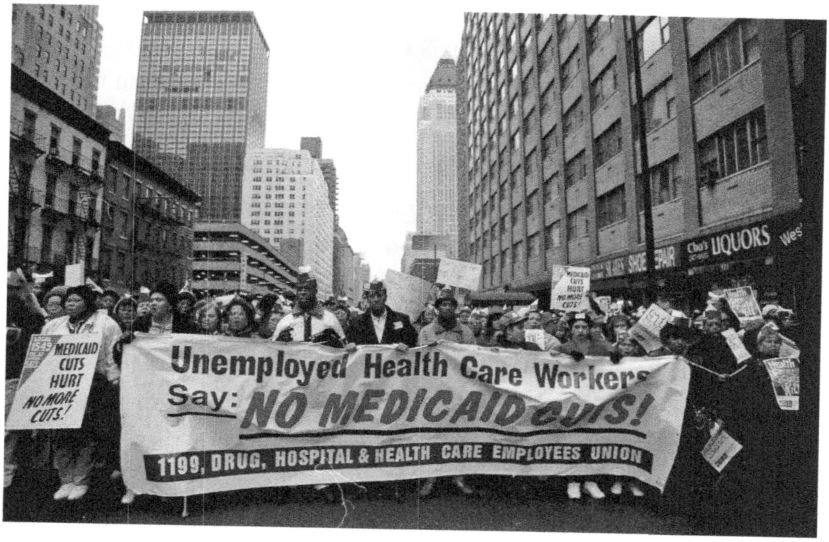
MEDICAID CUTS HURT NO MORE CUTS!
Unemployed Health Care Workers
Say: NO MEDICAID CUTS!
1199, DRUG, HOSPITAL & HEALTH CARE EMPLOYEES UNION
LIQUORS

FIGURE 2.2 Protesters in New York City marching against cuts to Medicaid on December 12, 1992.

Source: Bill Tompkins / Getty Images.

search the city's residents on the sole basis of "reasonable suspicion." In 2011, NYPD officers made nearly 700,000 such stops, nearly all of them of African Americans or Latinés. Advocacy campaigns by Communities United for Police Reform, founded in 2012, vowed to make police reform a major issue in the upcoming mayoral election.[57] At a press conference, one of the founders, Jumaane Williams, then a member of city council from Brooklyn, noted, "We represent the communities that stop-and-frisk and police accountability are huge issues in and what we're telling you is, these tools are being abused in our community, and they're not working."

The New York Civil Liberties Union, the Center for Constitutional Rights, Bronx Defenders, and other legal groups sued New York City to end the practice, charging it was discriminatory and unconstitutional. A 2013 federal court decision found that stop-and-frisk tactics violated the constitutional rights of minorities.[58] In his 2013 run for mayor, Bill de Blasio condemned stop-and-frisk, winning support from Black and progressive white voters—and the election. According to the American Civil Liberties Union, in 2017, the NYPD reported 11,629 stops, a 98 percent decrease from 2011, a tangible benefit of activists' success in the electoral arena.[59]

Critics have questioned whether David Dinkins's budget and policy decisions matched his public commitment to the city's public hospital system and whether de Blasio translated his opposition to stop-and-frisk before he became mayor to his actions on policing once he had the job. But whether elected officials' promises to advance the policy goals of activists reflect real devotion to their aims or merely the belief that it is in their best political interest to support the cause, either way activists bring new policy ideas onto the political and electoral agendas. In both these examples, activists helped to shape the city's political discourse, influenced the actions of elected officials, and opened windows for more substantive policy changes.

HOW ACTIVISTS RIDE THE WAVES OF CHANGING POLITICAL ECONOMIES

Changing trends in New York City's population, economy, and politics shape the terrain in which activists and social movements plan and carry out their campaigns. Like surfers scanning the waves, savvy activists rely on astute analysis or good fortune to sight the whitecaps of change that can carry them forward—and avoid those that can dump them into the sea.

What questions have New York City activists and organizers asked about the changing political economy in which they operate, and what strategies have they used to answer those questions?

First, activists look for windows of opportunity. The political scientist John Kingdon postulated that windows of policy opportunity open when observers define a problem, identify a solution, and recognize a political climate that allows for action.[60] Kingdon believed that these policy windows open for only a short time, requiring advocates to monitor the problem, solution, and political streams carefully, taking decisive action when the situation is right.

Make the Road New York recognized that after the 2007–2009 financial crisis, New York businesses were hiring more low-wage workers and fewer who earned enough to support their families. They also realized that growing numbers of the low-wage workforce were recent immigrants, settling in the very New York City communities where MRNY was organizing. In this same period, the group allied with several major labor unions to work together to win higher wages and better labor protections for these workers. Throughout the second decade of the twenty-first century, MRNY used these converging windows of problem (growing low-wage labor), solution (new forms of labor organizing), and political opportunity (the growing power of revitalized labor movements) to win legislative and legal victories and political and public support to improve the living and working conditions of low-wage workers.

Second, activists assessed how changes at the state, national, and global levels influence their prospects for campaigns centered in New York City. WE ACT for Environmental Justice, for example, was founded in 1988 to overcome environmental threats to the well-being of residents of Harlem. As WE ACT identified local problems—a new polluting sewage treatment plant on the Hudson River or several Harlem-based bus depots for diesel-fueled buses—its leaders and members learned that the causes of Harlem's environmental problems often started outside Harlem, in decisions made in Albany or at city hall or in the corporate boardrooms of waste disposal companies. To abate these threats to their community's health, they needed to be able to operate at local, citywide, state, and national levels.

At the local level, two of WE ACT's founders, Vernice Miller, a longtime community leader, and Peggy Shepard, then a young community activist with roots in local politics and the civil rights and women's movements, used their connections to West Harlem tenants' associations, civic groups, and the local Democratic Party to mobilize opposition to the treatment plant and to enlist elected officials in their campaigns.

At the municipal level, WE ACT joined other environmental justice (EJ) groups to organize the New York City Environmental Alliance, a citywide network of EJ groups, mostly in low-income communities of color, which could exchange information, plan strategy, and advocate with the city council and mayor.

In 1994, to move to the national level, Shepard, then the executive director of WE ACT, and other environmental activists from around the country persuaded President Bill Clinton to sign an executive order that mandated that the US Environmental Protection Agency and other federal agencies take action to identify and reduce the "disproportionately high and adverse human health or environmental effects on minority populations and low-income populations."[61] New federal environmental laws mandating safer disposal of toxic and hazardous materials created the need for more and safer toxic waste and garbage facilities. Existing sites, concentrated in low-income communities of color, were leaking and unsafe. These developments created the opportunity for a national EJ movement to react to disproportionate impacts. By creating a platform that could bring EJ activists from around the country to Washington, these groups could bring national influence on their local campaigns and inform federal initiatives with insights from local successes.

In these ways, WE ACT, originally neighbors and activists, joined to protect their own community, became a municipal, regional, and national force for environmental justice, using its multiple networks to gather the evidence and political insights needed to plan effective, often winning campaigns at multiple political levels.

A third question activists sought to answer as political economies changed was how to predict which powerful actors were likely to support or oppose the policy goals they pursued. Understanding the motivations and stakeholders of both allies and adversaries enables social movements to frame their messages, chart strategies, and create winning coalitions.

A brief example illustrates this point. In 2022, together with other housing organizations, Housing Justice for All released *Pay to Play*, a report that assessed the real estate industry's influence on two bills, Good Cause Eviction and a repeal of the fifty-year-old law exempting property taxes on new construction in New York City.[62] The report found that between 2018 and 2022, three major lobbying groups representing New York City's biggest and richest property owners, the Rent Stabilization Association, the Community Housing Improvement Program, and the Real Estate Board of New York, had spent almost $19 million on lobbying, litigation, and public relations to advance their agenda in Albany.

Most of their campaign contributions went to New York State Senate candidates, both Republicans and Democrats, many outside of New York City, effectively giving landlords a powerful voice in the legislative body in order to defeat or water down pro-tenant legislation. By revealing the multiple ways that the real estate lobby sought to influence legislators and by "naming and shaming" the lawmakers who accepted these contributions, Housing Justice for All was able to focus its attention on supporting candidates who went on to defeat some of the landlord-friendly politicians.

PROFILE: MAKE THE ROAD NEW YORK

For twenty years, Make the Road New York has decided which issues to take on and how to mobilize its constituents for winning campaigns based on its assessment of opportunities to take advantage of New York's changing political economy and the shifting roles of the players who shape it. An examination of how this group translated changes in New York's politics and economy into changes in goals and strategies provides additional insights into this process.

MRNY represents immigrants, people of color, and working-class families in New York City and State, with sister organizations in Connecticut, New Jersey, Pennsylvania, and Nevada. Founded in 2007 by the merger of two groups with roots in New York City's immigrant communities, MRNY organizes to expand workers' rights, improve health care, protect immigrant and civil rights, advance environmental and housing justice, and advocate for police reform and rights for transgender and lesbian, gay, bisexual, and gender-nonconforming groups.

MRNY's name comes from a poem by the Spanish poet Antonio Machado—"wanderer, there is no road, the road is made by walking."[63] By using this tag, the group signaled its practical approach to organizing—find the path to a better world by joining with others to build it, a clear difference from the more ideological nationalist and anticolonial roots of the Young Lords.

To make progress on its comprehensive and ambitious policy agenda, MRNY leverages the assets it has developed over the years. Its 25,000 dues-paying members make it one of the largest activist organizations in the city,[64] and the largest nonunion membership organization of immigrants.[65] In 2023, MRNY had revenues of $31.8 million, a staff of 220, and about 200 volunteers. Unlike some activist organizations, MRNY operates in multiple arenas where policy gets made—city and state legislatures, elections, and courts, as well as in the streets, workplaces, and community spaces where people gather (see figure 2.3).

These experiences and assets give MRNY members and leaders, in addition to a cadre of trained community organizers, deep knowledge of a wide repertoire of tactics and strategies to advance its policy goals. MRNY tackles the multiple problems that its members experience in their daily lives. It reaches out to its constituents based on their ethnic and political identities as immigrants, residents of geographical neighborhoods, and workers in low-wage and often precarious industries. Recognizing the importance of an inclusive approach to diverse communities, MRNY also promotes the needs and aspirations of its constituents who are women or LGBTQIA. Rooted in the multiethnic communities of Brooklyn, Queens, and Staten Island, MRNY appeals to New Yorkers who came to the city from regions around the world including Latin America, Southeast Asia, and the Middle East.

Jane McAlevey, the late author and activist, and others have catalogued some of the successes and limitation of MRNY campaigns, providing useful evidence for a retrospective review.[66] In 2009, in response to growing deportations of undocumented immigrants and federal harassment of their families, MRNY launched campaigns to reverse the federal Immigration and Customs Enforcement (ICE) practice of deporting

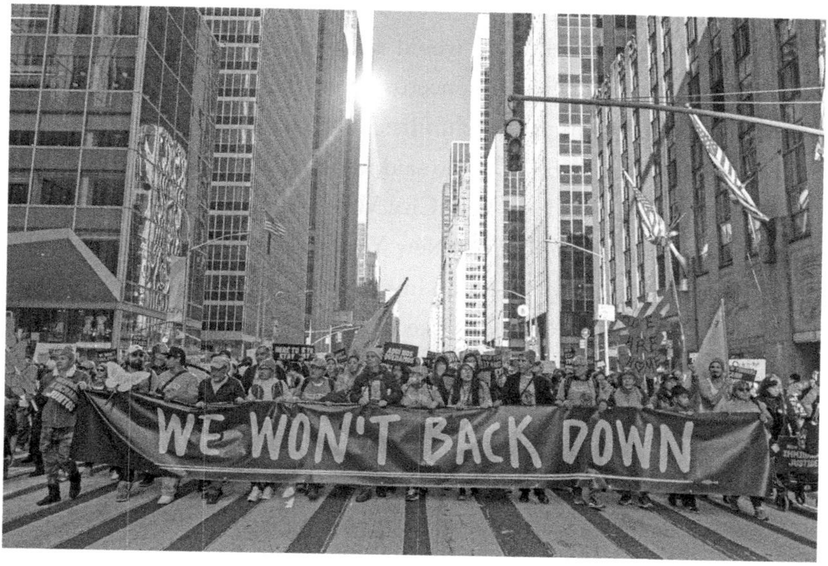

FIGURE 2.3 Make the Road New York members take over Fifth Avenue in Manhattan a few days after Donald Trump won the 2024 presidential election.

Source: Make the Road NY. https://docs.google.com/document/d/1G7iOy5HLloe-EG1kgQeov7Ypta8k896Nv8SVzbMFaqY/edit?tab=t.0

immigrants who had ended up in jail. Between 2004 and 2008, the New York City Department of Correction sent more than 13,000 undocumented immigrants from Rikers Island, the city's jail, to ICE detention centers outside New York.[67]

"When we first decided to launch this campaign [to convince New York City and State to stop cooperating with ICE], everyone said, 'You are fucking crazy,'" Javier Valdes, the campaign leader and an MRNY co-executive director, told McAlevey.[68] But MRNY members reported that their own families and friends were being deported, even when they were later found to be innocent of the charges against them. These personal experiences convinced the group to act.

In 2011, after several years of campaigning, community education, legislative advocacy, and the creation of a coalition of more than thirteen organizations, MRNY convinced New York Governor Andrew Cuomo to announce that New York State would no longer cooperate with ICE to deport detainees.[69] "There are concerns about the implementation of the program as well as its impact on families, immigrant communities and law enforcement in New York," Cuomo said, echoing MRNY's charges.

Several months later, New York City Mayor Michael Bloomberg signed a city council law to prohibit the New York City Department of Correction from using city funds to detain immigrants, ending the city's collaboration with ICE. As MRNY Co–Executive Director Valdes observed, "By signing this bill into law New York once again takes a step to protect immigrant families. As we continue to fight for family unity and immigration reform, we are proud that our city leads the way towards a system and country we want."[70]

These victories show that through its coalitions, its press coverage, and its moral credibility as an organization rooted in New York City neighborhoods, MRNY, with its allies and the communities it had mobilized, acquired the political muscle to influence elected city and state officials to support their demands. By helping to make valuing of immigrants an accepted belief, MRNY altered politics in New York, an illustration of the reciprocal interactions between mainstream politics and activist movements.

It is also true that both the first and second Trump administrations again made immigrants the targets of federal policies, requiring MRNY to take on this work again. These new attacks on immigrants also show the fragility of activist victories. With shifts in politics and the economy, politicians and their supporters return to tested methods of building political support by demonizing populations they disrespect. In 2017, MRNY helped to organize the airport demonstrations that opposed President Trump's so-called Muslim ban, which prevented people from several Muslim-majority nations from visiting the United States.[71] Nationwide demonstrations and successful lawsuits subsequently limited the scope of the ban. In 2024, MRNY assisted immigrant youth to join demonstrations in support of legal action to extend Deferred Action for Childhood Arrivals, a policy that allows some individuals who were physically present in the United

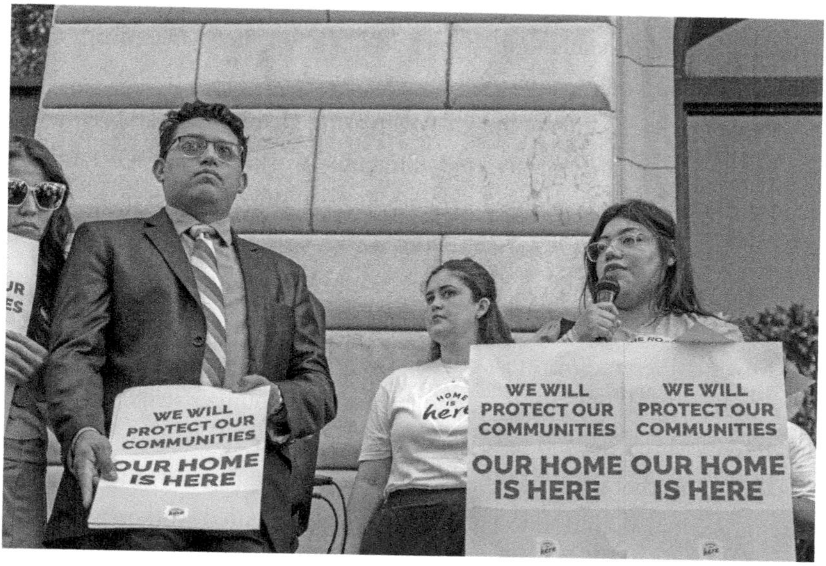

FIGURE 2.4 In October 2024, immigrant youth organized by Make the Road share their stories outside of the US Court of Appeals for the Fifth Circuit in New Orleans, where the future of the Deferred Action for Childhood Arrivals program was being argued.

Source: Make the Road NY. https://docs.google.com/document/d/1G7iOy5HLloe-EG1kgQeov7Ypta8k896Nv8SVzbMFaqY/edit?tab=t.0

States in 2012 to obtain a two-year period of deferred action from deportation (see figure 2.4). In 2025, MRNY's sixteen years of experience challenging ICE informed the collective response of the city's activists to President Trump's aggressive enforcement of his new immigration policies.

On the labor front, MRNY organized workers at grocery stores and car washes in Bushwick, Brooklyn, two of the many categories of precarious workers whose numbers were increasing in New York. These newly formed worker organizations then supported the group's campaign to pass new city and state laws to prevent wage theft, a success that enabled the MRNY to reach more immigrant workers and establish partnerships with influential unions like the Retail, Wholesale and Department Store Union.[72] Eddie Ott, an influential New York labor leader, noted that MRNY's "union-friendly approach and their demonstrated ability to turn out large numbers of their members for events in NYC set them apart from every other group in New York City."[73]

Ten years later, during the COVID-19 pandemic, an MRNY survey found that its members, often undocumented workers, and their families, reported overwhelming job loss and loss of life. Ninety members of MRNY died from COVID-19, making the harm painfully conspicuous. In response to the resulting flood of grief, MRNY helped to organize the Fund Excluded Workers Coalition. To achieve its goals, the coalition organized rallies and a protest outside the governor's office, blocked traffic on two New York City bridges, and led a moving hunger strike that lasted for twenty-three days. These actions, and the more than two hundred organizations that joined, helped to persuade the state government to allocate more than $2 billion to ensure that undocumented workers were also eligible for pandemic relief benefits.[74]

MRNY also mobilized to address health and health care directly. It was a leader of the Coverage for All Campaign to expand health-care coverage to immigrants regardless of their immigration status. The campaign failed at the state legislative level, but it did help to persuade the city's public hospital system to establish New York City Care, a program to provide free or subsidized health care to uninsured and undocumented New Yorkers. MRNY also helped to convince New York State to maintain Medicaid eligibility for DREAM Act recipients, regardless of changes in the federal rules. As an illustration of their skillful combination of direct services and policy advocacy, MRNY hired bilingual community health workers to provide in-home and community services and health education to immigrant families, enabling more people to use the access to care they had won.[75]

To achieve its successes in restricting ICE, protecting the rights of immigrant workers, and expanding access to health care, MRNY learned how to leverage New York City's key assets.[76] It built on the city's history of progressive policies supported by earlier elected officials such as Mayor Fiorello La Guardia and President Franklin Roosevelt, whose support for La Guardia made the city a showcase for protecting vulnerable populations against damaging market swings.[77] It forged ongoing alliances with New York's powerful labor unions and chose to work in communities with a high density of union members. It acknowledged the multiple identities of its constituents—as immigrants, people of color, workers, women, young and older people, LGBTQIs, and residents of a neighborhood—and sought to engage people based on all those characteristics, not forcing them to choose one over the other.

Unlike some of the late 1960s radical groups like the Young Lords Party, MRNY chose to work both inside and outside traditional politics, elections, and the party system. This choice gave Make the Road a wider selection of tactics and strategies than a commitment to using only strategies outside mainstream politics would have provided. MRNY worked closely with the Working Families Party (WFP), a progressive political third party first organized in 1998 by a coalition of New York labor unions, community organizations, and others. This alliance was facilitated in 2023 when WFP hired Ana María Archila as its codirector for New York State. She is a longtime activist and the cofounder and former co–executive director of MRNY.[78] Showing its skills at avoiding partisan wrangling, Make the Road also worked with the New York Democratic Socialists of America (DSA), the other major progressive political party in New York, to win approval of the state's Excluded Workers Fund that supported low-wage workers ineligible for federal pandemic relief and the 2019 New York State housing law reforms.

Through its endorsements, campaigns, and community education, WFP, MRNY, DSA, and other allies elected a cadre of more left-wing city and state legislators. These politicians brought new ideas and new voices to city hall and Albany that helped to move policy debates and laws on immigration reform, workers' rights, protection of renters, health care, and policing in more progressive directions.

WFP, DSA, and MRNY recognized that their goal was to build power, and they actively sought out opportunities to advance this aim. As Sochie Nnaemeka, WFP's former New York State director, explained, "I do think there are these moments that progressives and the left can plug in and raise the stakes of a contest. Whether we can maintain access to reproductive care in New York state, talk about a different approach to public safety, maintain access to public benefits, and push back on fascist-leaning electeds, we have to recognize the power that we have."[79]

These groups also realized that the changing political economy required policy action at the state and national levels as well as in New York City. As urban scholar Peter Dreier has noted, "cities by themselves cannot capture enough of the wealth generated within their borders to significantly reduce concentrated poverty. We need metropolitan-wide as well as federal policies to do that."[80]

To realize this aim, MRNY established affiliates in Connecticut, New Jersey, Nevada, and Pennsylvania, looking to establish models for policy and organizing that could both win local victories and support regional and national action to address the problems they identified. A few early leaders of MRNY later created a national organization, the Center for Popular Democracy, which supports and strengthens democratic people's organizations around the country. Its mission is to build the power of communities to ensure an inclusive, equitable society—"where people of color, immigrants, working families, women, and LGBTQ communities thrive together, supported by a resilient economy and political institutions that reflect our priorities."[81] Similarly, the Working Families Party and DSA established affiliates or endorsed candidates in other states.

In summary, MRNY shows that activist groups can survive and thrive in complex and rapidly shifting political and economic circumstances. The group has done this by firmly rooting itself in multiple cohesive communities, carefully listening to the concerns and aspirations of these constituents, and skillfully building coalitions that bring together diverse communities to pursue their shared goals. MRNY builds power to win short- and long-term victories and relies on the wisdom of activists with prior movement experiences and the passion, commitment, and life experiences of its newly recruited members and leaders.

Whether it would have been possible for MRNY to have evolved in a more hostile environment, one with fewer cohesive immigrant communities, fewer union members, higher levels of political resistance, or a less favorable history of progressive activism, is unknowable. Its capacity to identify and leverage the assets of New York City is itself a tribute to the skills of its members and leaders.

The emergence of a more progressive wing of New York's Democratic Party and of new third parties in turn gave MRNY access to the city's legislative and electoral arenas, enabling the group to win a more influential voice in shaping policy. Changes in New York City's people, economy, and politics laid the foundation for the rise and success of MRNY. Its many campaigns and its political actions in turn changed New York, opening new doors for the voices of immigrants, low-wage workers, and people of color.

Both the Young Lords and Make the Road New York confronted the multiple health-related problems that made life difficult for poor and working-class New Yorkers—inadequate, unaffordable, and unsafe housing, abusive policing practices, and lack of affordable health care for those at highest risk of medical problems. Both groups articulated a comprehensive vision of a different world where social justice, dignity, and respect were goals that motivated concretely focused collective action and political organizing. And both contributed a record of successes and failures that continue to inspire and inform health activists in New York City and beyond.

Unlike the Young Lords, MRNY has so far shown the ability to grow and change with changing times and to expand to new cities and states, an achievement that offers hope for future activists. In my view, this accomplishment reflects MRNYs deep roots in multiple New York City communities, its ample toolbox of tactics and strategies, and its careful assessment of changes in New York's politics and economy. Its pragmatic commitment to making its political road by walking it gives the group a flexibility that enables it to change with the times.

Both the Young Lords and MRNY changed New York and were in turn transformed by the city. The Young Lords showed the potential for mobilizing community-based activism that took on daily living conditions that undermined health while calling attention to citywide, national, and global policies that shaped health, a vision of activism that still resonates. However, changes in the city's and nation's government and economy in the 1970s made the organization's strategies and style less effective and less sustainable.

MRNY showed it is possible to build alliances among key sectors of the city's population—low-wage workers, immigrants, people of color, residents of low-income neighborhoods, and LGBTQI residents—and bring their collective voices into neighborhood and citywide politics. The challenge facing health activists in the coming years is to forge these sometimes transitory alliances into enduring organizations that have the power to win lasting changes in the city's living conditions and its population's well-being.

3

HOW ACTIVISTS DEFINE THE PROBLEM

To achieve their policy goals and choose the appropriate strategies and tactics for that purpose, activists need to define the problem they seek to fix. These choices are grounded in organizers' analyses of the political and economic circumstances in which their campaigns play out, a process described in the previous chapter.

In New York City's campaigns to improve well-being and living conditions over the last sixty years, activists have defined problems at the community, municipal, and national levels and they have used a variety of formal and informal methods for problem identification. They have used health, social justice, human rights, and other lenses to investigate these problems, yielding differing insights into their causes and solutions.

A closer look at campaigns to improve the city's housing illustrates how activists and reformers have organized to improve housing, and how landlords and real estate developers have resisted efforts to limit their power or profits. These clashes have shifted from battles over improving conditions in tenements, building more affordable housing for working-class New Yorkers, and creating enough high-quality public housing, to fights on controlling rents, preventing lead poisoning, and expanding the rights of renters and homeowners vis-à-vis landlords and developers.[1] Each of these changing goals required a precise definition of the problem.

Part of defining the problem is considering the extent to which housing problems are also health problems. The decisions of activists and their supporters influence how they frame their messages, choose allies, and monitor success. Why should New York City's housing movement also be considered a health movement? Growing evidence and the day-to-day experience of New Yorkers demonstrate that a roof and walls that keep out rain, cold, and excess heat; protection from exposure to lead poisoning, mold, rats and roaches, or other toxins; buildings and homes that prevent falls, injuries, and fires; and homes with enough space for residents to avoid infecting each other with communicable diseases are foundations for physical health.

Similarly, rents that leave enough income for food, health care, and other essential needs, coupled with building and neighborhood conditions that do not force apartment dwellers to isolate themselves and their children behind locked doors, protect public health and public safety. The assurance that one will not face the housing instability that unaffordable rent increases, eviction notices, or landlord harassment often cause are foundations for mental health.[2]

To ground this examination of how activists define problems at the intersection of housing and health in the real world of New York organizing, I begin with a profile of Housing Justice for All.

PROFILE: HOUSING JUSTICE FOR ALL AND ITS CAMPAIGNS FOR EVICTION PREVENTION

Housing Justice for All (HJA) was created in 2017 at a meeting of grassroots community groups committed to taking on the power that the real estate industry wields in New York. A statewide coalition of more than eighty groups representing tenant and homeless New Yorkers, HJA is "united in our fight for housing as a human right."[3] First known as the Upstate Downstate Alliance, HJA's early name communicated its definition of the problem: the need for housing activism that brought together organizations based in New York City with those in upstate and suburban communities. For many years, state legislators saw housing reform as a New York City issue. By creating an alliance that brought together groups from across the state with different sets of interest around a shared agenda, HJA was able to expand both the constituency for reform and its own power.[4]

HJA took on this problem by recruiting organizational members from throughout the state, including, for example, the Peekskill Coalition for Equitable Housing from the Hudson Valley, People United for Sustainable Housing Buffalo, the Nassau County Democratic Socialist Alliance from Long Island, Cityroots Community Land Trust from the Finger Lakes, Citizen Action for New York, a statewide group, and dozens of housing groups in New York City.[5]

These partners then launched a statewide campaign to address another problem that HJA had identified: the lack of tenant voices in the state legislature, a body with significant influence on housing policies and regulations in the city and state. For several years, thousands of members of the HJA organizations wrote to their legislators, testified at hearings, and attended demonstrations in Albany. In May 2019, more than 1,500 tenants rallied in support of HJA's comprehensive package of housing bills at the state capitol, joined by Senate Deputy Leader Michael Gianaris, a sponsor of one of the bills, shown in the image on the cover of this book.[6] In this and other actions, HJA built on more than sixty years of activism to improve the healthfulness of New York's housing (see figure 3.1).

Like Make the Road NY, HJA also worked to support progressive candidates and to encourage its members to vote. In the 2018 state elections, with the Working Families Party and the New York Democratic Socialists of America, HJA and other activist groups helped elect several new senators and assembly members and helped to defeat more conservative Democratic officeholders who had supported the Republicans, a position less popular with New York State voters two years after Donald Trump had first become president.

One of the newly elected senators was Julia Salazar, a former housing organizer and the first member of DSA to win a seat in the state legislature. DSA is a nationwide socialist organization. Its New York City

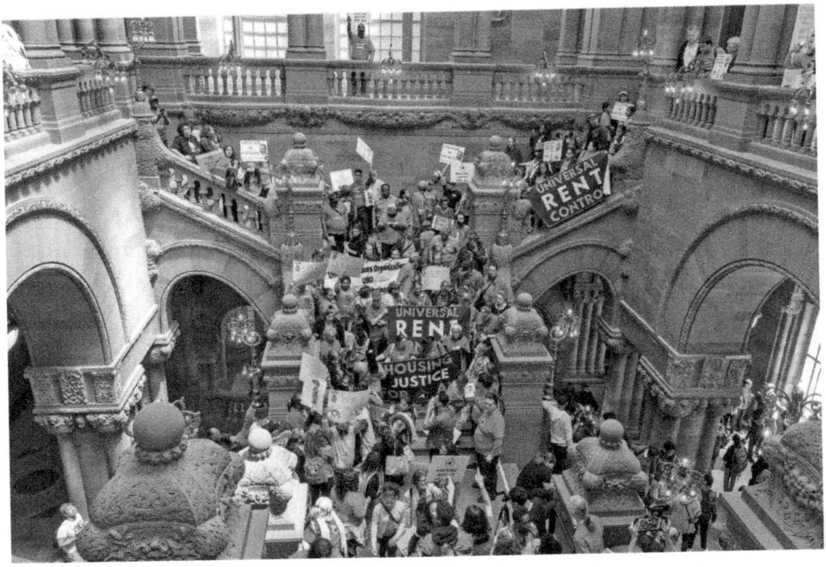

FIGURE 3.1 In June 2019, Housing Justice for All, a statewide coalition of more than 80 organizations that represent tenants and homeless New Yorkers, demonstrated inside the New York State legislature in support of Universal Rent Control and other housing reforms. The new rules that passed marked a significant victory for the 2.4 million people who live in rent-regulated apartments in New York City.

Source: Housing Justice for All

chapter organizes to win city and state electoral and legislative fights that benefit the city's multiracial working class.

Soon after her election, Salazar wrote and introduced the Good Cause Eviction bill, a part of HJA's package of housing reforms that seek to make it harder for landlords to evict tenants.[7] Salazar became an important and influential ally of HJA, helping the group to find that voice in the legislature it had been lacking. She was reelected in 2020 with 97.5 percent of the vote in the general election. In 2024, Salazar told a reporter, "I think that there's evidence that progressives and the left in New York are really thriving and have thrived even in the face of very well-funded opposition,"[8] a success she attributed to the alliance between

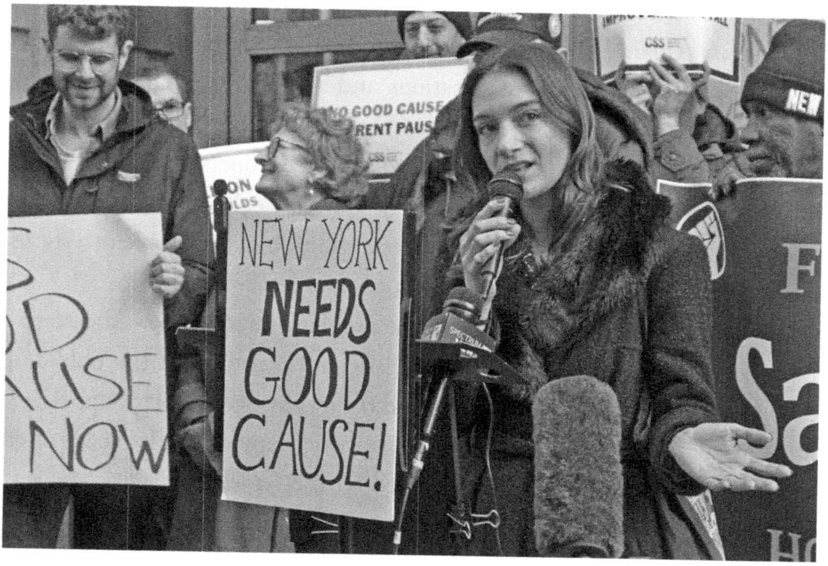

FIGURE 3.2 At a rally and press conference in Brooklyn in 2024, New York State Senator Julia Salazar, lead Senate sponsor of what became the Good Cause Eviction Law, demanded that the state take action on the housing crisis.

Source: Luis Rodriguez for the Community Service Society. https://www.caribbeanlife.com/intensified-calls-for-passage-of-good-cause-eviction/

the Working Families Party, DSA, and statewide grassroots coalitions like HJA (see figure 3.2).

Housing activists also recognized that a major obstacle to their goal of preventing evictions and implementing other housing reforms was the disproportionate power in Albany of the landlord and real estate sectors. To follow up on its 2022 report *Pay to Play*, which assessed the real estate industry's influence on two housing bills (described in the previous chapter),[9] HJA published a 2024 report that found that in the last five years the top real estate lobbying firms in New York State had spent $13.6 million on lobbying and met with lobbyists and their staff more than 1,200 times, with members of the governor's staff 1,240 times, and with city and state housing agencies almost 1,000 times. By publicizing the outsized contributions and extensive interactions between real estate industry lobbyists and elected officials in Albany, HJA educated voters and advocates and shamed the legislators who had these conversations and accepted the industry's campaign contributions. Significantly, these educational campaigns denormalized voters' tolerance of landlords and developers as the dominant influence on housing policy in New York State. By calling attention to this reality, HJA hoped to win support for its definition of the problem: a status quo that gave too much power to landlords and developers.

A related clash over definition of the problem emerged from the acceptance among many legislators, journalists, and members of the public of the industry's portrayal of landlords and tenants as two equal groups fighting for their rights and needs in a pluralistic democracy. In 2023, after some of HJA's proposals were defeated in the legislature, Cea Weaver, Housing Justice for All's campaign coordinator, observed, "the fact that Good Cause and the Housing Access Voucher Program got where they did—as leading priorities for Albany in negotiations this year—is proof of how far the tenant movement has come. The real estate lobby may have killed the bills for now, but they will never kill our determination to win."

Weaver noted that housing affordability consistently polls as a top issue of concern for New Yorkers and that "voters will be going to the polls with record high-rent burdens, unstable housing, and in far too many cases, no housing at all. They will be looking for representation that addresses these foundational concerns."[10] By defining the problem not as two equal groups competing in a democratic system, but as a handful of companies and individuals from the 1 percent using their wealth and power to undermine the housing rights of millions of New Yorkers, HJA and Weaver hoped to portray its members as Davids fighting against the real estate industry Goliath.

The group's choice of name provided another opportunity to frame the problem. By making housing justice for all its goal, HJA asserted that housing is a right, not a market commodity. This linked HJA with the environmental justice, climate justice, and sexual and reproductive health justice movements, all of whom insisted that pursuing health and justice were inextricably linked. The Urban Institute has defined housing justice as activities that ensure that "everyone has affordable housing that promotes health, well-being, and upward mobility by confronting historical and ongoing harms and disparities caused by structural racism and other systems of oppression."[11] For health activists working across issues, defining the problem to be remedied as injustice offered a bond that could build the power of multiple groups.

Changes in the political economy since the 1970s also led the housing activists who preceded Housing Justice for All to alter their definitions of the problem. This process influenced the activist landscape in which HJA operated.

New York City's fiscal crisis of the mid-1970s, described in the previous chapter, the election of Ronald Reagan as president in 1980, the promotion of neoliberalism with its recipe for austerity, privatization, deregulation, and distrust of government, and ruling elites' ideology of market supremacy forced activists grounded in the movements of the 1960s and early 1970s to confront other ideas and political forces.

Writing in 2019, housing activist and scholar Oksana Mironova described the shift in this period from "expansionist" housing organizing to "defensive" organizing. Expansionist housing activism, she wrote, uses community rights to "back up moral, legal and policy claims to public and private resources, or for expanded protection by the state." Defensive struggles, on the other hand, Mironova defined as "those where the end goal is to defend an individual or a group, program, policy or law against government or private action."[12] This shift from offense to defense occurred in housing, but also in other streams of health activism such as health care, policing, and food. The nature of the problem—in this case inadequate access to affordable housing—remained the same, but the changing zeitgeist, the invisible forces that dominated the characteristics of a given era, required activists to adapt their definitions of the problems they attacked and the solutions they proposed in response to the evolving political economy.

The legislative successes of HJA and its allies and Zohran Mamdani's successful 2025 campaign for mayor, in which he ran on the issue of housing affordability, may signal a window of opportunity for another shift in the prospects for housing activism in New York.

***

For as long as New York City has had a housing movement, the tendency of different sectors to create siloed campaigns and alliances has plagued both HJA and other housing activists. Renters and their organizations pursue rent control, public housing residents seek improvements in public housing maintenance and resist privatization of public housing, homeless groups—yet another stream of housing activism—advocate for supportive housing, improvements in shelters, and new housing for those without. Identifying this siloization as a problem and developing strategies for a more unified housing movement are key priorities in New York as well as across the country. "What we need," writes urban planner Cassim Shepard, "is a nationwide program of housing reform backed by a mass social movement."[13]

HJA has taken steps to create Shepard's solution to the problem of siloed responses to the nation's housing crises: Its partners include groups working on public housing, rent control, homelessness, and prevention. Its newsletters, events, electoral work, and presence in the state capitol have created a space for activists from across the state and housing issue groups to exchange ideas, debate strategy, and forge shared policy agendas. Its legislative packages provide housing and other activists an arena for shared action. These activities build the potential for a more unified movement, a path that health movements in other streams of activism could learn from. To build on this opportunity, in 2025, HJA created a new organization, the New York State Tenant Bloc, a 501(c)(4) organization (meaning it can support candidates), that plans to exert influence in New York elections and support candidates who back tenant-friendly policies.

What do we know about the successes of HJA to date? And to what extent have their definitions of problems contributed to—or limited—these victories? First, since 2019, several new city and state laws have been passed to limit evictions and specify the procedures landlords must follow to evict a tenant. These include the following measures:

- In 2017, New York City enacted Local Law 136, which made the city the first in the United States to provide access to free legal services to all tenants facing eviction proceedings in housing court or the public housing authority. In 2023, according to a report by the National Coalition for the

Civil Right to Counsel, 84 percent of the city households represented in court by lawyers were able to remain in their homes, preserving tenancies and promoting the preservation of affordable housing and neighborhood stability.[14]

- In 2019, the state legislature and governor approved new rent laws that strengthened tenant protections and limited landlords' rights to raise rents or deregulate their properties. The real estate industry fiercely opposed the bill. John Banks, the president of the Real Estate Board of New York, noted, "There was a path to responsible reform that would have protected tenants as well as owners, jobs and revenues, but Albany chose not to take it."[15]
- In 2020, the state legislature passed, and the governor signed, what *The New York Times* called "one of the most comprehensive antieviction laws in the nation," designed to help New Yorkers cope with the loss of jobs precipitated by the COVID-19 pandemic.[16]
- In 2022, New York City passed a law that ensures that all New York City residents over the age of sixty are entitled to counsel when facing eviction, regardless of their income level.[17]
- In 2024, the state legislature passed the Good Cause Eviction law protecting tenants from unjust evictions and unreasonable rent increases. The new law applied to unregulated rental units in New York City and in any local municipalities in the state that opt in. It does not apply to public housing or rent-stabilized or rent-controlled apartments.[18] A similar bill had failed to pass in 2022.

What was the impact of these new laws? A 2025 report by Princeton University's Eviction Lab found that the eviction-filing rate in New York City was well below the national average in every borough except the Bronx, but even there the rate had been cut in half since the pandemic started. In four years, the number of evictions that New York City landlords filed in housing court fell from 15,000 per month in 2019 to 9,300 per month in 2024.[19] Every family not evicted because of this decline had the potential to avoid homelessness, maintain custody of their children, and escape the stress of eviction, at least for a time.

While several factors contributed to this decline, the new laws that HJA and other housing groups succeeded in passing and their education of journalists, elected officials, and the public about the perils of eviction and the availability of legislative solutions no doubt contributed to this drop in eviction, an impressive health and social justice victory.

FRAMING THE PROBLEM

To define the problem they seek to fix, health activists must identify the causes of this problem and then determine what definition will best focus their capacity to act while also enlisting the broadest support for campaigns to mitigate this problem. To determine causes, campaign planners need the skills of social epidemiologists, investigative journalists, and systems scientists. To define the problem in ways that engage supporters requires the mindset of community organizers, public relations specialists, and social media influencers.

An examination of some of the ways that health activist groups in New York City have taken on these two tasks shows some of the methods they have used. The city's Young Lords chapter, for example, identified a variety of problems that motivated them to act—threats to children's health, unsanitary living conditions, and inadequate housing. They defined these problems based on members' own life experiences and their interactions with community residents while organizing their campaigns. Their articulation of each problem in turn shaped the solutions they proposed, the strategies and tactics they used to achieve their goals, and the coalitions and alliances they created or joined.

Housing Justice for All defined its problems as the disproportionate political influence of real estate developers and landlords and, especially after the onset of the COVID-19 pandemic, the growing threat of eviction facing New York's renters. Their members' experiences interacting with legislators in Albany and their analyses of campaign contributions from the real estate sector informed the understanding of the first problem. The growing number of residents coming to HJA member organizations for help with responding to eviction notices during the first phase of the pandemic led the alliance to recognize the salience of taking on the rise of evictions.

To make informed decisions on the definition of the problem they will choose, activist groups ask three common questions:

1. How can we best align our health and social justice concerns about this problem?
2. How can we best balance our actions to address the local dimensions of this problem with its national and global dimensions?
3. What definition will best target the actors with the power to make the changes we want and facilitate maximizing support from the public for our solution?

Their decisions on these questions provide the road map activists use to plan effective, practical campaigns.

<u>Balancing health and social justice.</u> Activist groups like the Young Lords and Make the Road New York viewed the problems they took on as both health and social justice problems. Their experience as organizers led them to believe that residents who understood both dimensions were more likely to be engaged and to act than those who did not. Deciding how best to frame their understanding of the connections between these two dimensions influenced how they communicated with their supporters and the broader public.

The health frame invites participation from all those who face that threat or worry about its impact on their children, family, or community. It taps into the near universal human concern about health and the desire to protect one's own health and that of family, friends, and neighbors. It encourages the consideration of changes in policies, institutions, and behaviors that cause the problem, thus offering multiple opportunities for action. Notably, the health frame offers the potential for less adversarial, less political, more universal messages. Who could explicitly advocate for more disease or poorer health?

The social justice frame also has benefits. It appeals to supporters' sense of fairness, their desire to be treated with respect and dignity, and their aspirations for more just and equitable communities and societies. It has the potential to broadcast a vision of a better society, the belief that another world is possible.

For tactical and strategic reasons, activist groups may choose to emphasize one or the other of these frames for different constituencies or at various stages in their campaigns. In their different ways, Make the Road New York, the Young Lords, and HJA were skilled in blending concerns about health and social justice, as various statements from these groups illustrate.

From the Young Lords 7 Demands shown at a demonstration outside Lincoln Hospital in 1970:

> We want total self-determination of all health services through a community-worker board to operate Lincoln Hospital, this Board must have the commitment to serve the people.[20]

From a 2020 Make the Road New York report on the impact of the COVID-19 crisis on working-class, immigrant, Black and Brown New Yorkers:

> Our communities are reeling from COVID-19 and the crisis it has unleashed. . . . Far too many members and their loved ones have contracted the virus and died. We hear daily from workers who have lost their jobs, are excluded from accessing Unemployment Insurance and all other income supports, and do not know how they will be able to buy groceries or pay the rent. We hear, too, from front-line workers who face the risk of contracting the virus at their work sites, where they labor without adequate protections.[21]

From Monique Chandler-Waterman, member of the New York State Assembly from East Flatbush, Brooklyn, rejecting a proposed housing deal that would gut rent stabilization and good cause eviction:

We should not have to . . . make the choice between healthy groceries, prescribed medication, or paying rent or the mortgage."[22]

By linking the health and social justice dimensions of the problem they have defined, these quotes show how activists created multiple pathways for potential supporters to join campaigns to confront these problems. They also show how activists provide public health professionals with a language and framing that make social determinants of health an actionable target for ordinary people, a goal health professionals have struggled with.

Tackling local, national, and global causes. "Wicked problems," those that "lack obvious solutions and face real-world constraints that prevent easy fixes,"[23] usually have contributing causes at the local, national, and global levels. Activists seeking to solve these complex challenges must decide which levels of cause to target as their campaigns unfold.

Choosing local problems as the priority has advantages as doing so creates an accessible and familiar arena of action. Mobilizing local communities to win the power needed to achieve victory may require fewer resources and less time than getting results at the national or global levels. However, an exclusive focus on the community level risks falling into what organizers have called "the local trap,"[24] a mistaken belief that problems with national and global causes can always be solved at the local level.

A focus on national causes creates the potential for finding new and powerful allies and winning solutions with a broader health or social justice impact. But this choice requires more resources and time and is less feasible for groups that lack national experience and networks. When the national scene is dominated by empowered political forces opposing improvements in health or social justice—as was the case, for example, in the early days of the Reagan and Trump presidencies—activists sometimes choose to work at other levels until local action or changes in the political economy again support national action.

For some wicked problems—reducing carbon emissions, improving the quality and lowering the price of the world's food, or ensuring access to essential medicines for all—global action is essential. It is the global political economy that has created these threats, and ultimately only global action can bring about the needed changes. Successful global activism has the potential to save millions of lives and change the global political discourse. For example, the 2003 Framework Convention on Tobacco Control, the global treaty to limit the power of the tobacco industry in setting policy, challenged the tobacco industry around the world,[25] and international efforts to divest from the fossil fuel industry encouraged many investors not to invest in the fossil fuel companies contributing to the climate emergency.[26] Similarly, national activism to make essential HIV medicines more available in South Africa and Brazil inspired global action to achieve this goal more widely, an effort supported by ACT UP in New York City.[27]

HOW THE CLIMATE JUSTICE MOVEMENT DEFINED ITS PROBLEMS ACROSS LEVELS

To better understand how activist movements make these choices, I examine how New York City's climate justice movement defined problems that enabled it to move between and sometimes combine work at the local, national, or global levels. After Superstorm Sandy flooded and flattened many parts of Lower Manhattan, Brooklyn, and Queens in 2012, activists from the 2011 Occupy Wall Street action joined with others to create Occupy Sandy, a group formed to assist neighborhoods to recover from the storm's damage and to call attention to the growing threat that weather changes associated with climate change posed to New York City. Occupy Sandy organized several activities that highlighted its understanding of both hyperlocal and national problems that contributed to storms such as Sandy and their harmful consequences.

In the flooded Rockaways community in Queens, Occupy Sandy's food distribution centers provided food to residents in neighborhoods where stores had been shut by the storm. Sandy activists called these services mutual aid, not charitable donations, to distinguish their group from the mainstream relief organizations who had been slow to begin operations in flood-damaged neighborhoods and often used a charity frame for their support.[28] This concept of collective action to address hunger during crises reemerged after the COVID-19 pandemic, again in concert with more radical acts and a rejection of outside charity.[29] Numerous city community organizations provided food to newly unemployed neighbors, delivered food and other supplies to overburdened health-care workers, and mobilized in support of a moratorium on evictions during the pandemic. By asking community residents to help their neighbors recover from a disaster, Occupy Sandy made it easy for people to volunteer, thus providing a first step for what might become more direct activism.

Occupy Sandy volunteers also helped people to remove mold and mud from their homes and trained neighborhood residents to do this work safely, stepping in to fill gaps in municipal services and in the process illustrating a more responsive and bottom-up approach to crises. While some of Occupy Sandy's actions (for example, its cooperation with municipal agencies including the police) disturbed more radical members of Occupy Wall Street, its goal was to show that residents acting together at the local level could provide an alternative to top-down government responses. For other activist groups across issues and decades, the question "How can we show city government how to do its job better?" served as a useful prompt for defining an actionable problem.

In 2014, the People's Climate March attracted 300,000 climate activists from around the country to the streets of New York City, just ahead of the United Nations Climate Summit, also held in the city. On the day of the march, Mayor Bill de Blasio released a report called *One City: Built to Last* that outlined the city's long-term plan to respond to climate change. In it, the mayor wrote,

> Global climate change is the challenge of our generation. New Yorkers are facing the risks of rising sea levels, increased temperatures and heat waves, and increasing frequency of intense storms. The damage caused by Hurricane Sandy in 2012 provided tragic evidence of these risks. Almost two years later, we are still recovering. . . . We are faced with an

> existential threat, and inaction is not an option. New Yorkers will rise to the challenge. We will build on progress we have made to become more resilient to a changing climate and to mitigate the harmful greenhouse gas emissions that contribute to climate change. We are committing to reduce our emissions by 80 percent below 2005 levels by 2050, making us the largest city in the world to commit to this goal.[30]

The combination of well-defined threats to the city's future, strong media interest, activists, and communities mobilized to protect their neighborhoods, as well as the visible activities of several coalitions of labor, environmental, climate justice, and faith organizations convinced the mayor he could and should act. The portrayal of the problem as global, national, and local provided additional impetus for action since New York City mayors pride themselves on being at the forefront of solving the world's urban problems.

The Dirty Buildings Campaign of Climate Works for All, one of the coalitions to emerge to confront the climate crisis, took up another level of organizing.[31] In New York City, buildings are responsible for 70 percent of greenhouse gas emissions. To reduce high levels of carbon emissions from large residential and commercial buildings in New York, the campaign first helped to pass Local Law 97 in 2019. Known as the Dirty Buildings Law, it required buildings of more than 25,000 square feet to reduce greenhouse gas emissions by 40 percent by 2030 and 80 percent by 2050.

Campaigners emphasized that full implementation of Local Law 97 would create 141,000 jobs to implement energy-efficiency upgrades, support new opportunities for workforce development for low-income and women workers, and reduce air pollution and thus asthma-related medical visits and hospitalizations. By defining the multiple harmful health, environmental, social justice, and employment consequences of energy-inefficient buildings, the Dirty Buildings Campaign supported the creation of multifaceted alliances. It also enabled tenant, neighborhood, and citywide activism. After the law was enacted, the campaign continued to mobilize its partners to support full enforcement and adequate funding and to contest efforts by building owners to challenge the law in court.[32]

In sum, New York's climate justice movement defined the problems it confronted in ways that emphasized the role of intersecting global, national, and local determinants and the health, environmental, and equity consequences of rising carbon emissions at each level. This enabled activists to articulate the economic, social, health, and environmental costs and benefits of proposed responses to the problem and to frame their campaign messages in ways that supported and strengthened cross-cutting coalitions. This approach also enabled interested individuals and organizations to join climate justice actions to pursue their sometimes divergent interests, attracting more and more diverse supporters than would a single focus on, for example, flood relief or dirty buildings.

Targeting the right actors and engaging the right supporters. A good definition of the problem helps activists decide who to target in their campaign—government or market actors, local or national players, wealthy, powerful actors who can set an example for others, or sleazy ones who are easy to vilify? In making these decisions, campaign organizers consider both who has the power to fix the problem they have identified and what power activists will need to mobilize to convince this actor to do what they want. The ideal choice—seldom realized—is to target an actor who already has the power to fix the problem and to enlist a base of supporters who have already assembled the political clout to bring about the desired change. In the real world, the political context often complicates these choices, requiring activists to make difficult compromises.

A few examples from campaigns seeking to reduce childhood lead poisoning in New York City that followed the Young Lords' Lead Offensive (described in chapter 1) illustrate these dynamics. Although New York City's 1960 ban on the use of lead-based paint in new residential dwellings was one of the first in the nation and protected future generations, the rule left most of the city's low-income children in jeopardy as they lived in old buildings with flaking or chipping paint.

In 1969, Jack Newfield, a writer and editor at *The Village Voice*, an influential liberal weekly, wrote a series of columns on lead poisoning that told the stories of several children who had suffered permanent brain damage from lead poisoning. His target for action was the mayor. A political scientist who studied these lead campaigns wrote that these articles were "the most important catalyst of public pressure and bureaucratic response" because *Voice* readers were New Yorkers who had influence on John Lindsay, the incumbent mayor who was endeavoring to carve a path for liberal Republicans.[33] By showing he cared about Black and Latiné children, Lindsay hoped to build support in these communities.

By 1970, in response to the combined pressure of multiple groups urging the city to do more on lead poisoning, the NYC Board of Health altered the health code so that the city could force landlords to repair apartments where lead-poisoned children lived. Reelected as mayor, Lindsay appointed a health commissioner who happened to be an expert in lead poisoning, and she created a new Bureau of Lead Poisoning Control to coordinate screening, education, and case follow-up, an example of activism and electoral politics leading to improvements in municipal services.[34]

In 1982, after a decade of activism and legislative advocacy on lead poisoning, New York City adopted one of the first laws in the nation requiring building owners to remediate lead paint hazards in apartments of young children before they become poisoned. Local Law 1 of 1982, one of the nation's strongest lead poisoning–prevention laws, emphasized primary prevention. Landlords were responsible for remediation of the lead hazard, but they also faced civil penalties if a child was found to be lead poisoned.[35] But the change in the law by itself was not enough.

A decade of devastating cuts in city health and housing services because of the 1975 fiscal crisis led to new cases of lead poisoning and thus to new rounds of activism. A 1983 survey found that only about a third of preschool children in the city's high-risk neighborhoods had actually been screened for lead, as medical experts recommended.[36]

In that year, several community organizations, health professionals, and housing activists (including the author) created the New York City Coalition to End Lead Poisoning (NYCELP). The coalition's review of the city's lead programs faulted the mayor and the city's Health and Housing Departments for failing to act to prevent lead poisoning. A week prior to the release of the report, city officials announced the creation of a new interagency task force on lead poisoning and asked the NYCELP to delay release of its report. After much discussion, the coalition decided to release the report, believing that defining the problem as city inaction could generate additional political pressure for the city to act more effectively. Once the report was released, city officials refused to meet with the NYCELP.

As a result of this attention, the New York City Council and Board of Estimate allocated additional funding for lead poisoning. However, the Health Department decided to use these resources for a program to educate parents about how to remove lead paint dust from their apartment, rather than to require landlords to remove lead or increase enforcement actions. In response, the NYCELP sued the city for failure to enforce lead paint rules in the city's health and housing codes, again targeting the mayor rather than a single city agency for action.[37] The lawsuit resulted in court orders directing the city to fully and properly implement the 1982 law.

By 1999, however, seventeen years after Local Law 1 of 1982 was passed, several court orders increased pressure from the real estate lobby, and a 1996 New York State Court of Appeals decision that reinforced building owners' ongoing responsibilities led the city council to roll back its prior lead poisoning laws. The council enacted Local Law 38, which shifted much of the responsibility for controlling lead poisoning back to tenants.[38] By contesting activists' assignment of responsibility for lead poisoning prevention to city government, these actors hoped to create solutions that would cost less for the city and landlords.

In response to the scaled-back law, several organizations, including the New York Public Interest Research Group and the New York Coalition to End Lead Poisoning, filed another lawsuit against the city in which they charged that Local Law 38 inadequately protected children. In 2000, the New York Supreme Court struck down Local Law 38 and briefly reinstated Local Law 1 of 1982. In 2004, the New York City Childhood Lead Poisoning Prevention Act (Local Law 1 of 2004) went into effect, replacing the 1982 law.[39]

The new law named the Department of Housing Preservation and Development as the agency responsible for implementing and enforcing the law, recognizing housing as the fundamental cause of childhood lead poisoning in New York. It also directed the Department of Health to promulgate, interpret, and enforce some rules relating to the law, an example of the multiagency approach needed to successfully resolve many social causes of ill-health. In part because of stronger laws, between 2005 and 2012, the number of lead-poisoned children in New York City fell by 68 percent.[40]

Over the next two decades, lead poisoning periodically returned to the city and state policy agenda. One problem was the persistence of lead poisoning in the public housing operated by the New York City Housing Authority (NYCHA). In 2018, the Council of Presidents of New York City Housing Authority's Tenants Councils sued NYCHA for failing to provide health and hot water and failing to comply with federal and state law by not conducting timely lead paint inspections and failing to notify residents when the potentially hazardous paint was found in their apartments.[41]

"When we reach out to NYCHA to complain about our issues, we get shut down," explained Daniel Barber-Walker, president of the Citywide Council of Presidents and a lifelong resident of NYCHA's Andrew Jackson Houses in the Bronx. His goal was to force NYCHA to act. "We have let other people speak for us for too long. The fight has to come from the residents of public housing." In recent years, media exposés of the city's failure to act on lead poisoning in public housing led the Health Department and NYCHA to make additional efforts to protect children in public housing against lead poisoning.[42] As did Jack Newfield's *Village Voice* articles in 1969, investigative reporting can help activists to educate the public about the problems they have identified.

* * *

While journalists, reformist elected officials, and activists have often succeeded in identifying the government actors responsible for the problems they address, they have sometimes found it harder to identify and publicize the business actors. In the case of lead poisoning, targeting individual landlords for failing to act to prevent lead poisoning has been difficult. In 2020, however, New York State Attorney General Letitia James filed a lawsuit against Chestnut Holdings of New York, Inc., a property management corporation that manages more than 6,000 apartments in 134 buildings, mostly in the Bronx. James, a longtime progressive elected official in New York, has ongoing ties with several activist groups. The suit charged Chestnut with failing to comply with provisions of New York City's lead poisoning–prevention law. "All New Yorkers—in every city, village, and town across this state—have a right to live in homes that don't make them sick," said the attorney general. "I am committed to ensuring that landlords follow the laws to protect young children from lead poisoning."[43] In a 2021 settlement, Chestnut Holdings agreed to pay $300,000 to the Office of the Attorney General for initiatives to protect children from lead poisoning and ensure that all of its more than 6,000 apartments throughout New York City are in full compliance with the law.[44] This rare case shows the potential for deterring lead poisoning though legal action.

In important ways, the sixty-year fight against childhood lead poisoning has been a public health success. Deaths and hospitalizations from lead poisoning have been all but eliminated. Children's blood lead levels have declined significantly, and the number of children screened has increased. However, lead poisoning remains a major environmental threat to healthy child brain development and future learning and low-income and Black and Latiné children continue to experience higher levels of lead poisoning than better-off and white children. The story of health and housing activists' ongoing fights to end lead poisoning shows the importance of careful and ongoing analyses of which actors, over time and across communities, are responsible for what manifestations of the problem. These investigations in turn shape the strategies campaigns use to force these actors to fulfill their responsibilities to protect children's health.

But the history of lead poisoning control tells another, more discouraging story. For public health professionals, lead poisoning is a completely preventable problem. The exposure is known, methods to test children and buildings for lead are readily available, procedures for removing lead from buildings were long ago developed, and cities have had more than a hundred years of experience in using different strategies to prevent lead poisoning. Yet, as City Council Speaker Corey Johnson acknowledged at a city council hearing in 2019, the Childhood Lead Poisoning Prevention Act, enacted in 2004 with the goal of eliminating childhood lead poisoning by 2010, had failed, as had a long string of previous laws.[45] Like the ongoing battles to limit evictions in New York City, the failure of the city's government, activists, and voters to reduce the influence of landlords to shape the housing conditions and experiences of residents highlights the challenge of defining problems that require transformative changes in power relationships.

When activist organizations propose to take on problems that they have defined clearly and compellingly, they build a foundation of success for engaging supporters, choosing allies, selecting strategies and tactics, and measuring success, as seen in later stages of campaign implementation discussed in subsequent chapters. And when they propose tackling problems that are vaguely defined or not appealing to supporters, they make each of these tasks more difficult.

4

HOW ACTIVISTS DECIDE TO TAKE ON THE PROBLEM THEY IDENTIFY

Once activists have identified a problem they want to solve and mapped the political and economic forces they believe have shaped the landscape in which they will act, how have they decided which solutions to pursue to solve the problem they have named? In this chapter, I explore how activist groups and social movements make these decisions. I also consider how health activists think about power—the power of their opponents and their allies, and the power they will need to implement their proposed solutions. Through a profile of the AIDS Coalition to Unleash Power (ACT UP), one of the most successful and controversial activist organizations in New York City's recent history, I ground this exploration in practice.

PROFILE: THE AIDS COALITION TO UNLEASH POWER

ACT UP was created in New York City in 1987, six years after the US Centers for Disease Control (CDC) reported the first cases of what was eventually called AIDS, or the acquired immune deficiency syndrome, in Los Angeles and then New York City. By 1983, researchers had identified the human immune deficiency virus (HIV) as the cause of "HIV syndrome," the precursor to AIDS. Over the years, ACT UP expanded nationally and globally to fight for increases in research and improved prevention and treatment services for AIDS. Many ACT UP founders had also helped to create the Gay Men's Health Crisis (GMHC) in 1982, a New York City organization that continues to provide services for people with HIV and to advocate for policies that support AIDS prevention and treatment. They left GMHC because they believed a more activist, confrontational organization was also needed.

ACT UP also mobilized to ensure equitable access to prevention and care for HIV and to urge government action to meet the basic needs for food and housing for people affected by AIDS. ACT UP also tackled the stigma, discrimination, and poverty that burdened people with or at risk of AIDS and HIV. To achieve the multiple goals it identified, the group worked to change the policies, institutional practices, and beliefs that obstructed progress on the treatment and prevention of HIV infection.

Activists and others concerned about AIDS first created ACT UP to confront the emerging health and social crises posed by the AIDS epidemic. New York City was the epicenter of the national AIDS epidemic, a place with high concentrations of gay men and men who have sex with men, injecting drug users, female partners of men in these groups, and sex workers, but also of low-income people, people of color, and immigrants—all groups with various vulnerabilities to this new threat to health.[1]

In response to the waves of fear and terror that AIDS provoked in the communities most affected, ACT UP chose not to emphasize a single solution to the epidemic but rather to pursue the multiple paths that its members identified in their encounters with AIDS and its social responses. Their decision to focus on activism, rather than solely on medical services, to realize their many goals was facilitated by the fact that by 1987, GMHC and many other AIDS service organizations, some government-run and other nonprofits, were providing some level of services to the various communities most affected by AIDS.

Three specific campaigns illustrate ACT UP's range of responses. In 1988, ACT UP sponsored Seize Control of the FDA, a Washington demonstration that briefly shut down the US Food and Drug Administration and led to major changes in the way the agency reviewed and approved new drugs. Later the same year, ACT UP organized a demonstration at the New York Stock Exchange on Wall Street to protest the high price of AIDS drugs and the greed of pharmaceutical companies and to demand faster approval of new drugs. Stop the Church was a 1989 demonstration at St. Patrick's Cathedral objecting to the Catholic Church's role in interfering with abortion and AIDS policy and promoting stigma against gay people.

Brief descriptions of these campaigns, three of the many initiatives ACT UP sponsored in its most active years, set the stage for examining how the group decided to organize these campaigns and what remedies they proposed. These accounts are based on the extensive reports on ACT UP by activists, scholars, and the media,[2] and especially on Sarah Schulman's definitive book *Let the Record Show*, a comprehensive portrait of the organization.[3] Schulman, a writer and AIDS historian, was an active member of ACT UP and other reproductive rights, lesbian, and AIDS organizations who, with colleagues, interviewed 188 ACT UP members to record their accounts of the group's work.

"Seize Control of the FDA." Early one October morning in 1988, 1,500 protesters—people with AIDS, their friends, and queer activists from all over the country, arrived at the headquarters of the FDA in Rockville, Maryland. They were protesting what they saw as the failure of the FDA to approve medications to fight AIDS. The disease had already killed at least forty-five thousand Americans in less than a decade. The demonstrators carried posters with a red handprint and the words "the government has blood on its hands; one AIDS death every half hour," and, as they lay on the ground to block entrance to the FDA, they chanted, "Fifty-two will die today / Seize control of the FDA!" (see figure 4.1).[4] The day before ACT UP had sponsored a demonstration at the Washington, DC, office of the U.S. Department of Health and Human Services (HHS) under the banner "Health Care Is a Right."

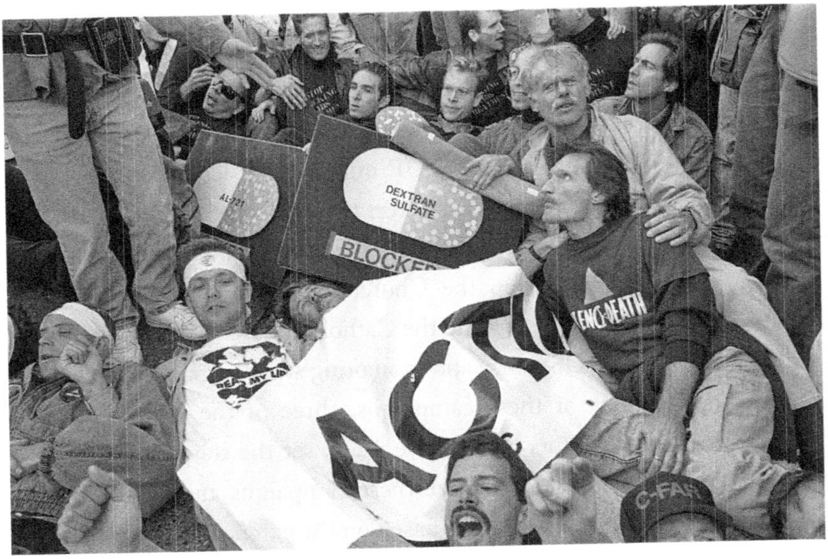

FIGURE 4.1 ACT UP (AIDS Coalition to Unleash Power) protesters at the headquarters of the Food and Drug Administration (FDA) on October 11, 1988, in Rockville, Maryland. The action, called Seize Control of the FDA, shut down the FDA for the day.

Source: Catherine McGann / Getty Images.

By moving their protests from New York City to the center of the federal government, protestors were insisting that AIDS was a national problem that required national solutions. In an interview with Schulman, Ann Northrop, a lesbian ACT UP activist who helped plan the FDA action and a former reporter and Vietnam-era antiwar activist, observed that ACT UP believed that change failed to happen because there was no pressure on people in power to make change. "So the strategy was," wrote Schulman, "to bring things out in the open so that people would be horrified, and so that people in power would be embarrassed and would make change out of that embarrassment."[5]

Soon after the demonstration, which attracted national and international media coverage, the FDA changed its rules on the use of experimental drugs,[6] permitting an experimental AIDS drug to be widely distributed while it was still being tested to determine if it was safe and effective. For people with AIDS, especially advanced AIDS, the change promised quicker access to potentially lifesaving drugs.

In its campaign to make effective HIV drugs more available, ACT UP followed an "insider/outsider" strategy, one that many activist campaigns have used effectively. Schulman defined it as the strategy in which one arm of a movement works directly with government or corporate officials to negotiate agreements while another arm uses disruptive strategies such as demonstrations or civil disobedience to put public pressure on decision-makers to make the changes the group seeks.[7]

At the FDA, and in its Wall Street action, ACT UP staged public demonstrations that sought to shame their opponents in the national and international media. At the same time, ACT UP members mastered the complex science of testing AIDS drugs, then met privately with FDA and National Institutes of Health officials as well as with staff from Burroughs Wellcome (the company that made several AIDS drugs) to persuade them to act more quickly based on the available science.

In effect, ACT UP members had identified two different causes for the lack of progress on developing new AIDS treatments. The first was a failure of scientific leaders to boldly apply emerging evidence to the task of offering immediate—not far-distant—ways to save the lives of people with AIDS. By reviewing that evidence with senior scientists and communicating their sense of urgency directly, ACT UP members sought to influence the decisions made inside the agency offices.

Other members believed that only outside pressure from politicians, the media, and the public would change the funding levels and the practices of FDA, HHS, and CDC. They took to the streets to pursue these goals. Within ACT UP, some members argued that this combination of strategies was more effective than either alone, while others feared that outside pressure tactics risked alienating powerful potential supporters or that insider tactics might compromise ACT UP's capacity to confront and challenge those in power.[8] By pursuing both, ACT UP hedged their bets, a strategy with both risks and benefits.

Zap at the New York Stock Exchange. New York City activists have long used places like Wall Street and the New York Stock Exchange to symbolize the role of capitalism in creating social problems. During the Vietnam War, Yippie activist Abbie Hoffman dropped dollar bills onto the trading floor of the stock exchange, leading the brokers and traders to leap into the air to grab the dollar bills floating down, delaying trading for a while, and winning international media coverage for the antiwar movement's message that Wall Street profited from the war.[9]

In 1975, ten thousand New York City workers and their supporters, led by Barry Feinstein, head of Teamsters Local 237, and Victor Gotbaum, executive director of District Council 37 of the American Federation of State, County and Municipal Employees, demonstrated outside First National City Bank on Wall Street to make the case that Wall Street should not benefit from the city's financial hardships and the city's budget should not be balanced "on the backs of the workers" and the city's residents.[10] These and similar protests attracted media attention and enabled activists to propose that fixing the ills they had identified required tackling the role of the market economy in promoting inequality and poverty.

ACT UP's 1989 Zap on the New York Stock Exchange targeted Burroughs Wellcome, the maker of AZT. AZT—also known as Azidothymidine—was one of the first antiretroviral drugs used to treat HIV infection. After initial enthusiasm, both researchers and activists realized that AZT needed to be used in combination with other drugs to effectively slow HIV infection. In the drug's first year on the market, the company expected to generate profits of $230 million selling AZT at a price of $10,000 per person per year, making it at the time one of the most expensive drugs ever.[11]

In the subsequent dizzying consolidation of the global drug industry, Burroughs Wellcome was bought in 1995 by Glaxo, later GlaxoKline-Smith, now GSK, the British-based multinational pharmaceutical and biotechnology company. For many people with AIDS, early reports on the benefits of AZT made them feel this was their best hope for surviving the disease. ACT UP's campaign to lower the price of AZT was one of the first of many global actions to force the pharmaceutical industry to lower prices.

At the stock exchange, borrowing from Abbie Hoffman's tactics, ACT UPers threw fake $100 bills onto the trading floor from a balcony. On the back of each bill, the activists had written "FUCK YOUR PROFITEERING, WE DIE WHILE YOU MAKE MONEY." The demonstrators also unfurled a huge banner saying, "Sell Wellcome."[12] Some traders attacked the demonstrators. Once again, the action attracted broad media coverage. Three days later, Burroughs Wellcome lowered the price of AZT by 20 percent.[13]

Underlying ACT UP's desire to lower the price of AZT and other AIDS drugs was an analysis that the price of drugs was, ACT UP members wrote, "inordinately influenced by the interests of major pharmaceutical companies" and that government research priorities had become "tied to corporate profit interests primarily through direct and indirect conflicts of interests by members of NIH [National Institutes of Health] policy-making committees and rank-and-file Principal Investigators."[14] The result of this entrenched system, argued ACT UP, is a "research agenda both public and private skewed towards drugs likely to receive FDA approval."

Later, in 1994 and 1995, ACT UP worked with New York Congressman Jerry Nadler and others to support the AIDS Cure Act, legislation designed to reduce corporate influence on the AIDS research agenda. The House failed to vote on the bill. In the longer run, however, Zap the Stock Exchange and other ACT UP actions focused attention on the pharmaceutical industry's windfall profits and raised public and media attention on the need for stronger federal regulation of Big Pharma. In the early 1980s, Merck, Pfizer, and other drug companies consistently topped *Fortune* magazine's Most Admired Businesses list.[15] But by 2019, public opinion polls showed that pharma was one of the lowest-rated industries in the United States, with 31 percent more Americans having a negative view than a positive one.[16] This declining political support for Big Pharma's agenda contributed to subsequent partially successful advocacy by activists and sympathetic politicians to lower the price of insulin, COVID-19 vaccines, and other products. These developments illustrate the potential for social movements to change harmful business practices and de-normalize the pursuit of profit at the expense of public well-being.[17]

Stop the Church. On December 10, 1989, more than 4,500 people participated in a demonstration at St. Patrick's Cathedral, making it the largest ACT UP demonstration to date. St. Patrick's was the biggest Catholic church in the United States and the seat of the Archdiocese of New York, led by Cardinal John O'Connor. Organized by ACT UP and WHAM!, Women's Health Action and Mobilization, the action challenged the Catholic Church's opposition to abortion, AIDS education in the public schools, clean needle exchanges for drug users at risk of HIV infection, gay rights, and its continuing stigmatization of gay people.

WHAM!, a group organized by reproductive health activists and ACT UP members, opposed the 1989 US Supreme Court decision *Webster v. Reproductive Health*, which upheld a Missouri state law that banned federal funds for abortions or abortion counseling.[18] By joining with ACT UP to sponsor Stop the Church, WHAM! activists highlighted the adverse impact of the church's desire to have its beliefs on sexuality determine public policy for all citizens, especially harming women and gay and lesbian people. The activists' proposed solution to this problem was to de-normalize the church's active involvement in setting public policy on public health issues.

According to *The New York Times*, the 400 police officers who guarded St. Patrick's on that day arrested 111 people, including 43 inside the church.[19] Those arrested were charged with blocking traffic or disrupting a religious service. Many of those arrested were carried out on stretchers because they refused to stand up. In a message distributed at the action, ACT UP and WHAM! explained their purpose:

> We do not challenge anyone's right to worship as they choose. However, recent actions by the Catholic church go beyond its constitutionally protected right to worship. The church, through its immense political power, restricts access to information that can save lives and access to health care, including abortion. . . . These actions of the church ensure the spread of HIV [the virus thought to cause AIDS], deny women

> control over their bodies and endanger all our lives. The intrusion of [Cardinal] O'Connor and the church hierarchy into politics and public health guarantees that ALL people will suffer from the murderous policies of the church.[20]

Some ACT UP members objected to the demonstration, fearing it would alienate potential supporters or imply that the group opposed religion. Others ardently supported the action. Victor Mendolia, a gay ACT UP activist, told Schulman that the Catholic Church has caused "more death and destruction and more chaos and problems on the planet than anything else,"[21] so he was eager to confront the church. Maxine Wolfe, an influential ACT UP leader with previous experience in civil rights, reproductive rights, and socialist activism, put it simply: If the church takes actions that seek to influence public policy, she told Schulman, "I don't care where you are, I'm going to come and get you, and you can't hide behind the church."[22]

By calling out the opposition of the Catholic Church and Cardinal O'Connor to sexual rights and freedoms and access to information and care, ACT UP members were saying, as Victor Mendolia put it, "we are the ones fighting for people's lives, and they are the murderers."[23]

Larry Kramer, a founder of Gay Men's Health Crisis, one of the first AIDS services and advocacy groups in New York, and later a cofounder of ACT UP, called Stop the Church "the most successful demonstration" in ACT UP's history. "I remember going to the meeting after it," he told Schulman. "Everybody was terrified because it had been in the paper and every editorial page had dumped on us. . . . I remember saying 'Are you crazy? They're afraid of us now! That's the best thing that could have happened to us.'"[24]

HOW ACT UP DECIDED

In each of these campaigns, ACT UP members identified a problem and took action to address it. Its process for making these decisions illustrates

ACT UP's commitment to participatory democracy. But it also shows the group's struggles to develop governance processes that enabled it to efficiently recognize and act on evolving political opportunities while keeping its members fully engaged.

In its early years in the late 1980s, ACT UP attracted hundreds of people to its weekly meetings, where it debated strategy, educated participants about HIV policy and scientific issues, and planned actions. Every Monday night for about seven years, ACT UP members from across its constituencies came to these meetings, expecting to voice their opinions and ready to debate differences between and among these constituencies, a key tenet of ACT UP's culture.[25]

To be sure, there was conflict. Some constituencies within ACT UP felt excluded, and no space was immune from the heavy hands of racism, misogyny, and homophobia that have long interfered with open activist discussions. But by holding regular open meetings, ACT UP created a space for all its members—Black, Latiné, and white gay men, cisgender and lesbian women (many with experience in earlier women's health activism), people with AIDS and their partners and relatives, drug users, and concerned citizens. At these meetings, participants learned about the AIDS epidemic, debated ideas, planned actions, flirted, and shared their fears, grief, and outrage.[26] From its start, ACT UP acknowledged that activists were motivated by ideas, beliefs, and emotions, all recognized as essential ingredients for successful campaigns.

Early in its history, ACT UP decided to encourage members with shared goals for action to come together and, with relative autonomy, plan strategies to pursue those goals. Some ACT UP members questioned whether this almost anarchic structure diminished its efficacy, and others left the organization because of the never-ending debates. A few questioned whether the image of inclusiveness masked a narrower focus. Most ACT UP members were white gay men, the stereotype of AIDS activism. Charles King, a gay white ACT UP member who later helped found Housing Works, an offshoot of ACT UP that served homeless people with AIDS, told Schulman, "I never thought that ACT UP itself was really about poor people and poverty. ACT UP, at its core, was gay men and their allies fighting for their lives. . . . The core of ACT UP saw homophobia and that was all they saw, and they never saw the other connections."[27]

Unlike members of the Young Lords or Make the Road New York, who primarily defined their identities by class and race/ethnicity, most ACT UP members identified as gay men or men who had sex with men, a characteristic that forged a powerful bond with others as well as a potential barrier to engaging different groups. From the start, however, ACT UP also included lesbian and straight women, drug users, and people of color. Many of its members had experience in prior movements, bringing a wide repertoire of strategic and tactical organizing experience to ACT UP campaigns.

ACT UP's participatory, at times anarchic, decision-making processes enabled the organization to move on many fronts. Its working groups included the Majority Coalition (for people of color); Black, Latino, Asian Pacific Islander, and Women's caucuses; and Committees on Treatment and Data, Needle Exchange, Media, Outreach, and Health Insurance.

Over the years, several organizations including the Treatment Action Group, Gran Force (an art collective), Black AIDS Mobilization, and Housing Works worked inside ACT UP to develop other approaches to AIDS activism. Sometimes in partnerships and sometimes in conflict with ACT UP, some became independent organizations. Like the Young Lords Party in the 1970s and Make the Road New York in the 2010s, ACT UP became a major supplier of experienced activists who went on to serve and lead the activist campaigns described elsewhere in this book.

Another strength of ACT UP was its innovative use of media to advance its goals. With participants and support from New York City's arts, publishing, advertising, financial, and other well-off sectors, ACT UP had access to the skills, money, resources, and political networks that helped it reach local, national, and international media. These skills enabled ACT UP to promote its definitions of problems and solutions to wider audiences.

Long before the advent of social media, ACT Up devised ways to get its ideas and images, steeped in outrage and humor, in front of the eyes of millions of New Yorkers. Its powerful slogans (e.g., Silence = Death) and images (see figure 4.2) and its use of art and mainstream media engaged emotions and generated indignation. To call attention to Mayor Ed Koch's unwillingness to take action to prevent AIDS, ACT UP produced posters designed to fit on subway overhead ad slots saying, "10,000 New York City AIDS Deaths. How'm I DOIN?,'" Koch's signature greeting to voters. Another criticized New York City Health Commissioner Stephen Joseph for his adjustment of official city AIDS rates. ACT UP's innovations in communication—pithy slogans, street posters, disruptive demonstrations—continue to influence activism today.

Two weeks after the 1989 Stop the Church action, veteran NBC New York reporter Gabe Pressman asked Cardinal O'Connor, "Don't you think it odd that you continue to open up hospices for people [with AIDS] to die yet you oppose condoms and safe sex education?" ACT UP activist Victor Mendolia observed, "that question would never have been asked (previously). In New York, the press did not ask questions of the cardinal."[28]

When ACT UP believed that *New York Times* science reporter Gina Kolata distorted research findings on the benefits of certain AIDS drugs, its members made stickers saying, "Buy Your Lies Here" to place on newspaper vending machines.[29]

HOW ACT UP CHANGED NEW YORK

ACT UP's policy wins on more rapidly testing and bringing to the market new HIV drugs and its successes in reducing stigma against people with AIDS and forcing policymakers to increase support for the housing, food, and health-care needs of people at risk of HIV were lasting contributions to the health of the people of New York City and beyond. Its new tactics, strategies, and the leaders for health and social justice activism it trained provided ongoing resources for New York City activists. Together, these contributions make ACT UP one of the most successful and best recognized of New York City activist organizations.

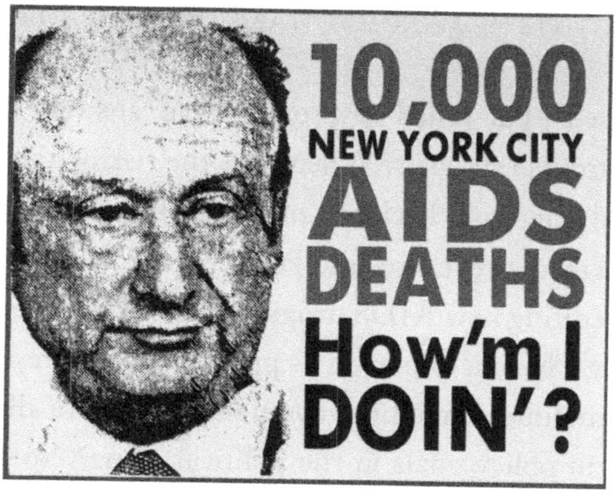

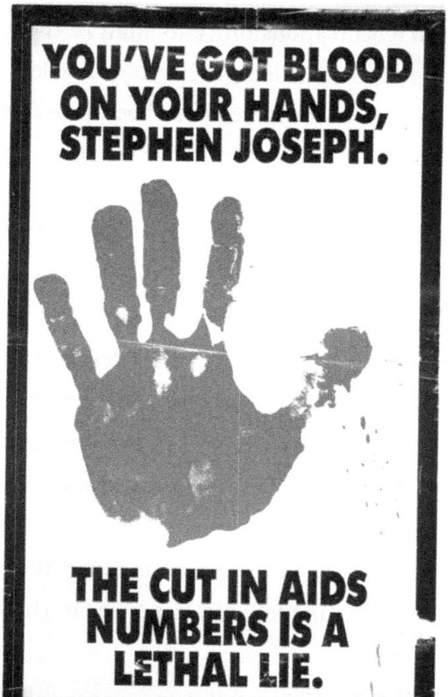

FIGURE 4.2 Two ACT UP posters, one from 1986 targeting Mayor Ed Koch for his lack of action on AIDS, and the other from 1988 accusing New York City Health Commissioner Dr. Stephen Joseph of altering New York City's count of AIDS cases.

Source: "ACT UP New York, 10,000 AIDS Deaths. How'm I doin'?" poster, 1989. Created by Richard Deagle for ACT UP's Target City Hall demonstration, 1989. Courtesy ACT UP New York, Manuscripts and Archives Division, New York Public Library. https://digitalcollections.nypl.org/items/510d47e3-5f5f-a3d9-e040-e00a18064a99; https://www.icp.org/browse/archive/objects/youve-got-blood-on-your-hands-stephen-joseph

ACT UP raised—but failed to provide clear answers to—questions that continue to trouble activists. When does the risk of alienating potential supporters or triggering backlash outweigh the potential to generate public debate and media coverage, also key activist goals?[30] Did ACT UP's insistence on expediting new AIDS drugs weaken FDA's oversight authority and enable Big Pharma to pursue its profits more aggressively? Did its participatory, sometimes anarchic governance structure diminish ACT UP's power to win policy goals in the political arena? No activist group can solve every problem it raises, but activists and scholars who have the benefit of hindsight have a responsibility to analyze the costs and benefits of the decisions that activists made in the heat of battle.

ACT UP's achievements would not have been possible without the lessons from previous cycles of activism and the ongoing support from activists in the gay and lesbian, women's, civil rights, labor, and health-care movements. And like the Young Lords Party, but unlike Make the Road New York, ACT UP was most active for less than a decade, limiting its power to follow through on its victories and defeats.

Finally, by its resistance to some ACT UP demands, the persistence of widespread homophobia and stigmatization of people with HIV in the city and beyond, and the reluctance of many city political leaders to take up the problem of AIDS, New York City also changed ACT UP. The organization became more impatient, exacerbating divisions within the group, and limiting its capacity to take on the more fundamental causes of New York City's sometimes inadequate responses to the AIDS epidemic.

TAKE ON BIG PROBLEMS OR SMALL ONES? HOW ACTIVISTS DECIDE

ACT UP members were inspired by the values and beliefs that emerged from the 1960s movements and the evolution of the gay rights and lesbian movements of the 1970s and, of course, by their fears about AIDS for themselves and their communities. The problems it chose to address were those caused or exacerbated by the AIDS epidemic and the pervasive stigma against those at highest risk. Even during these struggles, many AIDS activists recognized that the fundamental causes of the problems they confronted went deeper than the human immunodeficiency virus. But by focusing on the AIDS epidemic, ACT UP members could tackle what was dominating their lives.

Some ACT UPers recognized the limits of this framing. Getting drugs into bodies was both an ACT UP slogan and a policy priority. Mark Harrington, an ACT UP member and founder of the Treatment Action Group, has observed that ACT UP may have been "in too much of a hurry" to get untested drugs approved, opening the door for drug makers to seek quick approval of inadequately tested drugs.[31] Gregg Gonsalves, another ACT UP member who then became a global health researcher at Yale University, regretted ACT UP's limited attention to promoting universal health care, especially after President Bill Clinton failed to win over drug industry support for change, showing the limits of Washington politics.[32]

ACT UP's focus on getting immediate help for people with HIV infection was perhaps its greatest strength, but it was also a significant weakness that sometimes led it to step back from advocating more transformative changes. As Schulman wrote, "while activists were able, in a sense, to beat HIV, they could not beat capitalism."[33] In other words, ACT UP was unable to transform the profit-driven actions of drug and health-care companies, the inequitable access to housing, food and health care, or the unwillingness of public officials to allocate the public resources needed to make the full range of AIDS prevention and treatment available to all who needed it. Every activist movement in New York City and the United States and every public health campaign must decide if, how, and when to tackle the system of capitalism—or even to use the word in its public messages, a topic that has provoked sharp debates over the years.[34]

For those who believed that capitalism was the fundamental cause of the most serious local, national, and global health problems, any solution that did not have as its goal transforming modern capitalism was an unacceptable compromise. For those who believed that this system was inevitable, immutable—or the best an imperfect world could come up with—seeking to transform capitalism was a quixotic, impractical, or undesirable aim.

All social movements must decide how to divide their focus between the immediate manifestations of the problem its members choose to address and their fundamental causes. Founded in 1999, Voices of Community Activists & Leaders (VOCAL-NY) emerged from housing, drug users, and policing reform groups as well as from ACT UP. While ACT UP put AIDS at the top of its problem list, VOCAL-NY sought to integrate lessons from previous activism on AIDS, drug use, homelessness, and policing. It proposed more fundamental causes of New York City's continuing health and social crises than AIDS alone: inequality, poverty, and racism.

VOCAL-NY describes itself as "a statewide grassroots membership organization that builds power among low-income people affected by HIV/AIDS, the drug war, mass incarceration, and homelessness in order to create healthy and just communities."[35] Its strategies include community organizing, leadership development, advocacy, direct services, participatory research, and direct action.

In 2016, the group played a key role in developing and then advocating for New York State's Plan to End AIDS, which insisted that additional funding for supportive housing and food assistance for people with HIV and drug users would enable people with or at risk of HIV to take their anti-HIV medication and remain noninfectious.[36] When Governor Andrew Cuomo failed to adequately fund the proposed new housing units, VOCAL-NY members seized a suite near the governor's office and refused to leave until he restored funding. They occupied the space for twenty-four hours and six were arrested. Some funding was ultimately restored,[37] and a subsequent study showed that homeless people with HIV in New York City who received housing support were more likely to be engaged in care and to have higher levels of viral suppression than those without such support.[38] In the view of VOCAL-NY's members, this finding demonstrated that taking on more fundamental causes could lead to measurable health benefits.

In 2021, to showcase its broader analysis, VOCAL-NY proposed a Caring and Compassionate New Deal for New York City. As Paulette Soltani, the group's political director, explained, "the plan is based on a simple premise:

we can address poverty and public health concerns by providing people the housing, social services and care they need—and by divesting from policing and incarceration. Now, we are calling on the City Council to deliver a down payment toward that vison in the City's budget."[39] Illustrating VOCAL-NY's focus on advocating for policy changes that better meet the daily needs of its constituents, in 2025 the group released a report, *Wi-Fi for All: The Need for Wi-fi Access in NYC's Shelter System*, in support of proposed city and state laws that would require all city shelters to provide wi-fi.[40]

In that same year, after Mayor-Elect Zohran Mamdani announced his intention to end the city's sweeps of homeless encampments, Noam Cohen, a VOCAL-NY homelessness union leader, posted on Instagram, "Sweeps as an approach to homelessness is just wasting millions of dollars moving people out of sight and out of mind, so I'm looking forward to this new administration prioritizing housing and services instead."[41] Like ACT UP, VOCAL-NY also advocated a global perspective on fighting epidemics. In 2013, the group called on the World Health Organization to ramp up its programs to control hepatitis C, an infectious disease threatening drug users, people with AIDS, and others around the world (see figure 4.3).

With the benefit of hindsight, activists and scholars of activism can compare the benefits and costs of ACT UP's more focused approach to reducing the impact of HIV with VOCAL-NY's broader view of the necessity of reducing poverty and inequality and meeting basic needs for housing, economic security, food, and public safety. This broader view also characterized the Young Lords Party and Make the Road New York, each of which identified deep economic and political inequalities as the root causes of the specific problems they were seeking to remedy.

Since its founding, VOCAL-NY has been less visible than ACT UP in its heyday and seems to have had a smaller impact on policy. But twenty years after its founding, VOCAL-NY is still an active organization, one that is expanding into other states and taking on new issues—better services for those with hepatitis C, actions to reduce mass incarceration, and new efforts to expand the capacity of its members to participate meaningfully in American democracy.[42] Whether its commitment to building a mass movement that unites various constituencies harmed by the current

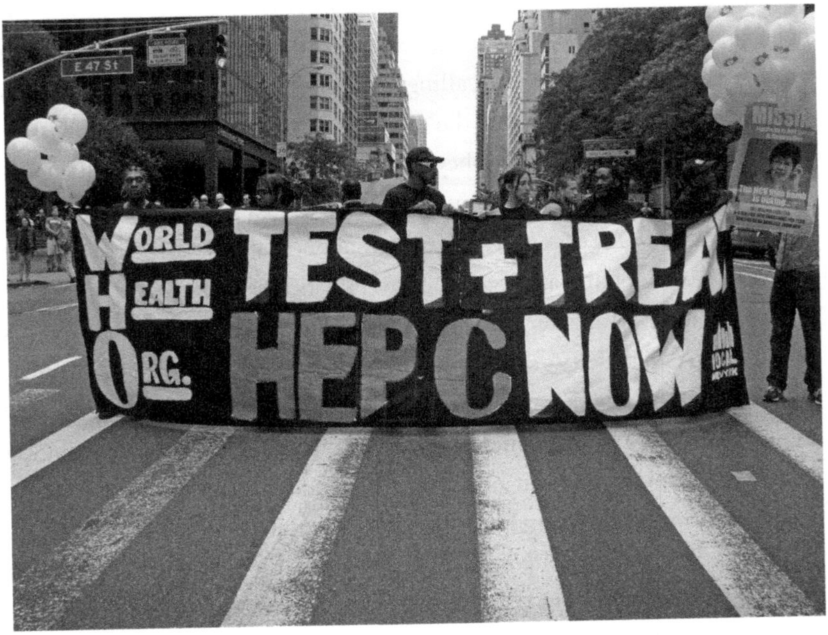
E 47 St
WORLD
HEALTH
ORG.
TEST + TREA
HEP C NOW
VOCAL

FIGURE 4.3 A 2013 demonstration in New York City by VOCAL-NY, an organization founded by ACT UP members, calling on the World Health Organization to ramp up its programs to control hepatitis C. Both VOCAL-NY and ACT UP linked their efforts to combat AIDS, drug use, and hep C in New York with the global efforts to control these health crises.

Source: VOCAL-NY, Creative Commons License. https://creativecommons.org/licenses/by/4.0/deed.en

political economy will ultimately enable VOCAL-NY to have a more lasting impact than an organization focused on responding to a single epidemic, however devastating, remains to be seen.

No simple algorithm can tell activists whether and when to frame the problem they seek to fix as rooted in the deepest structures of our society or as amenable to quicker, more achievable solutions. Rather, planners of health campaigns need to consider the strategic pros and cons of broader versus more focused definitions of the specific problem they address and the solutions they propose. One tool that activists have used to assist in these deliberations is power mapping.

MAPPING POWER AND MOBILIZING POWER

"To win a campaign," the authors of *Beautiful Trouble*, a toolbox for activists assembled by ten grassroots groups, write, "you need to correctly identify who has the power to fix the problem you wanted fixed. Then you need to pressure them to make the right decision."[43] These two decisions—ascertaining which individuals and organizations have the power to resolve the problem activists have chosen and what strategies and tactics will lead these power players to do the right thing—define the subsequent success or failure of health campaigns.

Power mapping, an exercise to identify powerful relevant potential allies and opponents, is one tool campaign organizers use to make these vital decisions. In a typical power mapping, activists locate the potential institutions and individuals who support or oppose their campaign along two axes. The first ranks these actors on how influential they are in contributing to the desired goal; the second on how strongly they are likely to support or oppose the campaign's goals. By allying with the most influential and supportive actors and planning how to overcome or isolate the most influential and least supportive players, planners of activist campaigns can draw a road map for the strategies, alliances, and coalitions they should pursue to win.[44]

A few examples illustrate how some New York City activist groups have used power mapping. WE ACT for Environmental Justice, profiled in chapter 5, is based in Harlem but operates citywide and nationally. Through its Food Justice Initiative, WE ACT assisted parents of public school students to improve the food served in their schools. Based on its belief that schools stigmatized poor students of color by serving them the cheapest, most highly processed, worst-tasting food in public schools (the problem), the group organized workshops for parents of three Upper Manhattan public schools to build a vision of what parents want for school food (the goal).

With these parents, WE ACT analyzed the school food system to understand what power they needed to leverage to achieve their vision. They investigated the corporate supply chain of school foods and their ingredients and identified the manufacturers and locations of the food New York City schools purchased.[45] WE ACT organizers and parents used this information to formulate their demands on the city's school food system, goals that shaped the subsequent campaigns to improve school food in New York City, profiled in chapter 6.

Three organizations seeking to prevent evictions of New York City tenants having trouble paying their rents provide another example of power mapping.[46] Right to Counsel, a group advocating for all tenants to have the right to legal representation in the city's housing courts, and JustFix, an organization that creates tools to fight displacement and promote policies that supported healthier housing conditions, partnered with the New York City chapter of the AntiEviction Mapping Project to produce the Worst Evictors Map.[47] This tool maps the landlords who have evicted the most tenants in New York City, enabling housing activists to choose the most egregious offenders in their neighborhoods—and to partner with tenants' groups from other neighborhoods taking on the same landlords. To link this tool to the alliance's mission, the producers of the map ask, "When we see empty glass condo towers towering over our city while hundreds of thousands of families face losing their homes during a global pandemic, we ask ourselves: Who are we building the city for and how? And what kind of city do we want actually to live in?"

Power mapping can help activists to identify who has the power to fix the problem they have identified. But to pressure those actors to make the right decision, as the *Beautiful Trouble* authors explained, requires activists to mobilize their own power and leverage the power of their allies to achieve this goal.

Social movement scholars have suggested various ways that activists can think about power. Steven Lukes, a sociologist now at New York University, has proposed a three-dimensional view of power.[48] The first dimension is overt power, typically displayed in the presence of conflict in decision-making situations. This form of power is used to win by prevailing over others. Covert power, the second dimension, is used to control what gets decided, by ignoring or sidetracking existing articulated injustices. The third is the power to shape desires and beliefs, thereby averting both conflict and grievances. When the opponents of activists have consolidated their control of the third dimension of power, these powerful actors can severely constrain the opportunities for activist campaigns to win their goals.

To overcome this weakness, John Gaventa, another sociologist, asked, "how do relatively powerless groups develop the capacity for agency and action which in turn give new possibilities for emancipation and freedom in their lives?"[49] His answer is to deepen our understanding of power, moving beyond "power over" to "power to," "power with," and "power within." "Power for," argued Gaventa, provides a logic for the transformative power activists can mobilize to bring about desired changes, transforming them from subjects of other players to actors.

ACT UP used the ideological and cultural power its campaigns had won for them to challenge the moral authority of the Catholic Church to set public policy, of Big Pharma to decide what drugs to produce and how much to charge, and of Mayor Ed Koch to determine AIDS policy for New York City. Each of these powerful actors, ACT UP argued, were compromised by their unwillingness to act for the public good rather than their own institutional interests. By itself, ACT UP clearly lacked "power over" the church, Big Pharma, or the mayor. But the group could add its ideas to the public debates on AIDS in New York City and the nation and it could propose alternative morals and values that made it easier for AIDS activists to mobilize the political power needed to win specific victories.

Some activists are hesitant to consider their own power, understandably preferring to win over supporters with their moral arguments and scientific evidence. But as the novelist Alice Walker has observed, "the most common way people give up their power is by thinking they don't have any." By making an inventory of all their sources of power, activists can choose when to leverage which of these assets.

In their guide for organizers, movement activists and scholars Deepak Bhargava and Stephanie Luce describe two forms of power they believe are especially useful for activists. "Solidarity power" describes the ability to form associations, networks, and alliances with groups with shared interests. "Disruptive power" defines the ability to resist or refuse to cooperate with the status quo.[50]

The Young Lords' alliances with the Black Panthers, women's groups, health-worker organizations, and other constituencies demonstrated the power of solidarity, as did Make the Road New York's ongoing coalitions with the labor movement, immigrant and immigrants' rights organizations, and LGBTQI groups. Both used this power to claim the right to speak for and act with more than only their members. The constituencies they spoke for, whatever their limitations in wealth and political influence, represented broad cross sections of the city's population. Sometimes speaking at the community level and sometime at the city or national levels, the Young Lords and ACT UP claimed that in a democratic society, it should be the majority of residents, not powerful business and political elites, who decide how people live and how their rights to well-being and respect are protected.

The Young Lords and ACT UP also used disruptive power to win attention and force political leaders to react. By burning uncollected garbage in the streets of East Harlem and seizing and using the city Health Department's tuberculosis and lead poisoning testing equipment, the Lords won media attention, responses from elected officials, and community support, victories that might have been difficult with more polite tactics. ACT UP's actions at St. Peter's Cathedral, on Wall Street, and at the FDA disrupted business as usual for the targeted organizations, won media coverage, offended their opponents (and some supporters as well), and demanded a response to their rebellious but righteous moral arguments.

Based on their studies of several social movements in New York and elsewhere, Frances Fox Piven and Richard Cloward, radical scholars of social movements, argued that disruptive social movements were more effective in extracting concessions from political elites. Unruly campaigns were harder to co-opt with modest concessions, and they had the capacity to leverage the greatest assets of poor people, their ability to withhold consent from participating in public processes and to disrupt business as usual.[51]

Power mapping also requires activists to look at the power of their opponents. Dominant institutions use visible power, hidden power, and invisible power to achieve their goals.[52] By investigating and revealing these forms of less visible power, planners of campaigns can identify unseen targets. In their 1981 book examining the causes of the city's 1975 fiscal crisis, *The Permanent Government: Who Really Rules New York?*, the reporters Jack Newfield and Paul Du Brul claimed that an elite group of unelected power brokers control New York City both politically and economically.[53] They show how the decisions of mostly faceless bankers contributed to the city's fiscal crisis—"New York didn't jump; it was pushed" into its predicament, they wrote.[54]

By revealing the identities of these decision-makers and the human consequences of their decisions, activist groups may not have been able to reverse the decisions of business elites at that time, but they did focus more public scrutiny on these often previously hidden actors. Perhaps they also laid the foundation for the later Occupy Wall Street movement and the resurgence of a national movement focused on greater equity that led to Bernie Sanders's presidential campaign and the election of Alexandria Ocasio-Cortez, Zohran Mamdani, and other progressive New York City, State, and national legislators.

In summary, activist groups have charted the power of their allies and opponents to provide the evidence they needed to plan winning strategies to remedy the problems they identified. They have used these insights to target and isolate the upholders of the status quo they seek to change and to identify the partners with whom they can accumulate the power they need to realize their goals.

A SEQUENCE OF CAMPAIGNS OR A MOVEMENT OF MOVEMENTS?

A dispassionate history of health activism in New York City since the 1970s shows a recurrent sequence of mostly unconnected campaigns tackling a multitude of problems, some playing out at the community level, some at the municipal, and a few with ties to statewide or national campaigns. Punctuating these campaigns are the occasional flares of broader national social movements—the labor, civil rights, women's, environmental and climate justice, and LGBTQI movements. These movements have fought for more fundamental transformations, but their power waxes and wanes with changes in the political economy and their skills and capacity to bring benefits to their supporters.

A fundamental difference between these two flows of activism is their definition of the problem. Most health campaigns identify a specific problem and a specific fix. Most social movements define deep-seated injustices that will ultimately require transformative changes. By exploring when and how these two streams do and do not intersect and reinforce each other, activists may be able to find synergies that can build their power in ways that increase their impact on health and health equity.

What specific strategies can activists use to better align single-issue health campaigns with broader social movements working to change the ways that power, wealth, and access to the resources that support health are distributed? I give a few examples here but return to this fundamental question in chapter 10.

Of course, specific health campaigns and social movements are not separate entities. They are intertwined, sometimes acting separately, sometimes in close constructive collaboration. Social movement organizations, formal groups that emerge from and shape social movements, translate the goals and vision of social movements into actions that advance movement goals.[55] Each of the organizations I have profiled—the Young Lords Party, Make the Road New York, and ACT UP—is a social movement organization. Each was connected to several broader national movements and each sponsored numerous health campaigns, sometimes as the lead and sometimes as part of a broader coalition.

Specific health campaigns or movement organizations decide whether and how to pursue such linkages. These decisions determine both the power they will need to achieve their goals and the power they can muster for that purpose. ACT UP, for example, designed its Stop the Church campaign to limit the Catholic Church's interference with public policies on AIDS and abortion. The group partnered with WHAM!, a women's organization, to bring the potential power of two constituencies, gay and lesbian people and women supporting reproductive rights and their respective social movements, into their campaign. By linking two issues—opposition to the Supreme Court's *Webster* decision on abortion rights and the Catholic Church's antagonism to AIDS education in public schools—and two constituencies, ACT UP and WHAM! had a wider reach and more power than either alone.

In its campaign to end ICE deportations of jailed immigrants, MRNY started its work on its own. The group's commitment to this issue came from the personal experiences of its members and their families. But over time, through a combination of national debates that pushed the immigration issue onto the nation's political agenda, the forceful advocacy of other groups like the Dreamers (undocumented immigrants brought to the country as children, raised as Americans, and now seeking legal status), and MRNY's skills in bringing together diverse constituencies, they generated the power to win victories. Thirteen organizations joined Make the Road's campaign in 2011 to convince New York State's governor and the city's mayor to enact new policies to end automatic deportation of immigrants.[56] In its 2025 policy statement, MRNY wrote about its broader goals of linking organizations working on multiple issues:

> As the Trump administration ratchets up plans to weaponize the military to deport and tear apart families, eliminate constitutional protections, and put more money and power in the hands of billionaires, it will be up to our elected officials in Albany to defend vulnerable New Yorkers from these devastating policies. We can create a New York in which everyone thrives—whether your family arrived last week or generations ago. With new policies that force billionaires to pay what they owe, we can fund programs that give each of us the skills and opportunities to succeed.[57]

These two examples illustrate the benefits and risks and the implications for power strategies of wide versus targeted campaign goals. Had ACT UP decided only to pursue its support for honest, comprehensive AIDS education in New York City schools, one of the aims of its Stop the Church campaign, it might have won additional allies and alienated fewer New Yorkers. By making the power of the Catholic Church to shape public policy its target, ACT UP had the potential to engage more constituencies but also challenged one of New York City's most powerful institutions, one with many allies across class, racial/ethnic, and gender characteristics.

Taking on the church allowed ACT UP to propose a vision and moral framework that could appeal to the many New Yorkers alienated by the church's conservative politics and morals. It also identified specific policies that could be changed if activists convinced elected leaders that the political risks of opposing these reforms were greater than the risks of inaction or support for Cardinal O'Connor.

For MRNY, the decision to challenge the deportation of jailed immigrants was far riskier than simply supporting the more mainstream, acceptable demands of the Dreamers, who wanted legal status for the children of undocumented immigrants. But as federal actions to demonize immigrants increased, even more during and after the elections of Donald Trump in 2016 and 2024, Make the Road's boldness put it in front of the growing opposition to anti-immigrant sentiment and policies. Their choice of this problem gave the group a bigger voice and wider visibility in the communities it sought to mobilize throughout the city.

Did ACT UP and Make the Road New York make the right decisions in their choice of targets? Monday-morning quarterbacking, especially by academics or others not engaged in a particular campaign, can be both irrelevant and unseemly. Thus, I believe the lesson from these stories is that by careful advance consideration of their choices on identifying problems, proposing solutions, and analyzing the power dynamics of their campaigns, activist groups can make more informed choices. By taking up these questions at the start of their campaigns and consulting their supporters, activists and social movements can decide their strategies and tactics, build more powerful coalitions, and reduce the risk that unintended consequences stemming from their choices derail their campaigns.

5

HOW ACTIVISTS ENGAGE PEOPLE IN THEIR CAMPAIGNS

Should ACT UP have focused on mobilizing people with HIV infection? Or should the group have made their priority all those at higher risk of infection or all the people who care about someone with AIDS or all gay men? Should the Young Lords Party have concentrated on mobilizing Puerto Ricans dissatisfied with their life circumstances in the neighborhoods where the party already has organizers? Or should it have sought to reach all Puerto Ricans, or even all people of color, in New York City?

For health activists seeking to bring about changes in policies, institutional practices, or public opinion, answers to such critical questions of who to engage and mobilize can determine their success or failure. A passionate, committed core of advocates, people whose life experiences and beliefs motivate them to make the proposed goal a priority, provides a foundation for wins, while lacking such a base can diminish the prospects for sustainable campaigns.

Identifying these individuals and groups and then recruiting them for action constitute a starting point for the implementation of activist campaigns. Marshall Ganz, the veteran organizer and trainer of activist leaders, suggests that the first question organizers should ask is "Who are my people?" He notes that these core supporters are "both the source of the needed change and the resources that will be used to create that change."[1]

For some campaign planners, the choice of which populations to engage is easy: It is their families and neighbors, or those who struggle to cope with a common health problem, or their partners in previous battles. For others, the choice is more difficult. Some ACT UP members firmly believed that since gay men were at highest risk for AIDS, that group should constitute the core of its membership. Others felt strongly that an interracial, cross-class organization that included people of all genders and identities could have a much more powerful voice in shaping policy. While these are not mutually exclusive choices, an organization does need to decide where to put its resources and what mix of populations will best win its policy goals.

How activist organizations answer these questions determines the strategies they use to get started, the messages they bring to potential supporters, and the coalitions they seek to organize or join. This chapter begins with a profile of WE ACT for Environmental Justice, a Harlem-based group whose core supporters of residents committed to protecting their community expanded as the group gradually extended its geographic and environmental health concerns. Over time, WE ACT became a key player in the citywide and national environmental justice movements, enabling—and requiring—the group to develop new bases of support.

Activists' choice of who to appeal to with what messages is influenced by the ways racism, sexism, homophobia, and other forms of inequity shape the social and political context of a particular campaign. To assist activists to overcome these negative forces, I also consider how a few other New York City–based campaigns have used other engagement strategies to build power across racial/ethnic and class lines to set the stage for intersectional alliances that help them to accomplish their goals.

PROFILE: WE ACT FOR ENVIRONMENTAL JUSTICE TACKLES THE CUMULATIVE IMPACT OF ENVIRONMENTAL INJUSTICES

WE ACT for Environmental Justice, originally named West Harlem Environmental Action, was founded in 1988 to decrease environmental threats such as air pollution and other toxic exposures to the well-being of residents of Harlem. Its roots, however, are planted in the civil rights, community development, health, and land use struggles of the 1960s and 1970s. Its history illustrates the rise of the environmental justice movement in New York City and the nation in the 1980s.

Through most of the twentieth century, Harlem was home to the city's largest Black community and the cultural and political capital of Black New York. Harlem residents and activists played key roles in the city's housing, labor, women's, education, and health-care struggles and in both mainstream and progressive city politics. WE ACT emerged from this blend of neighborhood, citywide, and national politics, helping to add an urban stream of environmental justice (EJ) activism that flowed into the national EJ river that had its source in the Black South.

Like United Bronx Parents, a leader of campaigns in that borough to improve school food and fight school segregation in the 1960s and 1970s,[2] and UPROSE, an environmental justice group still active in Sunset Park in Brooklyn that began to focus on environmental causes of asthma, lead poisoning, and polluted waterways in the 1990s,[3] WE ACT started as a local community group that benefited from and eventually contributed to national movements. Its campaign to reduce the threats from a sewage treatment plant that the city government moved from the middle-class Upper West Side to the mostly African American Harlem community over the objections of residents shows how EJ activists mobilized their neighbors. After the campaign to block construction of the plant in West Harlem failed, activists turned their attention to reducing health harms from the plant.

Reducing hazards from the North River Sewage Treatment Plant. Every city needs to dispose of the waste flushed down its residents' toilets, washed down the sinks of homes and businesses, and drained by its stormwater drainage system. After cholera epidemics in the 1840s, New York City initiated construction of a sewage treatment system that now includes 6,600 miles of pipes to carry wastewater and stormwater to fourteen sewage treatment plants, which treat and then discharge the 1.3 billion gallons of wastewater produced daily into rivers and bays.[4]

In 1962, after decades of debates about how to modernize the city's outdated sewage treatment system and where to locate new plants, the New York City Planning Commission voted to move one of the planned new sewage treatment plants from Seventy-Second Street, on Manhattan's Upper West Side, to a site on the Hudson River in West Harlem. The planning commission, appointed by the mayor and the city's five borough presidents, makes decisions about the growth and development of the city.

According to Vernice Miller, a cofounder of WE ACT, the decision to move the proposed treatment plant to Harlem was made at a hearing closed to the public and with no testimony from community representatives.[5] The commission concluded that the site at Seventy-Second Street did not have the space needed for the facility. Since New York City Parks Commissioner Robert Moses was unwilling to explore alternative sites in that area, the commission concluded that use of the Seventy-Second Street site would be detrimental to "adjacent residential and cultural development" and might cause "undue traffic interference" with planned middle-income housing and cultural institutions in that neighborhood.[6] WE ACT planners believed the decision to move the plant from a mostly middle-class white neighborhood to West Harlem reflected the commission's racial biases.

By 1964, the city had completed its review and approved the new sewage treatment plant at the West Harlem site, known as the North River Treatment Plant. In 1968, the New York City Board of Estimate, the body that then approved mayoral budgets, held three required public meetings to discuss the budget proposal. The mandate for open meetings came from the 1968 New York State "Sunshine Law," which required public agencies to open all meetings to the public, providing a valuable new source of information for activists. These three meetings provided the first opportunities for the public to comment on the plant, and many community residents and public officials did so by vigorously opposing the proposed project, claiming it would threaten health, harm the environment, and widen racial inequities.[7]

The Board of Estimate approved the project anyway and allocated $164 million for its construction. To mollify community concerns, the city included funds to build a public park for Harlem residents on top of the sewage treatment plant. Construction began in 1972.

Continuing delays in moving from approval to construction to operation led the United States Environmental Protection Agency (EPA) to sue New York City in 1979, charging that the city was violating the federal Clean Water Act of 1970 by continuing to discharge untreated sewage into the Hudson River. The EPA won a court order requiring the city to begin treatment within seven years.

According to WE ACT's Vernice Miller, this rush to bring the North River plant online to protect the river led the city to make "irreparable errors in the design and construction of the North River Treatment Plant." Once the plant was in operation, it exposed Harlem residents to air pollution and foul odors. "This decision," she wrote, "was a total offense to the thousands of people whose lives would be forever changed by the plant and its operations,"[8] the very people WE ACT came to define as its core supporters.

The outrage that Miller and her neighbors experienced as the plant's emissions wafted over their apartment buildings after it began operations in 1986 led to the creation of WE ACT two years later. After almost two decades of prior efforts to block the plant, the group's founders had forged the connections to Harlem residents, city officials, and citywide and national environmental groups they needed to create an effective organization. They switched their focus to demanding that the plant operate safely and that elected officials refrain from imposing further environmental burdens on their community.

This battle also contributed to the development of two key precepts of the environmental justice movement in New York City and nationally. First, EJ activists argued that no community should experience a disproportionate burden of environmental hazards. The primary policy goal should be to prevent such exposures, an application of the precautionary principle, a core public health precept that says that facilities and policies should only be implemented after it is known they will not lead to harm.[9] A related goal should be to ensure that every community has a fair share of whatever burdens cannot be eliminated. The second EJ principle is that communities must have a voice in making decisions about their neighborhood's environment, summarized in the slogan "nothing about us without us."

As WE ACT's founders laid the groundwork for its 1988 debut, they worked to translate these EJ precepts into action that addressed residents' concerns about their community's environment. Vernice Miller and Peggy Shepard (another WE ACT cofounder who was a younger community activist with roots in local politics and the civil rights and women's movements), used their connections to West Harlem tenants' associations, civic groups, and the local Democratic Party to mobilize opposition to the treatment plant and to demand action to address their concerns. Shepard later became the executive director of WE ACT and continued to play an active role in multiple community struggles (see figure 5.1).

It was the women of West Harlem who daily experienced the noxious odors permeating their homes from the treatment plant, who led local neighborhood and tenants' organizations, and who usually had responsibility for caring for their children or grandchildren whose asthma or respiratory illnesses were exacerbated by the pollution. It is not surprising, therefore, that these women played a leading role in demanding action on the treatment plant. As the campaign developed, some men did join, persuaded by the organizers' message that the city was not hiring local workers or minority-owned construction, contracting, or engineering firms to do the work on the treatment plant.[10]

By its actions, WE ACT addressed the intersection of gender and race/ethnicity. As Miller and her colleagues observed,

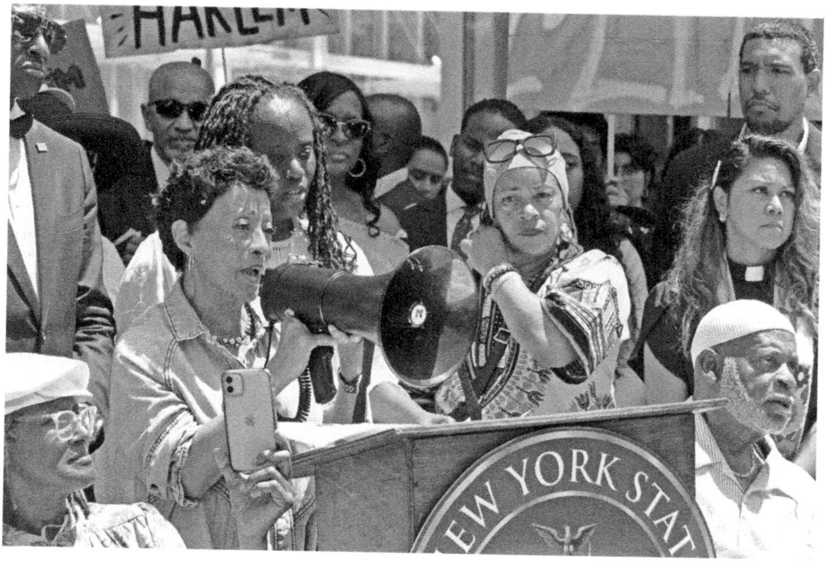

FIGURE 5.1 Peggy Shepard from WE ACT for Environmental Justice spoke at the Juneteenth Housing Justice for Harlem rally hosted by New York State Senator Cordell Cleare and other community leaders on June 19, 2024, calling for affordable housing and to defend Harlem from gentrification.

Source: WE ACT for Environmental Justice. https://weact.org/wp-content/uploads/2025/11/2026-Policy-Agenda-112025.pdf

> The process by which women in West Harlem challenged the racially based denigration of their community and the flagrant disregard for their quality of life involved a critical fusion of traditional gendered roles with a new activism and a willingness to confront the male-dominated political machine. The strength and wisdom of the senior women, combined with the conviction and drive of the younger women, empowered them to seek an effective means by which to continue their efforts and ultimately see their struggle to fruition. Women in West Harlem effectively asserted themselves in the political arena in an unprecedented manner and began the arduous, but necessary transformation of "old boy" politics.[11]

On Martin Luther King's birthday in 1988, West Harlem residents blocked traffic on two major highways in front of the North River Sewage

Treatment Plant. They demanded action to mitigate the impact of the plant, initiating a new direct, activist approach that characterized the soon-to-be-formed WE ACT.[12]

The West Harlem activists also built ties with elected officials who supported their goals. William Fitts Ryan, the progressive congressman for the area, had testified against the plant as early as 1968. So did Percy Sutton, a Harlem politician who was then Manhattan borough president and a member of the Board of Estimate. He said that the proposed plant was "an indignity imposed on the community . . . that make people feel they are not equal. . . . As the only Black representative on the Board, I am hurt, deeply hurt, that you do not understand what you are doing to Harlem."[13]

Nearly twenty years later, David Dinkins, Sutton's successor as Manhattan borough president and soon to be elected mayor, provided funds to hire Barry Commoner, a distinguished environmental scientist, to assess the environmental impact of the plant. Commoner's report found design defects in the North River facility and indications of harmful sulfur hydroxide and sulfur dioxide emissions, exacerbating Harlem's asthma epidemic.[14]

In 1992, utilizing yet another strategy of the EJ movement, WE ACT, in partnership with the Natural Resources Defense Council (NRDC), filed a lawsuit against the New York City Department of Environmental Protection and Mayor Dinkins. The suit alleged that the treatment plant was a public and private nuisance to the people who lived or owned property in West Harlem and that these residents had been prevented from enjoying the full fruits of their property because of the operations and malfunctions of the plant.[15]

The New York State Supreme Court rejected New York City's request to dismiss the case. On December 30, 1993, just hours before Rudy Giuliani was to be inaugurated as Mayor Dinkin's successor, WE ACT and NRDC reached a settlement with the city. The two plaintiffs were named as co-enforcers of the consent decree, giving WE ACT an ongoing voice in decisions about the plant. The settlement also required continuing monitoring of emissions from the plant as well as corrective measures by the city or state with substantial penalties if these were not implemented. Significantly, the agreement also established the North River Fund with public funding of $1.1 million to be used by WE ACT and NRDC to address community environmental and health issues in West Harlem.[16] These funds provided the activist groups with some of the resources they needed to continue to strengthen the community's power to protect its well-being.

Over the years, WE ACT took on other environmental threats to the health of Harlem residents. To reduce inequitable exposure to air pollution, WE ACT promoted the concept of "transit justice,"[17] an insistence that transportation policies and systems protect communities of color from exposure to higher levels of air pollution. WE ACT wanted to close some of the bus depots located in Upper Manhattan and noted that its communities were also home to a marine garbage collection transfer station, a diesel-fueled train line, two garbage truck depots, two parking lots for sanitation trucks, and a major bus station.[18]

WE ACT members believed that these multiple sources of air pollution contributed to local asthma death and illness rates five times greater than the citywide averages, and a hospitalization rate for asthma twenty-one times higher than in the city neighborhoods with the lowest rates.[19] Through its investigations of its own community, WE ACT grasped the concept of cumulative impact, the synergistic harmful effects of exposures to multiple toxins over the life course, a perspective that encouraged comprehensive and systemic policy responses.[20]

To mobilize community residents to confront these threats, WE ACT and NRDC created an educational campaign with the slogan "If You Live Uptown, Breathe at Your Own Risk," a message that was plastered in English and Spanish on bus shelters throughout the neighborhood. Residents were urged to send postcards to the governor and the Metropolitan Transit Authority (MTA; the agency that ran the city's bus and subway system) demanding a fair share of clean fuel investments for northern Manhattan.[21]

In 2000, after many years of unsuccessful negotiations with the MTA to relocate bus depots, WE ACT filed a Title VI Civil Rights Act discrimination complaint with the United States Department of Transportation. The complaint charged the MTA with racial discrimination for having located six of eight diesel bus depots in the mostly Black and Latiné communities of Upper Manhattan, exposing residents to higher levels of diesel exhaust, which contributed to increased rates of respiratory illness.

While the Department of Transportation investigation did not find that the MTA had violated civil rights laws, it concluded that the agency had failed to implement regulations that required it to assess the health impact of its practices, consider the health and environmental implications of its redesign of bus depots, or include community residents as equal partners in transportation planning.[22]

While the lawsuit was only partially successful, it helped to create political space for ongoing negotiations between WE ACT and the MTA. As Shepard explained, after the Department of Transportation ruling, when she called the MTA on a Saturday to complain about new bus routes, the MTA called her back on Sunday to assure her they were addressing the problem. "That's what access will do," she said.[23]

By identifying the multiple hazards facing their community and educating community residents and public officials about their findings, WE ACT helped to deepen public understanding of key concepts such as *cumulative impact*. Determining the most appropriate metrics for assessing cumulative impact (e.g., pollution levels from the combined exposure to traffic, waste facilities, heating systems, etc.) was a task for environmental scientists.

WE ACT showed that community residents could also contribute to data collection by training young people to collect exposure data—for example, sidewalk-level small particulate matter and diesel exhaust—not available through government sources, in the process educating young people to become environmental justice advocates (see figure 5.2).[24] This evidence helped explain the neighborhood distribution of air pollution–related disease.

WE ACT embraced another task needed to translate cumulative impact studies into policy. The group educated elected officials and community residents that the whole of harmful exposures across sources and

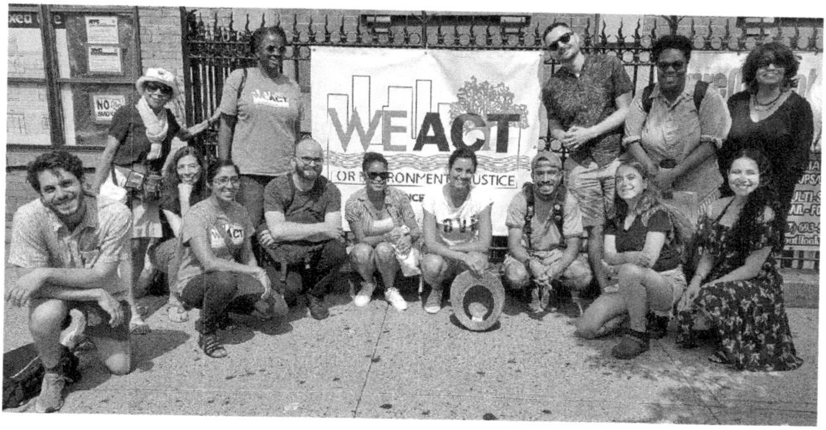

FIGURE 5.2 In the summer of 2019, WE ACT trained community members to become advocates to support its initiatives, help collect data, or lead their own community projects.

Source: WE ACT for Environmental Justice. https://weact.org/get-involved/ehjlt/

the lifespan was greater than any individual risk. By leading this education, WE ACT helped to build political support for more effective monitoring and regulation.

Building on this work, in 2022, WE ACT and other groups helped to convince New York Governor Kathy Hochul to sign landmark EJ legislation that ensures that cumulative impacts are taken into consideration in the state's environmental permitting processes when potentially polluting facilities seek permits in disadvantaged communities.[25]

Another concept WE ACT popularized was *environmental racism*, defined by Robert Bullard, a scholar and early leader of the environmental justice movement, as "any policy, practice or directive that differentially affects or disadvantages (whether intended or unintended) individuals, groups or communities based on race."[26] In this view, in the long run, protecting the health of communities of color will require dismantling these racist practices and policies.

Finally, a third concept WE ACT promoted was *environmental justice*, the insistence that all communities are entitled to equal protection of their environments.[27] This belief links the task of protecting health to the civil rights struggle and other social justice movements. Simultaneously, it highlights the potential for broader alliances and the necessity of developing strategies to win power to shape community environments. By identifying its core constituencies—those living in Harlem, concerned residents of other communities of color, and environmental and social justice activists—and the ideas that could move these groups to action, WE ACT built a foundation for success.

In sum, WE ACT contributed to improved health and health equity in New York City by introducing powerful new ideas into the city's political discourse. It mobilized the residents of Harlem to demand cleaner, safer, and healthier environments, actions that reinforced and sparked similar actions in other low-income communities of color in New York. WE ACT also instigated and supported the creation of citywide, regional, and national alliances to promote the goals of the environmental justice movement, thus building its power.

In turn, New York City had an impact on the goals and strategies of WE ACT by creating a political climate and networks that facilitated opportunities to join with other local and national groups to promote environmental justice, making it easier for WE ACT to expand its focus beyond Harlem.

New York is also a city with high concentrations of universities and environmental health researchers, giving WE ACT access to scientists who could provide the group with the evidence it needed to take into the political arena. To inform its local and national campaigns, WE ACT developed ongoing relationships with environmental and public health researchers at nearby universities. The group hired and trained young people to monitor levels of air pollution in Upper Manhattan and present their findings to the public and politicians.[28] Campaigns in areas without such concentrations of academics willing to partner with activists may have more difficulty bringing needed evidence into the public and policy arenas.

On the more problematic side, New York City's complex governance structure and politics make it hard to align community, municipal, and state priorities. Waste disposal, fossil fuel, and other polluting industries use their lobbying and campaign contributions to influence environmental and regulatory policy at all three levels. Like other activist groups, WE ACT often had to work for years to overcome these obstacles to achieve even the most basic reforms, and some of its campaigns failed to make meaningful gains.

ENGAGING SUPPORTERS IN HEALTH ACTIVIST CAMPAIGNS

How have other health campaigns in New York City taken on this task of engaging supporters? WE ACT based its appeal to its potential supporters on three of their identities. First, the group asked people to join as Harlem residents, those living in a shared geographic community with its own culture, history, politics, and self-identity. Second, the group appealed to supporters as African Americans, a people with a common history and connections to the national civil rights, labor, and environmental movements. This last bond grew in importance as more environmental activists began to embrace the environmental justice movement. Third, WE ACT recognized that women had a special role to play, given their history of activism, community rootedness, and exclusion from mainstream (male) politics.

Of course, these three identities overlap, so many of WE ACT's core supporters joined as Harlem residents, as African Americans, and as women. By providing these multiple entry points into activism, each resonating with shared life experiences of pride, outrage, and resistance, WE ACT translated Black feminist Kimberlé Crenshaw's intersectional theory into practice.[29] Its supporters did not need to decide which identity led them to action, as the three reinforced each other and offered multiple pathways into activism.

Sometimes, however, these identities did clash. Some men in Harlem, like men elsewhere, thought that it was a woman's job to protect their communities or families, not organize marches or block highways. Others thought that women did not belong in electoral politics, resenting Peggy Shepard's active role in local Democratic politics. WE ACT organizers were able to use gendered assumptions by appealing to men as breadwinners, pointing out that city government was failing to hire local workers to build the treatment plant, a missed opportunity for expanding employment. WE ACT cofounder Miller and her colleagues observed that Harlem women's commitment to reducing the community's high rates of asthma complemented men's commitment to creating more jobs, both vital community goals.[30] WE ACT provided spaces to discuss and debate these issues and thus created opportunities for forging identities that promoted community solidarity in opposition to the planned treatment plant—or at least identifying internal community conflicts that required discussion.

Another example of appealing to multiple cross-cutting identities comes from AIDS Counseling and Education (ACE), founded in 1988 by women incarcerated at Bedford Hills Correctional Facility, New York State's prison for women. ACE provided support for women with HIV and organized for improvements in their conditions and services. Over the years, ACE trained hundreds of women in prison to be AIDS counselors and peer educators, filling gaps in prison health services. ACE also pressured correctional officials to improve medical care and end misinformation about AIDS and the segregation of HIV-positive women.[31]

ACE appealed to supporters at Bedford Hills through their intersectional identities as people at risk of AIDS, women, people of color, and those ensnared by the war on drugs and mass incarceration. When Katrina Haslip, one of ACE's cofounders, was released from prison two years after founding the group, she created ACE-OUT, an organization that continued to provide "services and sisterhood" to women with HIV released from prison, adding yet another constituency.[32]

In recounting what she had gotten from ACE, Haslip emphasized its personal appeal to her:

> Somewhere behind a prison wall in Bedford Hills a movement or community was being built. . . . These women believed that none of their

> peers should be discriminated against, isolated, or treated cruelly merely because they were ill. . . . They believed it was necessary for this prison to build an environment of support, comfort, education, and trust. . . . I felt as if the women of ACE had built a cocoon around me, for me. I felt warmed by them and so totally understood. These were the women who understood my silence and yet felt my need to be heard.[33]

By offering supporters multiple entry points into activism, by having deep knowledge of the life experiences of these potential followers, and by framing messages that show how the proposed campaign goals can improve life circumstances, organizers of activist campaigns can more fully embrace their supporters and thus increase their base of support. Most important, by building the "cocoon" that makes supporters feel protected, cared for, and part of a group, organizations can win the trust that sustains ongoing engagement.

The requisite deep knowledge needed for such engagement can come from various sources. The organizers of WE ACT were themselves women living in Harlem, and the needed knowledge derived from their own collective life experiences and their ongoing relationships with family, friends, and peers. Similarly, the founders of ACE were women in prison, some with AIDS, living the experiences they sought to change.

IDENTITY POLITICS AND ITS ALTERNATIVES AS ROUTES FOR ENGAGEMENT

Movement scholars sometimes pose identity politics and political ideology as two alternative routes for engaging supporters with an activist campaign.[34] Identity politics describes the political mobilization of social groups whose claims are based on their identities as members of oppressed groups.[35] In ideological politics, people come together based on their shared beliefs about politics, power, and a vision of a better world.

Proponents of the identity route claim that it creates bonds between members of the oppressed groups that provide a powerful foundation for collective action. Critics warn that the focus on identity downplays fundamental structural forces such as economic and political inequalities or that it can undermine the creation of strong intersectional alliances.[36]

What the WE ACT, ACE and MRNY accounts suggest, however, is that organizers can engage people through multiple routes, including both identities and beliefs. Supporters joined these organizations based on their identities as Harlem residents, Black people, women, prisoners, people with AIDS, or immigrants. They also joined because they wanted healthier communities, more respect and dignity, and a fairer society. In each context, organizers struggled to find the right balance between identity and beliefs, and to frame messages that will appeal to each or both entry routes. To my mind, it is reassuring that practice-based evidence suggests that there are multiple routes to engagement, not a single formula, and that organizers can test and refine their strategies for attracting supporters, calibrating their approaches based on their successes and as circumstances change.

Over the years, organizers have developed various strategies for engaging supporters. MRNY uses what it calls the "high touch" model. Its leaders believe that its success in achieving its goals depends on its ability to "recruit, develop, mobilize, and retain members," as author-activist Jane McAlevey writes in her description of this model. She gives an example from a meeting she observed:

> Augusto, who was cochairing the meeting as part of such a leadership development assignment, asked for "silencio" and then approached each person in the room to ask them, "Que le gusta sobre este reunion and que no le gusta?" (What do you like about this meeting and what do you not like?) When he got to the third person, the front doors to the room opened and a few members began to carry in enormous pots of rice and beans. The fragrant smell wafting through the room was a challenge for Augusto at this point—almost two hours after the meeting began—but he pressed on with his questions undeterred. The answers he got were all variations on a theme: People liked being able to participate in the

> discussion and having a clear agenda; what they didn't like was "that this meeting is going on too long, look—see—our dinner is here and we should be eating it."[37]

"High touch" includes both insisting that each participant speaks and expresses their opinion and ensuring that they are offered food and other support that reinforces their identity.

Deep canvassing is another model for engaging participants more fully. Used in electoral campaigns, organizers seek to involve potential supporters in conversations where the organizers listen more and talk less, hoping to find common ground that can lead to further engagement. Showing Up for Racial Justice New York City used deep canvassing to begin conversations on reparations; in an assessment of this process, William Brennan and Margo Jackson concluded that such conversations can facilitate shifts in interactions with potential supporters.[38]

Through these and other methods, activist organizations seek to meet, engage, and enlist new recruits as ongoing supporters. Ultimately, their success will determine the organization's power to achieve its goals and its ability to sustain its accomplishments.

HOW ENGAGEMENT STRATEGIES CAN CHALLENGE OR REINFORCE RACISM AND SEXISM

No activist campaign—whether in New York or nationally—can escape the pervasive influence of racism, misogyny, homophobia, and other forms of domination that characterize the United States today. None can escape the deep rifts that these systemic forces have imposed on our society and on individuals, nor the deliberate efforts of opponents to foment these conflicts to divide campaign supporters by race, class, gender, sexual orientation, or gender identity. The ways in which an organization tackles this reality can shape its potential for success or failure. Get the engagement strategies across these lines right and a campaign can attract the supporters it needs and mobilize their power for action. Get them wrong and the result can be ongoing conflict, divisiveness, and defeat.

A few examples from the sexual and reproductive justice and police accountability movements in New York illustrate some of the ways that activists have confronted this task. The campaigns of these movements are profiled in more detail in chapter 9.

In 1974, ten women from Puerto Rican, reproductive health, health care, and legal activist groups in New York City formed the Committee to End Sterilization Abuse (CESA) to fight such abuse in Puerto Rico and New York City. In both these places—and across the country—women, especially Puerto Rican and Black women, had often been sterilized without their consent, following childbirth, or without being informed that the procedure was considered irreversible. The founders of CESA wanted to end these practices in New York City.[39] Led by experienced Puerto Rican and other women's health activists, CESA recognized that a broad coalition that included Latiné, Black, white, and other women as well as men was necessary in order to convince the city's public hospital system, and eventually the city, state, and federal governments, to end sterilization abuse.

But women from these different racial/ethnic and socioeconomic groups had different positions on the best tactics for combatting sterilization abuse and gaining access to legal abortion. As Dr. Helen Rodríguez, a Puerto Rican pediatrician and a founder and key leader of CESA, explained many years later,

> Women activists in the women's movement, who were primarily concerned with removing all legal obstacles to abortion, opposed the notions of guidelines, regulations, or legislation that in any way restricts access to sterilization. As we thrashed out the differences, we . . . began to listen to each other and to understand our personal experiences were different because our race, class or ethnicity exposed us to different institutions or practices. A basis for working together was solidly laid (for) identifying and understanding our commonalities.[40]

Rodríguez went on to beseech her listeners "to consolidate our ranks and focus our strength that we may create a universal equitable system fully consonant with our values of compassion and freedom." The fact that the Young Lords Party, whose former members were also part of CESA, had shown that it was possible for a militant Puerto Rican group to both forcefully oppose sterilization abuse *and* insist that all women should have the right to safe abortions further contributed to multiracial support for the new restrictions on sterilization abuse.

By 1975, CESA had helped to convince the New York City public hospitals to approve new guidelines that required hospitals to institute a thirty-day waiting period after women had given consent, to use a detailed and explicit consent form, and to provide counseling in the women's own language to those considering sterilization. CESA then helped to win approval for a city council law that required private and other New York City hospitals to follow the public hospital sterilization rules and for new federal health, education, and welfare regulations to end sterilization abuse in all hospitals in the United States that received federal funding.[41] By acknowledging class and race differences among its members and supporters in order to forge common ground, CESA was able to bring about important reductions in sterilization abuse.

The campaigns to end stop-and-frisk policing—and later to reduce city funding for the police—tell a more complicated story of how the racial divide can complicate engaging support. Stop-and-frisk describes the police practice of allowed officers to stop, interrogate, and search New York City residents on the sole basis of "reasonable suspicion." Critics charged that this practice violated the US Constitution's Fourth Amendment prohibition of unreasonable searches and seizures.[42] Despite Mayors Rudy Giuliani's and Michael Bloomberg's strong support for stop-and-frisk policing, activist campaigns against the practice succeeded in creating a multiracial coalition that significantly limited the practice. In 2013, a federal judge found the New York City Police Department's (NYPD) stop-and-frisk policy unconstitutional, ruling that it violated the constitutional ban on unreasonable searches and seizures.[43] Mayor Michael

Bloomberg, supported by police officials, announced he would appeal the decision.

In the 2013 mayoral election, Communities United for Police Reform, the multiracial alliance campaigning against stop-and-frisk, successfully persuaded many voters of color and some portion of white voters to oppose this form of policing. Bill de Blasio, a candidate for mayor, supported ending the practice and won both the primary and the general election with support from Black and white voters. In 2013, the NYPD reported 191,851 police stops; by 2016, the number had fallen to 12,404 stops.[44]

While over-policing had not vanished, the multiracial support for ending this visible practice had achieved a significant win. And the fact that homicide rates continued to fall after stop-and-frisk ended contradicted the main objection of its supporters. According to the investigative outlet *ProPublica*, by 2018, the number of homicides in New York fell to the lowest level since the 1950s.[45] The conservative publication *National Review* ran the headline "We Were Wrong About Stop-and-Frisk," noting that "major crime in New York City has continued to decline almost across the board in the four years of the de Blasio administration, to the lowest rates since New York City began keeping extensive records on crime in the early 1960s."[46]

In 2020, after the murder of George Floyd by Minneapolis police officers, a coalition of nearly one hundred New York advocacy groups, ranging from the Legal Aid Society to the Riders Alliance transit group, called on de Blasio to further reduce what they considered excess policing by cutting the police budget. "Historically, city government has spent far more on police than on public health, homeless services, youth services and other vital agencies," the groups wrote in a public letter. "We urge you to realign budget priorities with the understanding that safety for all is possible only when there is strong public health infrastructure, housing for all, quality education, environmental justice, food justice, transportation justice, [and] disability justice."[47]

A powerful right-wing campaign attacked the idea of defunding the police, and residents of many communities, Black, Latiné, and white, expressed ambivalence about defunding the police because of local crime and the absence of a compelling vision of other routes to public safety and violence prevention. Many activist groups calling for cuts in police funding were unable to develop an analysis and messages that might have created majority coalitions that could continue to fight for an end to police abuse and safer communities. In practice, few budgeting changes were approved, and when Eric Adams, a new mayor, and a former police officer, took office in 2022, he added new funding for the police.[48] He also failed to enforce police accountability rules.[49]

Given the deep roots of the structures and systems that maintain racial/ethnic, class, gender, and other stratification systems, no simple or single solution can surmount their power to divide supporters of activist campaigns. One lesson from the stories I recount is that acknowledging these divisions is a first step toward addressing them. As Helen Rodríguez from CESA observed, when activists of different classes, races, and ethnicities listen to each other, they create the opportunity to acknowledge and overcome these barriers.

A second lesson is the value of using what the activist-scholar Heather McGhee calls "sum of us" frames,[50] those that emphasize the collective benefits of proposed reforms for all groups, rather than the zero-sum messages that ruling elites often use to divide groups by race/ethnicity, class, or identity. These "sum of us" frames are more likely to win greater political support for their goals, as illustrated by the environmental justice movement's claim that reducing air and water pollution in the most affected communities improves environmental quality for everyone. Similarly, ending stop-and-frisk policing can increase trust in policing and make all communities safer, just as paying fast-food workers living wages grows the city's overall economy and makes fewer people at risk of homelessness, food insecurity, and vulnerability to disease outbreaks such as COVID-19—all threats to a stable and prosperous city for all.

FROM ENGAGING SUPPORTERS TO BUILDING COALITIONS AND ALLIANCES

Engaging supporters requires individuals to commit to taking action to achieve the goals a campaign has identified. But to accrue the power needed to win such changes, activist organizations need to move beyond the individual level. They need to forge the alliances and coalitions that unite their various constituencies of supporters and enable them to attain victories in the political arenas where policy decisions are made.

After they have engaged supporters, how have New York City activist groups achieved this aim? The Young Lords Party used powerful popular ideas such as creating neighborhood control of schools and health centers to establish bonds with various constituencies and organizations: Puerto Rican nationalists, advocates of community control of local institutions that made health-care, education, and housing rights for all, and labor groups that insisted that health-care and other workers must organize to win respect and power.

Promoting these ideas and taking action to turn them into practice allowed the Young Lords to work with, among others, opponents of school segregation, the Black Panther Party, the Puerto Rican independence movement, antiwar activists, groups seeking to curb sterilization abuse, and others. These multiple streams of activism broadcast a vision of a more just society, one where the abuses that disrupted the lives of many Puerto Ricans were reduced or ended.

For the most part, however, the Young Lords did not forge the deep organizational ties with other organizations that allowed them to win more substantial victories, counter police repression, or survive more than a decade. In her assessment of the demise of the Young Lords, historian Johanna Fernández cites several causes. In her view, relentless repression by the FBI and the police; the party's high demands on members, making participation difficult for many Puerto Ricans; their impatience for rapid victories; their ambivalence about whether New York or Puerto Rico should be the priority; and their moves away from democratic decision-making all contributed to their dissolution.[51]

Acknowledging the unfairness of hindsight, another critical reason for the Young Lords' short lifespan was its limited success in crafting ongoing and operational alliances with other activist and movement organizations. Perhaps its commitment to a centralized party structure, a characteristic that may have facilitated decision-making, also made the Young Lords less able to forge deep and lasting partnerships with other movement organizations.

Like the Young Lords, ACT UP also used confrontational tactics and radical rhetoric, planned its actions, and learned how to work closely with groups like WHAM!, Coalition for the Homeless, the HIV Law Project, the National Lawyers Guild, Gay Men's Health Crisis, and others. To be sure, ACT UP frequently had conflicts with these partners, but its personnel were also staff or members of these other organizations, serving as embedded liaisons between the two groups. And on specific campaigns, lawsuits, and actions, partners contributed expertise and resources that added to what ACT UP could provide on its own.

As in ACT UP, WE ACT members often belonged to other groups such as tenants' unions, neighborhood associations, and local political party clubs, giving WE ACT insider access to partners for its Harlem campaigns. Over time, WE ACT also joined coalitions with environmental justice groups in other neighborhoods. The Organization of Waterfront Communities, a citywide community-based coalition formed in 1996 after the Fresh Kills Landfill was closed on Staten Island, tackled the common threats waste transfer stations posed to the city's neighborhoods.[52] The New York Environmental Justice Alliance, founded in 1991 by WE ACT and several other grassroots environmental justice organizations from low-income neighborhoods and communities of color, provided the city's EJ movement with a visible voice that could use its collective power to influence city and state governments.[53]

At the national level, WE ACT Executive Director Peggy Shepard become the first woman to chair the National Environmental Justice Advisory Council to the Environmental Protection Agency in 2001; she used the forum to resist the George W. Bush administration's efforts to weaken the EPA and its environmental justice commitments. In 2012, WE ACT opened an office in Washington, DC, to advance the federal policy needs and interests of northern Manhattan and other communities combatting environmental racism.[54] In 2025, as Donald Trump endeavored to weaken the EPA, withdraw its regulations, and terminate its EJ initiatives, Shepard and WE ACT again provided a national voice for opposing these actions, speaking against these changes on CNN and other media outlets.[55]

FROM WHO TO WHAT

To launch campaigns to tackle the problems they have identified, health activist organizers need to identify their core supporters and recognize the life experiences and beliefs that enable a campaign to reach its followers. They then need to craft the messages and carry out the actions that will engage these constituencies in supporting the campaign's goals. To build the power they will need to achieve these aims, they next must forge the alliances needed to overcome the opposition of proponents of the status quo.

On the surface, these steps seem simple and straightforward. But as the examples of WE ACT, ACE, and other New York health activist campaigns described in this and previous chapters show, in order to make informed decisions on these tasks, organizers need deep knowledge of their potential supporters, a solid grounding in the history of their community or population, an up-to-date understanding of feasible communications strategies, and a grasp of the relevant changes in New York City and the nation's changing politics and economy.

On the one hand, activists could spend a lifetime studying these questions, delaying action as preventable health crises and social injustices unfolded. On the other hand, activists who have a game plan for uncovering what they need to know and clear priorities are more likely to make informed decisions than those without a plan. Finding the right balance between taking the time to learn what they need to know and deciding it is time to act is what makes organizing campaigns a learned skill, an art—and a formidable challenge.

In the next chapter, I move from considering *who* organizers of activist campaigns interact with to *what* they decide to do—the strategies and tactics that will convert goals into changes in policies, institutional practices, and public ideas.

6

HOW ACTIVISTS CHOOSE STRATEGIES AND TACTICS

Once organizers of activist campaigns have identified their problem of interest, mapped the political and economic context, pinpointed their proposed solution, and chosen key constituencies and allies, they must decide what they and other participants in the campaign should do.

In this chapter, I describe the strategies and tactics that health activist campaigns in New York City have used since the 1960s. I examine how activists decide what to do and how they consider the consequences of their choices. I also ask how the particular aims of advancing health and social justice—in comparison to other activist aims—influence the choices of strategies and tactics and how the setting of New York City shapes these choices.

To illustrate the range of strategies and tactics that health activists have used, I profile a few campaigns that have focused on providing and improving school meals in New York City. In the late 1960s and early 1970s, the Young Lords and the Black Panthers served breakfast before school to children in community centers in several New York City neighborhoods (see figure 6.1). They used this approach to demonstrate their

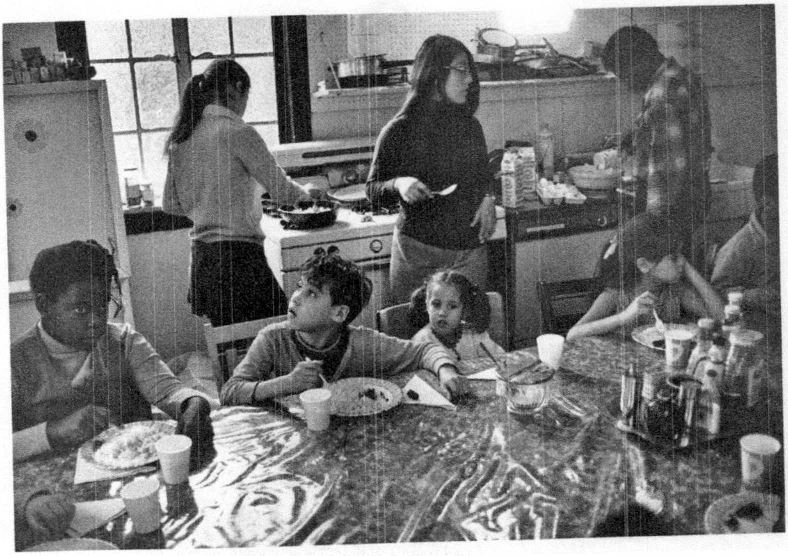

FIGURE 6.1 Young Lords members provide free breakfasts to children in East Harlem in 1970.

Source: Archives of the Puerto Rican Diaspora, Center for Puerto Rican Studies at Hunter College.

commitment to protecting children, serving people, and engaging their communities in radical politics.

United Bronx Parents (UBP), a multiservice community organization, also served breakfast to schoolchildren in the late 1960s and 1970s. To engage key actors in their campaign, UBP invited elected officials and community leaders to eat a standard school lunch and, as a contrast, served another meal to elected officials prepared in a school cafeteria by a local chef using fresh, healthy foods familiar to Puerto Ricans. Another time, in 1969, UBP parents dumped in front of the Lower Manhattan office of the United States Department of Agriculture (USDA), the funder of school lunches, plastic bags full of food discarded by children that they collected from school trash bins.[1] UPB chose this disruptive tactic to win media coverage and capture the attention of policymakers.

Almost forty years later, beginning in 2013, Community Food Advocates (CFA) organized the Lunch for Learning campaign, an effort to convince city government to provide free school lunches to all of New York City's 1.1 million schoolchildren. CFA assembled a coalition that brought together the constituencies most directly affected by the school lunch program as well as those that had the most power to influence the key decision-makers on school food in the city. In 2017, strong support from the city council, several labor unions, parent groups, and more than two hundred other organizations persuaded New York City Mayor Bill de Blasio to provide city funding to supplement federal funding to make universal free lunches a city policy. After several years of advocacy, New York Governor Kathy Hochul, in her 2025 State of the State speech promised to expand the city's free lunches to all schools in the state.[2]

These diverse and imaginative strategies and tactics, deployed over several decades to advance the goal of healthy food for all schoolchildren, illustrate some of the different approaches New York City activists have used to turn their political visions into new laws, budget allocations, institutional practices, and public ideas. They also show how long it can take to translate a simple idea—free school meals for all children—into a reality. What can activists and scholars of activism learn from these experiences?

STRATEGIES AND TACTICS FOR HEALTH ACTIVISTS

A starting point for this discussion is to define strategy and tactics. In their book *Practical Radicals: Seven Strategies to Change the World*, veteran activists and scholars of social movements Deepak Bhargava and Stephanie Luce propose that strategies describe an activist group's plan for accumulating the power it will need to achieve its goals, whereas tactics define the activities the group will employ to mobilize the needed power.[3] Based on their review of varied activist campaigns in different parts of the world, Bhargava and Luce identify seven power-generating strategies commonly used by activists: base building, disruption, narrative shift, electoral change, inside/outside campaign, momentum using mass protest to lead to narrative change, and collective care. Table 6.1 provides brief definitions and examples of campaigns described in this book that have used each strategy.

Most activist campaigns use two or more of these strategies. Make the Road New York, for example, uses both base building—creating a membership organization—and electoral change—allying with the Working Families Party, Democratic Socialists of America, and progressive Democrats to win legislation or city and state executive action to limit the power of federal immigration authorities. ACT UP used disruptive strategies in its Stop the Church campaign, created a narrative shift to advocate that new drugs for life-threatening illnesses should be previewed and approved more quickly than other drugs, and deployed the insider/outsider strategy by simultaneously meeting with FDA and drug company officials to review evidence on new drugs while also demonstrating outside the FDA's headquarters in Rockville, Maryland. These groups and others decided which strategies to use based on their explicit or implicit theory of change and on their assessment of the power needed to achieve specific goals.

Over the years, health activist groups have used an assortment of tactics to implement their strategies, as illustrated in the case profiles. In some cases, activists have simply stuck their hands into the tactics grab bag and pulled out a familiar or appealing action. In other cases, such as ACT UP's actions described in chapter 4, their choices have been informed by sophisticated power analyses and in-depth consultation with allies. By acquiring a deeper understanding of the pathways between strategy, tactics, and achievement of goals, activists can make more informed choices on what they do to accomplish their aims.

PROFILE: ORGANIZING FOR BETTER FOOD IN NEW YORK CITY SCHOOLS

For many years, New York City has had trouble meeting the most basic food needs of its residents. Between 2021 and 2023, nearly 1.2 million New

TABLE 6.1 Activist Strategies to Build Power

STRATEGY	DEFINITION	EXAMPLES OF NEW YORK CITY ACTIVIST CAMPAIGNS USING THIS STRATEGY
Base building	Organizing member-based mass organizations such as community groups or unions	Make the Road New York, Fight for $15, United Bronx Parents
Disruptive movements	Organizing designed to stop those in power from doing what they want to do	Welfare rights groups, stop Sydenham hospital from closing
Narrative shift	Organizing to change public understanding of major problems and their solutions	WE ACT, ACT UP, Occupy Wall Street
Electoral change	Organizing to win elections, approve referenda, or stop undesirable public policies	Housing Justice for All, Health Care for All New York, WE ACT
Inside/outside campaign	Working at the same time with political or other leaders, and employing outside pressure tactics such as marches, rallies, or demonstrations	ACT UP, WE ACT, Fight for $15
Momentum model (mass protest leads to narrative change)	Combining mass protests with narrative shift	Fight for $15, Close Rikers, end stop-and-frisk
Collective care	Providing care to people in need with the goal of changing and providing alternatives to established systems of care	Gay Men's Health Crisis, AIDS Counseling and Education (ACE) at Bedford Hills Correctional Facility, COVID-19 mutual aid groups, school breakfast programs

Modified from: Deepak Bhargava and Stephanie Luce, *Practical Radicals: Seven Strategies to Change the World* (New Press, 2023), 75.

Yorkers lived in households experiencing food insecurity or hunger, including 1 in 5 children.[4] Nearly 1 million New Yorkers have diabetes,[5] and in 2020, more than half (57 percent) of adults in New York City and a third (30 percent) of youth were overweight or obese.[6] Obesity and overweight, diabetes, and other conditions caused or worsened by diet are now the leading causes of preventable illnesses and premature deaths in New York City, and of the wide gaps in health between white New Yorkers and people of color.[7] In the last few decades, an active food justice movement has emerged in New York City, focusing on these and other problems that the city's food system and its political economy have been unable to solve.[8]

For more than sixty years, New York City activists have been attracted to mobilizing their communities to improve school food. What makes this such an appealing goal? First, most obviously, it is widely known that too many children in New York City experience hunger and food insecurity. Providing free, healthy food to the more than one million children in city schools is a practical way to reduce this problem that does not require transforming the food industry, ending poverty, or eliminating wealth inequality. Second, school food can bring together activists from education, poverty reduction, health-care, food, and civil rights movements, creating a shared meeting ground for multiple interest groups that can work together to improve children's lives. Third, while many organizations and government agencies play a role in school food in New York, one agency—the New York City Department of Education—has primary responsibility for implementing school food programs, making it a clear, accessible, and convenient target for focused activism.

Unlike housing developers and landlords, or the employers and businesses who hire workers, no single powerful constituency within New York City profits from the status quo in school food and lobbies aggressively to protect its profits, providing another reason why activists find it easier to win victories than if they were fighting powerful corporations. Finally, most funding for school food programs comes from the federal government (where special interests from the food industry do seek to influence decisions), making city and state officials eager to expand the program so as not to "leave federal money on the table." While some of the cuts in the 2025 and future budget bills signed by President Trump may lead to reductions in school lunch funding and thus change some of these dynamics, it is unlikely to end New York City's long march to improving school food.

Even though some entrenched institutions oppose school food reform, and multinational food companies profit from the school food status quo, their power to oppose change at the city level is less than in other activist domains. Finally, the goal of ensuring that no student is hungry and that all are food secure has a clear moral resonance. While conservative Republicans oppose most universal public benefits programs, including school food,[9] few New Yorkers would publicly argue that schoolchildren should be hungry.

In 1962, Michael Harrington published *The Other America*, an exposé of the continuing presence of poverty and hunger in the United States in the postwar era. Following the work of the civil rights movement, the book attracted the attention of President Kennedy and helped to create the moral and intellectual foundation for Lyndon Johnson's War on Poverty. This helped to spark an antipoverty and antihunger movement that broadened support for a national school food program focused on the well-being of children.[10] For some, providing the poor with food was more politically acceptable than providing them with income, housing, or jobs.

By the late 1960s, civil rights and other movements emphasized another angle—that healthy food should be considered a basic human right, rather than only a commodity distributed by markets that made profit the priority. By moving from charity to human rights, and by making the distribution of free, healthy food one more way for movements to serve and mobilize their constituencies, civil rights activists and their successors contributed powerful new frames for food activists, including school food proponents.[11]

The women's movement played a role in campaigns to improve school food as well. In her book *The Labor of Lunch*, Jennifer Gaddis describes how mothers and labor unions collaborated to organize and improve the pay for school food workers, creating new economic opportunities for women.[12] School food organizing offered women two benefits. First, free, healthy school food eliminates the task of making lunches to take to school from a mother's lengthy to-do list. Second, in our gendered society, women have always had the main responsibility for feeding their families, making mothers the frontline fighters for better school food, thus challenging traditional roles in which men were supposed to be the political activists.[13]

Over the years, campaigners for school food have used many strategies and tactics to expand the reach and quality of the program. Their efforts constitute a natural experiment testing the impact of these various approaches on the desired outcome of fewer hungry children and more well-nourished learners.

SCHOOL FOOD CAMPAIGNS IN THE 1960S AND 1970S: BLACK PANTHERS, YOUNG LORDS, AND UNITED BRONX PARENTS

The seeds of the organizing that led to New York City's 2017 decision to provide free school lunch for all children were planted in the 1960s by militant civil rights groups and the struggles to end school segregation in New York. New York's Black Panther Party and the Young Lords sponsored free breakfast programs in the late 1960s for several reasons. Providing free breakfasts for Black and Latiné children before they went to school demonstrated activists' desire to serve the people, humanized their image as revolutionary warriors, and offered opportunities to recruit new members.

In 1969, the two groups worked in tandem to provide free breakfasts at a social service agency in East Harlem, an example of the collective care strategy of organizing, and of narrative shift, by claiming that adequate food before school was a right, not a privilege offered to the deserving by charity. Unlike the more gendered activities of these organizations, both men and women prepared and served the breakfasts, challenging sexist stereotypes.[14] According to some scholars, the free breakfast programs of the Young Lords and the Black Panthers in New York, Oakland, and Chicago helped to put free breakfast in schools on the national policy agenda and contributed to public support for the expansion of a similar federal program a few years later.[15]

The Young Lords also insisted that the food they served had to meet high nutritional standards. Luis Nunez, a Young Lord and a former Vietnam medic who ran the group's kitchen, explained to the historian Johanna Fernández that the Young Lords' Ministry of Health consulted with nutritionists who set standards on "the right amount of starch, vitamins, and nutrients" in the breakfasts and other meals they served. Nunez said that one objective of the meals was to show children the "dignity and satisfaction" of eating like "a rich man" and to give them a chance to "feel what's it's like to eat . . . all sorts of things they don't get at home."[16]

In the 1970s, United Bronx Parents, a community organization founded in 1966, laid another foundation for the next fifty years of school food activism. UBP wove together the many strands of prior efforts that had motivated activists concerned about school food to create a cadre of activists, a series of message frames, and a repertoire of strategies and tactics that continue to be used today.

The leader of UBP was Evelina López Antonetty, a charismatic community organizer who demonstrates how activist leaders and campaigns of one era can contribute to subsequent mobilizations. Antonetty came to East Harlem from Puerto Rico when she was eleven. Her family members had been union organizers and Puerto Rican nationalists in Puerto Rico and New York. Like many New York City activists of the mid-twentieth century, Antonetty was a member of organizations affiliated with the Communist Party and a supporter of the antifascist forces in the Spanish Civil War. Her mentors included Puerto Rican nationalists and the East Harlem Congressman Vito Marcantonio, an Italian American member of the Communist Party–supported American Labor Party.[17] These exposures gave Antonetty a knowledge of activist strategies and tactics and commitments to community organizing and representing the needs and voices of working-class women and men, especially Puerto Rican New Yorkers.

From the 1960s through the 1980s, Antonetty and other members of UBP were immersed in ongoing national and local struggles to desegregate public schools. In New York, many civil rights activists, frustrated by the entrenched opposition to desegregation, turned their attention to increasing community and parental control of schools in New York's Black and Puerto Rican neighborhoods. These schools received less funding and were assigned more inadequately trained teachers than schools serving mostly white better-off neighborhoods.

In 1967, UBP received funding from private groups and the federal Office of Economic Opportunity, the agency responsible for implementing LBJ's War on Poverty, to train parents to advocate for changes in their children's schools.[18] Through this activity, UBP learned directly from parents about the appalling conditions in city schools, the disrespectful treatment of Black and Latiné parents and their children, and parental commitment to improving public schools. Many parents believed that better schools offered their children the most meaningful path out of poverty. Through its formal and informal training programs, UBP trained hundreds of parents. In the next decade, these men and women became the cadre of activists who helped to bring the fight for community control, improved education, and better school food to schools and neighborhoods throughout New York City.[19]

UBP added school food to their activist agenda for two reasons. First, parents and children complained about the poor quality of the food schools served: stale sandwiches, spoiled milk and food, unsanitary cafeterias, and no attention to cultural preferences. Equally important, parents felt they had expertise and worthwhile ideas for improving school food. Kathy Goldman, another leader at UBP, told Lana Dee Povitz, a historian of New York City's food movement, that one mother told her, "The principal may know more about reading and teaching, but when it comes to food, I'm just as much of an expert as he is."[20]

UBP recognized that food was both a means and an end. It was, wrote Povitz, a way of "bringing poverty-stricken families into the struggle for community control. Parents who were otherwise reluctant to be involved in 'educational' issues would see a change in school food . . . and feel empowered to work for other forms of social change. . . . Working to improve school food was also an end in itself, because decent and nutritious school food would benefit families in concrete and immediate ways."[21]

Two campaigns on school food illustrate the strategies and tactics UBP used to organize parents, mobilize power, and win concrete victories. In 1969 and 1970, UBP led a campaign to improve school lunches in city schools. After hearing a litany of complaints about school food from their parents, UBP and its parent organizers designed a study to monitor and evaluate lunchrooms in twenty-five South Bronx schools for eight weeks.[22] During this period, parents reviewed menus, level of food service, amount of waste, and cleanliness in the setup of kitchens and cafeterias, a good example of activists gathering evidence to make their case to the public. This report informed UPB's choice of methods used to pursue their goals.

UBP's approach to school food shared characteristics with the Young Lords' and Black Panthers' school programs, but it also differed in important ways. Like the two militant organizations, UBP was committed to both community service and political organizing. In addition, all three groups endorsed the idea that access to adequate food was a basic human right and that the failure to end hunger and food insecurity was an indictment of a racist and oppressive political and economic system. What was different was that the Young Lords and the Panthers embraced radical rhetoric and made revolutionary change their central goal. For UBP and Antonetty, the central goals were to win community control of the schools, ensure that families had enough to eat, and provide local jobs.[23] This base-building strategy put the daily survival of community residents first. As one indication of the connections between the two approaches, Antonetty served as a mentor and adviser for several of the Young Lords in the late 1960s and early 1970s, and later for local Congressman José E. Serrano.[24] The two nicknames Antonetty acquired—Hell Lady of the Bronx and Mother of the Bronx—demonstrate her multifaceted reputation.[25]

Two UPB tactics illustrate the group's creativity. When the group presented the findings of its study of school food to school officials, the Bureau of School Lunches failed to act. So UBP invited a group of elected officials to a lunch meeting. Due to Antonetty's extensive political network, state senators, assembly members, city council members, staff of the mayor, the governor, and Bronx Borough President Herman Badillo attended the event. As they showed up, they were greeted by hundreds of protesting parents, escorted onto school buses, and brought to the elementary school that had scored lowest on the UBP survey, where they were served a typical school lunch. One state legislator reported food poisoning after the event, a reminder of the perils of inadequate school food safety standards.

As the officials left the lunch, they were given an invitation to another event where UBP said "they would be delighted to serve you a 'real school lunch' the way it should be."[26] That meal, hosted by a Puerto Rican principal at a junior high school, included sliced pineapple and grapefruit sections, sweet potatoes, stewed beans, spareribs, black-eyed peas, and other Black and Puerto Rican favorites. The menu was printed in English and Spanish. More than five hundred people attended, showing UBP and the community that school lunches could be different.

Once again, the Bureau of School Lunches ignored community voices, deciding instead to emphasize frozen meal packs heated in convection ovens rather than prepared from scratch. To protest its anger with this decision and the waste it generated when many children refused to eat the meals—and to win media coverage—UBP dumped plastic bags full of food collected from school trash bins at the city's USDA offices.[27] This disruptive strategy focused the attention of the public and political leaders on the failures of the city's school food system. Articles on the weaknesses of the city's school lunches in *The Wall Street Journal* and *The Amsterdam News* amplified UBP's messages.

By 1971, UBP started to have more success in a second campaign to bring summer meals to school children. The New York City Board of Education had refused to apply for new federal funding for summer meals, claiming it had neither the capacity to run the program nor the level of support needed to open schools in the summer. The New York State Education Department suggested UBP take on the task. After some hesitation and deliberation, UBP agreed. Despite a variety of budgetary and logistical problems, that summer, UBP served 150,000 children a day in all five boroughs, providing a total of more than 6 million lunches.

UBP contracted with ARA Food Services (now Aramark), a national food service provider, to produce and distribute the food. Because UBP was the contractor, they insisted ARA hire community people to pack and deliver the food, ultimately creating three hundred full-time jobs for the summer. This arrangement foreshadowed both a later alliance between school food activists, the union representing cafeteria workers, and city schools that extracted concessions from for-profit companies to protect children's health.

Through these activities, UBP shifted the narrative from parents and children as subjects of school policy to parents and the community as actors, agents of change. Its tactics showed activists, community residents, and elected officials that parents could mobilize power in Black and Latiné communities, could put a seemingly mundane issue on the city's political agenda, and could win concrete victories that improved the well-being of their children.

CAMPAIGN FOR UNIVERSAL FREE LUNCH

New York City schools have long been the second-largest provider of free or subsidized meals in the nation, exceeded only by the US military. But on September 6, 2017, New York City Schools Chancellor Carmen Fariña expanded this role by announcing that public schools would make free lunches available to all 1.1 million children attending these schools, ending the practice of requiring some children to pay for their food. "This is about equity," Fariña said. "All communities matter."[28]

The decision to make free school lunches available to all children marked the culmination of the Lunch for Learning Campaign sponsored by Community Food Advocates, a food justice organization founded in 2010 to advocate for the improvement of public income and food support programs. According to Liz Accles, executive director of CFA, the success of the campaign brought impressive benefits to the children and people of New York City.

First, it gave all children at the city's public schools the opportunity to get free lunches, and, under a previously adopted program, free breakfasts every weekday during the school year. These forty free meals a month left families struggling to make ends meet with more money to cover necessities like food, health care, travel, and other essential needs.

Second, the new policy ended the stigma experienced by children who had previously received free meals when they had been offered only to low-income families, a stipulation that had left many low-income middle and high school students unwilling to claim the benefit because of teasing or ridicule from peers.

Free school lunches also increased the number of children who received school meals. In the first year after universal free lunches were instituted, 26,000 more children ate lunch in school every day, consuming 4.6 million additional meals that year.[29] This was especially helpful for children from families with undocumented individuals, who often feared submitting the required paperwork for enrollment in the lunch program. Since the undocumented were not eligible for SNAP, the federal program that enabled many low-income citizens to obtain free food from local supermarkets and groceries, free school food was particularly important for this population.

Finally, universal free lunches reduced the administrative burden on schools as they no longer had to collect and process documents from each student's family,[30] freeing staff to focus on more essential tasks.

LUNCH FOR LEARNING CAMPAIGN STRATEGIES AND TACTICS

CFA began its Lunch for Learning campaign in 2013. Over the next four years, the group carried out activities that can serve as a model for other health activist campaigns. Many of the activities and impact of the campaign were described in a 2021 article assessing the effort in the medical journal *Pediatrics*.[31] The article presented the unusual example of a formal evaluation of an activist campaign and demonstrated Lunch for Learning's skill in enlisting pediatricians and their professional organizations in their research, advocacy, and evaluation.

What did the campaign accomplish? First, the group assembled a coalition made up of the constituencies most directly affected by the school lunch program and those who had the most power to influence the mayor, city council, and the Department of Education, the key decisions-makers on school food in the city. The most affected group included parents, students, and teachers. The actors who had power comprised the unions or associations representing teachers, cafeteria workers, and school principals; elected officials and their staffs, including the mayor, city council members, and borough presidents; and organizations of pediatricians and other health professionals.

"Who were the folks that should be in the room who could bring voice, energy, specific expertise, and experience to the campaign?" CFA organizers asked.[32] They then invited these individuals and organizations to join. Unions, for example, had a big influence on New York City mayors, especially incoming Mayor Bill di Blasio, so they were invited to contribute their expertise and clout. Students could tell compelling stories about their experiences with school meals to their elected representatives, so they, too, were invited. According to Accles, more than two hundred organizations eventually signed on to the Lunch for Learning Campaign. Their participation in demonstrations at city hall and elsewhere kept the issue in the media and on the minds of elected officials (see figure 6.2).

Second, CFA organized a core group of key members of the campaign and met with them every other week for four years. Having a diverse but consistent core group to plan strategy and tactics helped to keep the coalition focused. "It's very hard to keep the momentum going, to keep energy going. Part of it is having people that have the ability to do that, because that's not always the case," Accles explained.[33] The campaign also stayed focused on universal free lunches, supporting groups working on related issues but not merging with them.

During those four years, the core group arranged to have parents, students, teachers, and others testify at every city council hearing on the topic, thus educating the council's members, telling stories about how school food affected their constituents, and showing the breadth and depth of their support.

A third activity was to conduct and present their own research to counter Department of Education misinformation. When some school

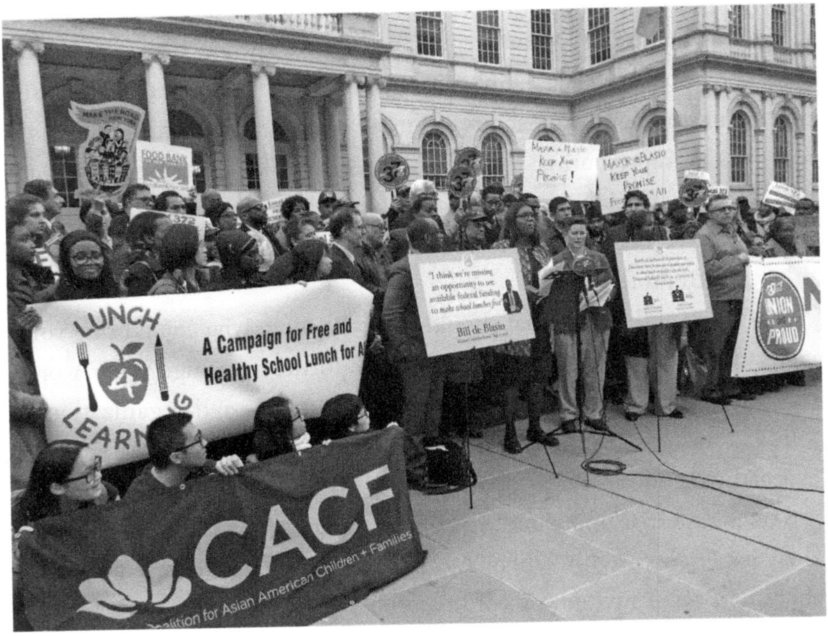

FIGURE 6.2 In 2017, with parents, students, elected officials, and school cafeteria workers and their union, DC 37, Liz Accles, behind microphone, the executive director of Community Food Advocates, the lead sponsor of the Lunch for Learning campaign, speaks at a rally in front of city hall to persuade Mayor Bill de Blasio to approve free lunch for all public school students in New York City. To the left of Accles is Tish James, then New York City public advocate and later New York States's attorney general.

Source: Lunch for Learning. https://www.fordfoundation.org/news-and-stories/stories/fighting-the-stigma-of-free-lunch-why-universal-free-school-lunch-is-good-for-students-schools-and-families/

officials argued that most low-income children already had access to free school lunches, CFA staff were able to use the department's own database to show that many schools with high proportions of low-income students had low enrollment rates in the previous, more limited free lunch program.

CFA attributed this lack of participation to these children's fear of stigma, symbolized by school children's derogatory label of school food as "free-free." Aminata Abdouramane, a senior at a Brookly high school in 2016, explained,

> I know this game all too well, as I was once that bullied student in the cafeteria. As a new freshman, I experienced the humiliation of having other students announce that I was in line for the "free-free." After a week of this nonstop bullying, I begged my parents to pack me lunch. On good days, I ate my lunch by myself, away from the cafeteria. But on bad days, when my mom didn't have money or time, I had no other choice than to go to the cafeteria and eat the "free-free."[34]

When school officials claimed they could not afford to make free lunches universal, CFA presented their own cost estimates, which were substantially lower than those of the Department of Education. This evidence strengthened the support of sympathetic city council members, who in turn increased pressure on the mayor to allocate the funds needed.

Finally, to ensure that their messages were focused and persuasive, with the support of a foundation grant, the campaign hired a communications firm to help them bring their message to the media and to elected officials. Ensuring that their health, educational, economic, and moral arguments were consistent, well crafted, and detailed enough to meet the needs of each constituency helped them to build political and public support for universal free lunches.

For several years, Chancellor Fariña opposed universal free meals, and until 2017, the mayor was not willing to overrule her, even though he had pledged to support free school lunches during his 2013 campaign. In 2014, Fariña agreed to free universal lunches in middle schools, but only expanded it to all schools in 2017 after new state funding became available. In addition, the city council had allocated more funding for school food and the mayor had endorsed the plan, putting additional pressure on the chancellor to say yes.

After its success, Lunch for Learning continued to monitor implementation and to assist the school system to improve school meals. When campaign planners learned about a new Department of Education plan to create "enhanced cafeterias" with diner-style booths, small tables, salad bars, and attractive colors, they enthusiastically supported the concept and helped to advocate for additional mayoral and city council funding for this innovation.

The COVID-19 pandemic totally disrupted school food, but it also led to a variety of federally funded innovations including "Meals to Go," where children and their families could pick up meals in front of the school to take home during pandemic-related school closures. When federal funding ended, CFA advocated for continued support for this program, a battle they did not win.

In 2022, together with another statewide coalition, CFA supported continuing the universal free lunch program instituted during the pandemic. The New York State Legislature approved and the governor authorized additional funding that allowed more than 160 school districts throughout New York State to provide free meals, but failed to establish the principle of universal free lunches throughout the state.[35] In 2024, a coalition of more than 200 city and state advocates again urged New York Governor Kathy Hochul to budget for universal free lunches throughout the state, a recommendation she did not approve.[36] But in 2025, Governor Hochul allocated $340 million in new state funding for school meals for every student in the state's public schools,[37] an important victory for the city and state activist coalitions who had been pressing for this change for years.

Lunch for Learning's success in winning free universal school lunch for New York City public school students was an impressive accomplishment, one that built on decades of prior activism described in this chapter and elsewhere.[38] United Bronx Parents and Evelina Antonetty contributed trained parent activists who spent years fighting for better school food, an understanding of the connections between better food and better education, and the power of parents and communities to mobilize against manifestations of racism and poverty in their daily lives. The Young Lords and the Black Panthers showed that feeding schoolchildren could be part of envisioning a radically transformed society and articulated the principle that having enough to eat was a basic human right.

Over the years, the campaigns to improve food in public schools helped to further the goals of other food movements. Their successes expanded the public sector in food, created practical alternatives to a market-driven food system, and highlighted a vision of a food system driven by human need rather than profit. UBP's core message, contained on a flyer Antonetty sent to all parents in the schools they worked in, was "Our children have the right to the best—the best food and the best education."[39] These simple but powerful words brought together parents who wanted better education and food for their children, those who wanted to desegregate public schools in New York City, and those who wanted to end child poverty.

School food campaigns also strengthened democracy and civic engagement. Thousands of parents and children participated in rallies, signed petitions, and learned about city politics, with the added benefit of winning their goal of free lunches throughout the school system and showing that activism could make a difference. Lunch for Learning also taught a lesson in government accountability. When Mayor de Blasio hesitated to implement universal free lunches in 2017, activists widely distributed a video of de Blasio endorsing universal free lunches at a 2013 mayoral forum on food policy organized by CFA and other food justice organizations. This message reminded the mayor that his 2017 reelection campaign might benefit from support from parents of school children and activists supporting universal free lunches.

In sum, by using every strategy listed in table 6.1 over the years, school food activists won major victories that improved school food, reduced food insecurity among schoolchildren, and expanded the public sector's role in food. They also showed that it can take decades to achieve relatively modest goals, the value of sustained and comprehensive strategies (versus quick-fix solutions), and the benefits of deploying multiple tactics selected to reach specific audiences and complete the step-by-step tasks often needed to secure victory.

CHOOSING STRATEGIES AND TACTICS

All activists must choose strategies and tactics, whatever their issue or setting. But health activists in New York City face two more specific questions. First, they need to ask how their goals of improving health and social justice, compared to other activist policy goals such as changing foreign policy or stopping the banning of books in school libraries, affect their choices of strategies and tactics. Second, they must consider whether their location in New York City creates distinct opportunities and risks in their selection of strategies and tactics, a question that activists in other places must also consider.

Health, defined by the World Health Organization in 1946 as "a state of complete physical, mental, and social well-being and not merely the absence of disease or infirmity,"[40] provides a powerful moral frame for action on several fronts. Many activist campaigns have the implicit or explicit goal of improving well-being. WHO's addition of the social determinants of health perspective in a 2008 report widened that frame even more.[41] With the growing recognition that housing, work, food, climate change, education, and other social factors play a major role in determining who is healthy and who is not, activists working on many issues can use the "health halo" to justify or explain their work. I use the term "health halo" to describe the credibility and appeal of an activity perceived to improve health.

Two strategies that Bhargava and Luce (see table 6.1) suggested, narrative shift and collective care, seem especially well suited for campaigns that center on health. Narrative shift seeks to change public understanding of major problems and their solutions. Many school food groups used a variety of tactics to develop this strategy. The Young Lords wanted to show the children they fed the "dignity and satisfaction" of eating like "a rich man" and a chance to "feel what's it's like to eat . . . all sorts of things they don't get at home."[42] UBP insisted that "our children have the right to the best—the best food and the best education."[43] Lunch for Learning demonstrated that schoolchildren, parents, teachers, and health-care providers wanted a voice in shaping how and what city schools feed their children, and did not want the Department of Education to make these decisions without consulting them.

In each case, the tactics that campaigners used to implement their strategies challenged the status quo. Their actions helped to shift policy debates on school food onto grounds more favorable to activists. The new narratives these groups promoted were that good, healthy school food should be a right, not a privilege; that complaints about school food were not because children were spoiled and picky, but came from those wanting the best for all the city's children; and that in a decent democratic society, parents, children, and school staff deserved a voice in setting school policies.

Governor Kathy Hochul illustrated school food activists' success in bringing their messages into the mainstream by echoing their message in her 2025 State of the State speech. "The research is clear," said the Governor, "good food in the lunchroom creates good grades in the classroom."[44]

Health activists often choose the strategy of collective care, which means providing care to people in need with the goal of offering alternatives to established service systems.[45] The Young Lords' and Black Panthers' free breakfast programs illustrate collective care. ACT UP members, sometimes working in collaboration with the Gay Men's Health Crisis, a more care-oriented AIDS group, directly supported people with AIDS while simultaneously advocating for stronger health and social assistance services. ACE (AIDS Counseling and Education at the Bedford Hills Correctional Facility, described in chapter 5) supported women struggling with HIV while in prison, and demanded more humane services for them. These campaigns gained credibility and authenticity by both caring for their participants and fighting for changes in policy and institutional practices. They also learned first-hand about the real needs of those they served.

The mutual aid campaigns launched during the COVID-19 pandemic in New York City offer a more recent example. These neighborhood-based groups brought food and medicine to homebound people, delivered personal protective equipment to essential workers in hospitals, and raised funds for unemployed workers, many of whom were ineligible for unemployment benefits or federal relief checks because of their immigration status or job title.[46] COVID-19 mutual aid was also an implicit critique of a government that had failed to anticipate or plan for a predictable epidemic, failed to respond quickly and effectively, and failed to protect the most vulnerable residents of the city and the nation.

In recent decades, service has claimed an ever-larger share of the New York and national economies, the number of older, ill, disabled, or very young people needing care has increased, and recurrent cycles of austerity budgeting have made safety net programs unreliable. These trends have made the collective care strategy the approach of choice for an increasing number of health activist campaigns.

As shown by the COVID-19 mutual aid groups, collective care strategies can engage multiple constituencies. These include people with a specific diagnosis or health vulnerability, family and friends who care for them, health professionals from home-care workers to nurses and physicians, and the many concerned individuals who feel compelled to act when a health crisis threatens their community. This strategy also communicates a vision of a better society, where people take care of each other and individual responsibility and collective action are two sides of the same coin, not opposites in conflict.

As the Trump administration cuts back safety net programs like SNAP and Medicaid, undermines the concept of collective caring, and pits vulnerable groups against each other, the strategic use of collective care approaches has attracted renewed interest as a useful political and moral frame for activism and economic development.[47]

Activists deploying collective care strategies also face several challenges. How can they find the right balance between providing care to those in need—a more than full-time task—and mobilizing for policy change? How can the unpaid volunteers who sustain collective care prevent burnout and cope with the pain and grief they witness daily? How can they partner with other groups to provide the information and resources people need to act collectively as well as individually?

In one such collaboration, the Right to Counsel NYC Coalition, which led the campaign to make it a right for tenants to have a lawyer when facing eviction in New York City, and Housing Justice for All worked with mutual aid groups to produce a tool kit on how to organize a rent strike during the COVID-19 pandemic.[48] More recently, immigrant rights and reproductive justice and abortion rights activists have combined providing care to people in need with political and legal fights against policies they believed damaged the well-being of their constituents.

In their discussion of collective care, Bhargava and Luce suggest several ways to strengthen its capacity to mobilize power more strategically and find answers to these challenging questions. They recommend that activists

- Use collective care models to turn emotion into power.
- Create pathways for new participation.
- Increase the capacity of participants to do political work.
- Prepare members to be ready to act when a movement surges.
- Help organizers find the equilibrium they will need to stick around for the long haul.
- Build ideological power explicitly by showing the potential and benefits of more democratic relationships and organizations.[49]

These recommendations, based on the authors' analyses of multiple activist campaigns, provide organizers of health campaigns using collective care strategies with practical steps they can take to use this approach to build power and achieve their goals.

Health activist campaigns have used all seven strategies listed in table 6.1. In choosing which to use and how to combine two or more strategies, campaign planners need to ask how their *health* goals should influence their choices. This will depend on their identification of the causes of the problem they seek to fix, the individuals and organizations they expect to enlist as supporters, and the current potential for change based on their assessment of the opportunities and obstacles presented by the current political economy, topics discussed in previous chapters.

The Lunch for Learning campaign, for example, decided that the array of constituencies they hoped to activate already supported the ideas campaign planners thought would bring universal free lunches to all New York City public schools. Three such ideas were that no child's learning should be deterred by hunger or food insecurity, that healthy school food supported the lifetime well-being of children, and that making the policy universal would be both politically and morally appealing and administratively efficient. By mobilizing those who already agreed with these health-related ideas to convince power brokers to act, Lunch for Learning built the power to get to yes.

Campaign organizers also need to consider how their health goals might influence their choice of tactics. While activists have long debated whether illegal activities, property damage, or even violence has any place in their tactical repertoire,[50] it is hard to imagine an explicitly health-focused campaign choosing to use tactics that physically harmed its opponents. Especially after the September 11, 2001, attack on the World Trade Center, any protest in the United States that included violence risked being called terrorism, a label that usually moved its perpetrators outside public understanding or sympathy. In recent years, the Trump administration has branded any vigorous opponents of its policies as terrorists and all its supporters, no matter how violent, as patriots,[51] a linguistic sleight of hand that activists must consider when choosing tactics.

After the demise of groups that advocated the strategic use of violence in the late 1960s and early 1970s, US activists pursuing health goals have generally avoided deliberately harming people. Breaking the law and seizing property or space, however, are tactics that have been used successfully over the years. The Young Lords seized—"liberated," in their words—unused lead poisoning and tuberculosis testing equipment from the city Health Department to use on the streets of East Harlem to screen for these two prevalent conditions.[52]

In 1988, the Association for Drug Abuse Treatment and Prevention announced its intention to distribute free needles and syringes in New York City to reduce HIV transmission via dirty needles. Defying New York State law, its executive director, Yolanda Serrano, said her agency was prepared to face prosecution and the loss of its financing and tax-exempt status "to protect the public and save lives," a declaration that was reported on the front page of *The New York Times*.[53] "Somebody has to take the first step," she said.

In 1990, ACT UP activists were arrested on charges of illegal possession and distribution of drug paraphernalia. In a landmark court case, the defendants were acquitted using a "public health necessity" defense. The court noted that although the defendants had in fact broken the law, their actions "sought to avoid the greater harm" of preventable cases of HIV infection.[54] Through these illegal tactics, activist groups helped to promote changes to the law on distributing sterile needles in New York City and elsewhere.

Protests after the 2020 death of George Floyd, an African American man who died after a white Minneapolis police officer pressed a knee on his neck for nearly nine minutes, led to weeks of civil unrest in New York City and around the nation. After a day of mostly peaceful demonstrations, reported *The Guardian*, roving bands of people smashed into stores in Manhattan and the Bronx, burned piles of trash, and in at least one case, attacked a police officer.[55] The police arrested more than two hundred people.

In that same period, New York City police beat up and arrested hundreds of other demonstrators. Eventually, more than six hundred of these protestors filed complaints or court cases charging police with illegal acts and unnecessary violence, leading to legal settlements in which the city paid the plaintiffs more than $25 million to resolve these claims.[56] Police use of unnecessary violence against protestors or those judged to be breaking traffic or drug laws is both a health and a criminal justice issue. Activists must balance the risk of normalizing police violence by *not* reacting to such incidents with the risk of provoking backlash by appearing to condone or not condemn what some will call activist violence.

A national poll conducted by CNN shortly after Floyd's killing found that 84 percent of Americans agreed that peaceful protests after police violence against African Americans are justified, while about a quarter (27 percent) said that violent protests in response to police harming or killing of African Americans are also justified.[57] Three years later, only 32 percent of those polled believed the earlier protests had been highly effective in bringing attention to racism against Black people, and even fewer thought they had improved police accountability or race relations. Black respondents were twice as likely to support the movement as white ones.[58]

A mix of persistent white opposition to antiracist activism, a vigorous conservative countermovement to Black Lives Matter, and many Americans' deep discomfort with civil unrest no doubt contributed to the decline in white support. The point here is that activist campaigners need to consider the short- and longer-term positive and negative consequences of their actions. Positive effects include greater attention to the issue and a greater willingness to support what are perceived to be effective solutions. Negative impacts may include potential backlash, media disapproval, and the possible alienation of some supporters by their choice of tactics. By considering possible responses, planners can make more informed choices about strategy and tactics.

No evidence can prove or disprove whether any specific tactic is never or sometimes justified or effective. Rather, activists, including health activists, must analyze their decisions on the continuum of disruptive, illegal, or violent tactics from moral, strategic, and philosophical perspectives as well as based on their own values.

New York City activists have used a wide variety of tactics to inform, educate, mobilize, disrupt, isolate, or ridicule opponents. The tactics that campaign organizers choose communicate many messages. They can evoke connections to other movements—for example, sit-ins, freedom rides, and marches to the civil rights movement; strikes and boycotts to the labor movement; or burning membership cards or die-ins to antiwar movements. By choosing tactics from the repertoires of prior movements, activists highlight their connections to the values and goals of those who preceded them.[59] Or, depending on the tactic, they can appear to be no different and no better than their opponents.

Activists also send a message through *where* they choose to stage their actions. A demonstration or sit-in at a corporate headquarters or a bank suggests who the group believes is responsible for the problem in question. Actions at medical centers or insurance companies locate the cause within the structure and financing of the nation's health-care system. Marches through the communities most affected by the problem invite residents to participate. Protests against opponents of vaccinations, deniers of climate change, or proponents of drug company deregulation can put a spotlight on those supporting health-harming policies.

By matching tactics to strategies and goals, selecting actions to achieve a specific purpose related to achieving the aims of the campaign, and targeting tactics to specific supporting and opposing constituencies, activists make choices that increase their chances of winning. And by establishing organizational processes in advance to make these decisions thoughtfully but expeditiously, campaign organizers can be ready to act as new opportunities or threats arise.

NEW YORK CITY INFLUENCES ON CHOICE OF STRATEGY AND TACTICS

New York City provides activists with one of the world's most visible stages. Campaigns have chosen their activities to take advantage of the limelight at the city's iconic sites. As the case profiles have shown, demonstrators have decided to perform at Wall Street, St. Patrick's Cathedral, Central Park, Washington Square Park, the Statue of Liberty, or New York City Hall. After 2016, the many properties owned by Donald Trump also provided places for protest. Each of these sites evokes the history of previous battles, attracts media attention, and elicits emotions from both New Yorkers and those who know the city from tourism, movies, or their own memories.

In the campaign to hold Purdue Pharmaceuticals accountable for its aggressive and misleading promotion of OxyContin, which contributed to the deaths one million Americans from overdoses from this drug and the epidemic of opioid use that followed,[60] the New York City–based national activist group Prescription Addiction Intervention Now (PAIN) sponsored demonstrations at the Metropolitan Museum of Art and the Guggenheim Museum, two internationally recognized art collections to which the Sackler family, the owners of Purdue, had donated millions of dollars. PAIN worked with Vocal-NY, TruthPharma, and other activist groups to educate Americans about how the Sackler family was using its immense wealth to sanitize its image and avoid responsibility for the deaths its drugs had caused.

On March 10, 2018, an army of protesters marched into the Temple of Dendur, the most popular exhibit at the Metropolitan, located in the Sackler Wing of the museum. The demonstrators chanted, "Sacklers lie! Thousands die!" and "Temple of Money! Temple of Greed!" They flung thousands of orange pill bottles into the Temple of Dendur's pool and carried signs demanding "FUND REHAB" and "SHAME ON SACKLERS."

Nan Goldin, a well-known artist, a founder of PAIN, and herself a former OxyContin addict, shouted, "We're here to call out the museums who allow the Sackler name to line their halls, tarnish their wings to honor the family who made billions off the bodies of hundreds of thousands." Then she dropped to the ground, followed by the other protestors who surrounded the temple's pool, filled with bobbing pill bottles and "dead" bodies.[61]

Media coverage of the demonstration sent these images around the world, leading to the removal of the Sackler name from this and other museums and to legal actions that resulted in a settlement with state attorney general for $6 billion to go to rehabilitation services.[62] More broadly, the PAIN protests promoted a national reconsideration of the role of the pharmaceutical industry in public life and the need for more stringent regulation. Using some of New York's iconic art institutions as a site to disseminate this message played an important role in the campaign's successes.[63]

As home to diverse populations, New York City also enables national and local demonstrations to show that Blacks and whites, young and old, gay and straight, middle class and poor, immigrants and native-born can join to demand public attention to their concerns. The New York City Climate Marches in 2014 and 2023, the 2018 Women's March in New York City, the 2020 Black Lives Matter demonstrations, and the 2025 demonstration to Stand Up for Science and No Kings Day opposing Trump's policies showed these movements attracted supporters across demographic characteristics and identities, counteracting the tropes of siloed activism. By mobilizing New Yorkers and attracting activists from outside the city to their protests, organizers can send images around the country and sometimes the world that show broad and deep support for their cause.

The salience of place to the choice of strategies and tactics is of course not unique to New York City. Washington, DC, Chicago, Los Angeles, the Dakota Access Pipeline in North Dakota, and Warren County, North Carolina, known as the birthplace of the environmental justice movement, and many other places are locations with rich histories of protest and iconic sites that symbolize particular disasters or protests. Like activists in New York, those in other places need to identify the sites that will amplify their voices and choose the strategies and tactics that will leverage these assets.

BEYOND STRATEGIES AND TACTICS

On the one hand, choosing strategies and tactics is the bread and butter of campaign planners and organizers. Based on their experiences, the responses to their previous actions, and their knowledge of the contexts in which they are acting, activists decide what to do next week and next year, immersing themselves in the details of their specific unfolding campaigns.

On the other hand, every decision they make is embedded in the history of previous activism and foretells a particular campaign's future steps. It is hardly surprising, then, that some activists get overwhelmed by this complexity and choose to focus only on the immediate demands on their attention, on tactics rather than strategy.

But as I have argued previously in this book, many of the factors that shape the success or failure of their campaigns are outside the control of activists. That is why focusing on what they *can* control—including the strategies and tactics they choose to use—is so important. By concentrating on what is in their power, activists can maximize their ability to influence the outcomes they pursue.

Based on this review of the strategies and tactics that activist campaigns in New York City have used to pursue health and social justice, I suggest five questions activists can ask to help them make these decisions.

1. Which strategies and tactics will most usefully build on our previous successes in campaigns on similar or related issues?
2. Which will emphasize, rather than distract, from our core messages and values?
3. Which will maximize our opportunities to win over additional supporters and persuade or isolate potential opponents?
4. How can we anticipate possible backlash to our strategies and tactics and make choices that prevent, minimize, or effectively counteract such reactions?
5. How can our strategies and tactics solidly link our health and social goals and our location in New York City?

By asking and answering these questions over the course of their campaigns, activists can ensure that their choices are informed by careful reflection, evidence from previous experiences, and consideration of their long- and short-term goals.

7

HOW ACTIVISTS FORGE RELATIONSHIPS WITH ALLIES AND OPPONENTS

While activists have substantial control over the strategies and tactics they use, external forces also determine their interactions with their allies and opponents. In this chapter, I look for patterns of interaction between health and social justice campaigns and key outside actors, seeking evidence as to which approaches to collaboration or confrontation are more successful in helping activists to achieve their goals.

The New York City campaigns described in this book repeatedly encounter many of the same institutional actors. A brief overview of the scope of activist interactions with seven of these key players—government agencies and politicians, businesses and trade groups, scientists and academics, community organizations and nonprofit groups, journalists and the media, philanthropy, and other social movements—provides the starting point for this chapter. The case profile describes the work of the close Rikers campaigns, an ongoing, decade-long effort to close the Rikers Island Detention Center, a complex of eleven jails located on an island in the East River between the boroughs of the Bronx and Queens. The profile examines how this series of campaigns interacted with the key players over the last decade.

For each actor, I consider three questions:

1. What do activist campaigns want from this actor?
2. What does this actor want from activists?
3. How do the external actors assess the risks and benefits of interaction?

By anticipating what allies or opponents are expecting in their interactions, campaign organizers and leaders can map their options and make informed choices.

KEY ACTORS IN ACTIVIST CAMPAIGNS

GOVERNMENT AGENCIES AND POLITICIANS

Every campaign described in *Fighting for New York* had some interactions with public agencies or politicians. Campaigners want support from government allies for legislation or budget allocations and for intelligence or information on future political developments. They also want politicians to use their bully pulpits to advance their campaigns' goals. Activists also want to know what resources their adversaries will use to block their campaigns, what compromises they might be willing to make, and their opponents' real and perceived vulnerabilities in the political arena.

In turn, government allies look to activists for political support, votes, and campaign contributions. They hope for endorsement of their other policy proposals ("you scratch my back, I'll scratch yours"), supportive testimony at legislative hearings, outreach to neighbors and friends, and for activists to use the media in ways that lead to favorable coverage. Elected officials opposed to activist demands seek to isolate or stigmatize opponents, find acceptable compromises, or co-opt or sway activists to support their opponents' point of view.

Most government agencies and politicians are risk averse. In general, they avoid interactions that might cause loss of political support, a drop in campaign contributions, or negative media coverage. If endorsing (or opposing) activists has the potential to build their base of political support, enhance their chances of reelection, or propel them to higher office, they are more likely to engage.

Government officials and elected leaders, like other populations, include those with deep values and strong moral principles and those who are mostly transactional, willing to do whatever they need to do to advance their interests. By understanding both the broader landscape of the political arenas in which they operate, and the specific character, values, and constituencies of the targeted officials, activists can develop an informed game plan for these interactions, one that is neither unduly cynical nor inappropriately idealistic.

A few examples from WE ACT for Environmental Justice's interactions with government officials and politicians illustrate these points. Both before and after its official launch, WE ACT leaders worked to support progressive Harlem Democrats and to oppose machine ones. These relationships helped to cement an ongoing relationship with Davd Dinkins, who, once he was elected mayor, provided formal and informal support to WE ACT. At the national level, WE ACT's ties with Democrats—and their connections to the national environmental justice movement—helped them to get the attention of President Bill Clinton and to play a role in setting EPA policy on environmental justice. For New York City politicians who wanted to be able to claim their Harlem roots, support from WE ACT provided a credible and reliable source of support as the group's older Black women members had long been community activists and leaders.

BUSINESSES AND TRADE GROUPS

Health-care, environmental justice, housing, and other activists in New York City frequently view health insurance companies, polluting industries, real estate developers, or other business sectors as their opponents, the actors whose practices they want to change to achieve their health goals. To realize this aim, campaigns seek to change harmful industry practices by pressuring companies directly or by reducing the influence of these industries on elected officials and legislators. They do this by publicizing industry-specific activities that harm health, shaming politicians who accept campaign contributions from these industries or endorse health-damaging business goals, or threatening boycotts or disinvestment drives.

In some cases, activists have formed alliances with specific businesses or trade associations, portraying them as high-road employers or businesses who set an example for others in the sector. By publicly aligning with such allies, activists seek to dispel the perception that they are anti-business and thus hope to win over other market-based actors. The Restaurant Opportunity Center, which organizes and supports low-wage and immigrant food workers in New York and elsewhere, used this approach to enlist in its campaigns for higher wages and benefits restaurants that already paid decent wages and treated their workers with respect.[1]

In their interactions with activists, business leaders hope to avoid threats to profitability, reputational damage, or uncertainty about regulatory or tax policy. To attain these ends, market-based actors search for acceptable compromises with their critics—or the capacity to co-opt, stigmatize, or politically isolate activists.

Business leaders' assessment of the risks and benefits of friendly or hostile relationships with activists depends on the broader political climate. In times when more liberal politicians are in office, such as David Dinkins, Bill de Blasio, Bill Clinton, or Barack Obama, businesses have made more efforts to find compromises, whereas under a Rudy Giuliani, the Bushes, or Donald Trump, they have been more likely to isolate and discredit their opponents, thinking victory in the political arena is an achievable goal. However, both Republican and Democratic politicians at all levels of government have chosen to ally with businesses rather than activists if they believe the pollical benefits of such support outweigh its costs.

Activists often work to discredit business opponents. Housing Justice for All, the statewide coalition of housing groups profiled in chapter 3, used its 2022 *Pay to Play* report to show how trade associations of real estate and housing developers influenced legislation on evictions and real estate taxes.[2] The report revealed to their supporters and the media the multiple ways in which the $19 million these three groups spent on lobbying, litigation, and public relations advanced the real estate industry's agenda in Albany. Through this report, Housing Justice for All and their allies made it more difficult for the sector to claim it had been acting in the public interest and contributed to defeating some of the landlord-friendly politicians in the state legislature and thus paved a path for more tenant-friendly regulations and laws.

In another effort to build the power needed to implement stronger statewide protection for tenants, Housing Justice for All, together with other housing groups, organized local groups in upstate cities to demand local rent-control laws. Their theory was that by building local support for tenant protection across the state, they would be better able to defeat the real estate lobby in the state legislature. In 2022, lawmakers in the small upstate city of Kingston, New York, passed its first rent-control law. "I think it helps dispel this false divide of housing affordability supposedly only being a New York City issue," said Jonathan Bix, executive director of For the Many, a Hudson Valley–based organizing group.[3]

SCIENTISTS AND ACADEMICS

Activists depend on scientists and academics to provide evidence that can advance their policy goals, assist them to design research and evaluation studies that can inform their campaigns, enhance their credibility in political and public spaces, and support their efforts to win public or private funding for their work. Health, environmental, nutrition, and medical practitioners and their professional organizations can also support activists through these roles.

Scientists and academics seek activist organizational partners that can enlist community residents, workers, young people, or other community residents in their research studies. In his book *Street Science*, environmental scientist and urban planner Jason Corburn describes examples of such studies in New York City, including community members and professionals who combined forces to document and reduce the risks from subsistence fishing from the polluted East River, the asthma epidemic in Latiné communities, childhood lead poisoning, and local sources of air pollution.[4]

Corburn asserts that street science—research in which community residents define the problems, gather evidence, and interpret findings—offers researchers new, more grounded methods and "open[s] up both problem framing and subsequent methods of inquiry to local knowledge and community participation." This offers scientists an additional understanding of problems than offered by traditional methods alone and thus a greater potential to generate useful solutions.[5]

Some researchers seek partnerships simply because they want access to data and research subjects they would have difficulty obtaining by themselves and expect to maintain full control of their studies. Others support the social justice goals of the campaigns they study and strive to establish mutually beneficial partnerships that advance the goals of each party. Whatever the motivation of researchers, activists need to negotiate agreements for these interactions that serve their needs.

Activists and researchers with experience in community research partnerships enumerate both benefits and risks from this approach. Benefits include a deeper understanding of the harms that community residents experience, access to informants who might otherwise be difficult to engage, and more community ownership of the findings and their use to improve health. The risks they have identified are the time it takes to establish such partnerships and to work out conflicts as they arise, and the possibility of either partner losing a voice in the process or disengaging from the partnership. Activists sometimes fear that researchers will gather data and leave, depriving them of the benefits of together interpreting and applying the findings to policy deliberations.[6] Researchers have sometimes found it difficult to communicate the limits of the data.

The case of Community Food Advocates (CFA), the organization that led the Lunch for Learning campaign in New York City described in chapter 6, illustrates some of the positive interactions between activist campaigns and researchers. CFA leaders recruited a team to document the implementation and impact of the campaign that included researchers from Columbia University Medical Center, Montefiore Hospital, Albert Einstein College of Medicine, and the Mount Sinai School of Medicine. Together with CFA staff, this team collected and analyzed data on school lunch participation from the New York City school system, key documents, and media reports to mark the campaign's milestone achievements, school cafeteria observations, and city budget analysis. Their findings were reported in *Pediatrics*, a well-recognized medical journal.[7]

CFA also partnered with the Committee on Nutrition and Obesity of the New York chapter of the American Academy of Pediatrics, providing a forum for pediatrician advocacy to improve child nutrition and well-being. Participating pediatricians provided compelling evidence through letters and in-person testimony to the city council and others to advance the campaign.[8]

COMMUNITY ORGANIZATIONS AND NONPROFIT GROUPS

Most activist campaigns also work closely with community organizations and nonprofit groups, a large and diverse category sometimes called civil society. Civil society groups are defined as institutions that advance the interests and will of citizens and operate outside of government and the market.[9] Some scholars consider activist organizations and social movements part of civil society, but here I distinguish between groups that have explicit social change goals and strategies, the topic of this book, and the non-activist civil society bodies that advance social interests by providing services, educating the public, or in other ways.

Activists look to community organizations, defined here as groups based in and serving a geographic community, for assistance in engaging community residents in their campaigns; educating activists about community history, needs, and desires; and providing their campaigns with human and material resources (e.g., space for meetings, financial support, access to social networks). Community organizations also provide credibility with public officials.

Larger citywide, state, or national nonprofit groups provide activists with similar assets, but on a regional or national scale. Their contributions include access to regional and national networks, a deep knowledge of municipal and state politics, and links to philanthropy and sometimes public funding. With their experience and credibility, nonprofits can also assist activists to broaden their coalitions, thus augmenting their power to achieve their goals.

What do civil society groups want from activist organizations? Community organizations usually have limited resources and capacity to take on more than a few issues. Partnering with activists expands their capacity and resources so that they can pursue broader goals, especially goals related to changing policy or institutional practices.

Many community organizations are limited in pursuing explicitly political strategies by tax law or their own values. For these groups, partnering with social justice campaigns offers them a less visible, less risky way to support social changes favored by their leaders or members. Partnerships with more radical groups allows them to say to elected officials that failing to address the issues activists raise may disrupt traditional politics.

Activist interactions with civil society groups carry both benefits and risks. For each party, successful partnerships expand their reach and capacity. They provide access to political support, new resources, and valuable strategic insights. But such alliances also pose risks. Negotiating and maintaining partnerships is time-consuming, diverting leaders and members from other critical tasks. Maintaining multiple partnerships with different types of civil society groups elevates the potential for conflicts, which can sap energy from a campaign. Every activist campaign struggles with when to compromise and when to stand firm. With multiple and diverse partners, it can be difficult to agree on a framework and process for deciding when to compromise with or confront their opponents.

A few examples of Make the Road New York's relations with civil society groups illustrate some of the ways that activist organizations manage these interactions. After MRNY decided to assist the low-wage immigrant workers it was organizing to form unions, its leaders decided they needed a union partner with the experience, skills, and networks necessary for their campaign. They reached out to the Retail, Wholesale and Department Store Union (RWDSU), an organization with long experience in union organizing, and invited them to join their ¡Despierta Bushwick! (Wake Up Bushwick!) campaign to organize supermarket workers to demand back wages their employers had withheld.[10]

As Eddie Ott, a longtime municipal labor leader, noted, "from almost day one, Make the Road caught the attention of New York City's unions, because the group's leaders understood a union contract could be a tremendous tool for their members. This union-friendly approach—and their demonstrated ability to turn out large numbers of their members for events—set them apart from every other group in New York City."[11]

MRNY also looked to its community partners, such as legal services, social services, and health-care providers, to serve as resources for its members. As Deborah Axt, a former co-executive director of MRNY, explained, "This is a place you come for safety, respect, to learn, to grow, to invest in becoming a leader yourself. . . . Of course, it is also true this is a place you can come when you have an emergency. You will be able to find lawyers here who are the best lawyers. . . . This trustworthiness and ability to intervene in emergency moments in people's lives matters a lot in creating that feeling."[12] For MRNY, its community partnerships enabled it to fulfill its vision of serving its members as well as keeping them engaged in its campaigns.

JOURNALISTS AND THE MEDIA

The media—newspapers, television, radio, and social media—are key resources for campaigns as they enable activists to communicate with their supporters and opponents beyond those they can reach in face-to-face interactions. But journalists and the companies that employ them are also actors who have their own goals, interests, and agendas. To set goals for their activities with the media, campaign organizers need to understand the overlap and differences between their needs and the priorities of media organizations.

Activists need mass and social media to reach current and future supporters, communicate with the larger public, publicize events, reach the eyes and ears of government and business decision-makers, and promote the big ideas that open doors toward long-term support. Earned media—the press coverage or publicity a group receives without paying for it—can be a precious resource for cash-strapped activist organizations. Trusted journalists can become key informants for activists, alerting them to new developments, unreported stories, or potential allies or opponents.

Media outlets and reporters need activists in order to learn about stories that can reveal the hidden shenanigans of elites, corruption, wrongdoing, or simply human interest. In some cases, activists are situated to become whistleblowers. Reporters also need activists so that they can cover both sides of stories about ongoing campaigns or conflicts between movements and government or business actors.

Activists and media representatives acknowledge risks as well as benefits from their interactions. Activists fear that reporters will misquote or misrepresent their words and actions, serving to reinforce their opponents' messages or attacks. They worry that the public airing of their grievances or their strategies may precipitate backlash, making them more vulnerable to defeat or loss of public support. Sometimes activists forget that most media outlets are now owned by big corporations or investors who might grab attention in any way possible to maximize revenues and profits or advance a corporate political and economic agenda. While reporters and their employers hold diverse political points of view, in the last two decades, the increasing consolidation of the media industry has made many outlets more conservative politically.

A few examples from the work of the campaigns to close Rikers, profiled in this chapter, show how activists and media interacted. In 2015, *The New York Times* published an opinion column by Neil Barsky, the founder of the Marshall Project, a nonprofit media outlet that reports on criminal justice, with the title "Shut Down Rikers."[13] Its placement in an outlet with local and national influence helped introduce this idea into the political mainstream. Brian Lehrer, the host of a nationally syndicated interview show on New York Public Radio, interviewed Darren Mack, a leader

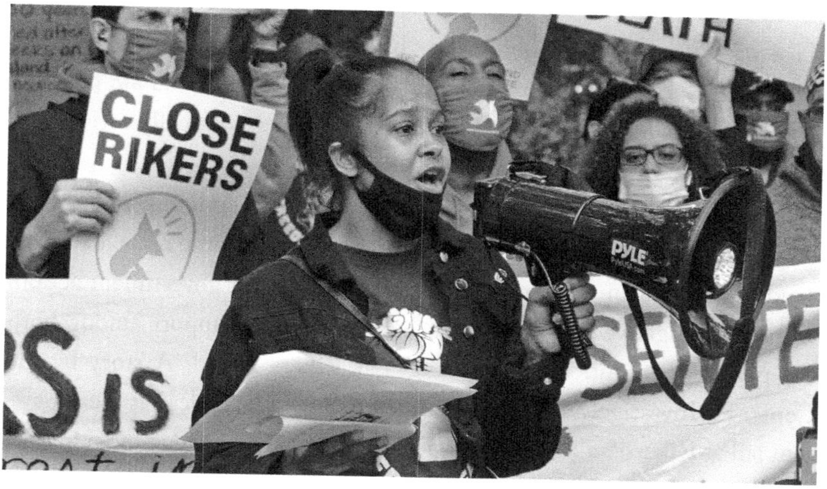

FIGURE 7.1 A January 6, 2022, Freedom Agenda demonstration in support of closing Rikers Island Detention Center.

Source: Photo by Jeroen Stevens, courtesy of Freedom Agenda and the Campaign to Close Rikers. https://fa.urbanjustice.org/wp-content/uploads/sites/22/2022/01/How-to-Advance-and-Strengthen-the-Plan-to-Close-Rikers-Interactive-For-Digital-01.06.2022.pdf

of Freedom Agenda and the campaign to close Rikers,[14] and in 2017, Bill Moyers, the public television journalist, produced and broadcast a film, *Rikers: An American Jail*, that brought the debate about closing Rikers to national audiences.[15]

In 2018, activists got media coverage in another way. #CLOSErikers campaigners protested outside the mayor's State of the City address at the Apollo Theatre in Harlem and broadcast a TV ad slamming de Blasio for boasting of New York as a "sanctuary city" while continuing to operate what they called "a notorious penal colony." As the mayor sought to burnish his national profile as a progressive, such coverage jeopardized these aspirations.[16] In the following years, multiple demonstrations kept questions about Rikers's future in the media and on the radar of elected officials (see figure 7.1).

Over the decade during which activists campaigned to close Rikers, reports on the movement's progress and obstacles also regularly appeared in the city's political journals, such as *City Limits*, *Gotham Gazette*, and *City and State*.[17] These publications have smaller circulations than *The New York Times*, *The New York Daily News*, or *The New York Post*, but they reach activists, legislators and their aides, and other politically active New Yorkers.

Investigative reporters, who seek to uncover wrongdoing, corruption, or government injustices, can often assist activist campaigns to reveal conditions that can spark public outrage and calls for government action. Three investigative reports in 2014 helped to build support among both the public and politicians for changes at Rikers Island. A story by the Center for Investigative Reporting on mental health services at the adolescent jail at Rikers;[18] a *New York Times* article based on a video of an inmate suicide at Rikers obtained by the paper;[19] and a *Times* exposé of a Department of Correction report on violence at Rikers that removed data on hundreds of fights that had been reported educated the public about the horrific conditions at Rikers and the culture of neglect.[20]

Through these interactions with the media and journalists, Close Rikers activists informed their wider constituencies about emerging issues and kept the fate of the jail on the agendas of the New Yorkers most likely to speak out on the issue. The cumulative impact of this ongoing coverage added pressure on politicians to take action.

PHILANTHROPY

Activists rely on philanthropy to fund their campaigns and therefore consider foundations and other donors to be key actors. To win funding, activist organizations need to get the attention of philanthropists, create opportunities to make their pitch, and then actually get support. In many cases, organizers then need to secure continued funding. Every step of this process requires a delicate dance, one in which the funder usually has the unilateral power to say yes or no to waltz, tango, or foxtrot—or to search for another partner.

What activists want from funders is obvious, but they must choose among different strategies as to how they pursue funding. Some foundations issue public calls for proposals on specific topics, providing activist organizations with the opportunity to apply. Some of these require only a short letter of interest, which foundation staff then screen to invite likely applicants, imposing less of a burden on activists than the full proposal other foundations expect. Activists experienced in fundraising learn how to calculate their odds of success for a specific request and choose not to submit for the less likely prospects. But less experienced activists may choose to apply for any opportunity, a kind of Hail Mary strategy that can divert staff resources from other tasks.

Other foundations accept proposals only from organizations that they invite to apply. This leads activists to search their networks for influential friends who can help them get an invitation, and for other ways to get the attention of funders, a process that can disadvantage new or less experienced groups. Some funders include community or activist representatives on their decision-making panels to provide additional viewpoints than those of foundation staff.

Philanthropies also need activists. Donors seeking to promote health equity or social justice, reduce climate change, end poverty, or dismantle racism must find and fund the activist groups that are key players for achieving those goals. Funders need to distinguish likely winners—groups that will succeed in their campaigns—from organizations that can alienate donors, board members, or the wider public. Since foundations retain the power to sign or not sign the check, their relationship with activists is profoundly unequal, a reality that colors their interactions.

Activists sometimes worry that the funder may impose conditions that divert the organizations from their goals or compromise their values. A specific fear is that funders will demand a comprehensive evaluation of their campaign, an assessment that they worry can take resources away from activism or force the group to document outcomes they do not think are important or force assessment before the activism can bear fruit. Funders, on the other hand, want to be sure that their support leads to the accomplishment of the goals they endorse. The reluctance of activists to evaluate may lead philanthropists to turn down funding requests. This conflict is discussed in more detail in chapter 9 on the evaluation of activism.

The campaigns to close Rikers provide some examples of these exchanges. In 2015, Open Philanthropy, a foundation whose main donors are Cari Tuna and her husband, Dustin Moskovitz, the cofounder of Facebook and Asana, awarded a $900,000 grant to JustLeadershipUSA and the Katal Center, sponsors of the first round of the campaigns to close Rikers. Foundation staff offered the following explanation:

> We see this as a high-risk, high-reward grant. We consider advocacy of this kind to be risky in general, and this will be the first large public campaign (to our knowledge) aimed at closing a major city jail. . . . There are many potential points for failure. However, we expect that a successful campaign would be a major step forward for criminal justice reform, potentially amplifying the message that large jails do not meaningfully increase municipal safety and that current incarceration practices have severe negative impacts, especially on the poor.[21]

In a conversation with foundation staff, Glenn E. Martin, the founder of JustLeadershipUSA, observed, "If there was ever a chance to close the facility, in the 100 year history of Rikers, the time is now."[22]

Chloe Cockburn, the foundation's program officer for criminal justice reform, estimated that the campaign had a 70 percent chance of persuading New York's leadership to make a commitment to close Rikers and outlining a plan. The likelihood of Rikers closing may be substantially lower, she wrote, given the many possible failure points and uncertainty about maintaining the necessary political momentum over the several years it will take to close the jail.[23]

The Lippman Commission, chaired by the former chief judge for New York State, Jonathan Lippman, was appointed by the New York City Council Speaker to provide advice on closing Rikers. The commission decided not to accept government funds, believing that such funding could alter the perception or reality of independence from the elected officials the commission wanted. Instead, they applied for and received foundation funding from, among others, the Ford Foundation, the Open Society Foundation, Trinity Church Wall Street Foundation, the David Rockefeller Foundation, the New York Women's Foundation, and the Brooklyn Community Foundation. Members of the commission included Darren Walker, president of the Ford Foundation, Peter J. Madonia of the Rockefeller Foundation, Ana L. Oliveira, chief executive officer of the New York Women's Foundation, and other philanthropic leaders.[24]

Lippman insisted that the decision to refuse public funding assured independence, but some abolitionist critics of the proposal to replace Rikers with new, smaller jails in the boroughs argued that major foundations supporting the commission were themselves actors with political positions.

Activists seeking to abolish mass incarceration, for example, criticized the Ford Foundation, one of the supporters of the commission. In 2019, fifty activists—including members of Decolonize This Place, Take Back the Bronx, and No New Jails—staged an action in front of the Ford Foundation to protest a statement from Darren Walker, who protestors claimed had voiced his support of New York City Mayor Bill de Blasio's plan to build new jails in the borough. Protestors opposed this proposal as just another form of mass incarceration.[25]

At the same time, some funders of the campaign to close Rikers cited their support as an example of their contribution to activism and social justice. The New York Community Trust, a funder of the campaign, claimed that, "thanks in part to advocacy from Trust grantees, the New York City Council approved an $8 billion plan to close Rikers and build four borough-based jails by 2027, and to reduce the city's overall jail population to 3,300."[26]

These anecdotes show that even actors that provide funding, an essential resource for activists, cannot escape the controversies inherent in activist interactions with outside institutions. Whether it is the strings funders attach to their financial backing, their support for other activities that activists consider problematic, or the perception of unilateral decision-making, social movement organizations often encounter dilemmas inherent in soliciting and accepting funds from another party.

PROFILE: CLOSE RIKERS ISLAND DETENTION CENTER

As the descriptions of these exchanges among various actors show, the proposal to close the jails housed within the Rikers Island Detention Center provoked intense controversy. Supporters of closure argued the complex was too big, too old, and too mired in its history of abuses to be reformed. Opponents insisted that this single facility was still essential to public safety in New York and no alternative was politically feasible in the current period. This profile of activist campaigns to close Rikers provides insights from these types of conflicts that can yield generalizable lessons. It illustrates the complex decisions activists must make in choosing how to interact with potential allies and adversaries.

In 1664, Peter Stuyvesant, the director general of the Dutch settlement of New Amsterdam (the precursor to what would become New York City), bestowed an island in the East River between what is now LaGuardia Airport in Queens and Hunt's Point in the Bronx to Abraham Rikers (originally spelled "Ryckens"). Rikers built a house and farm on the land that had belonged to the Indigenous Lenape people, and his family lived on the land for several generations.[27] During the Civil War, the island was used as a military training ground. In 1884, the family sold the island to the city, and in 1932 New York City built its first jail there, designed to relieve overcrowding at the Welfare Island jail further south on the East River. The facility, which opened in 1935, consisted of seven cellblocks for 2,600 inmates.[28]

Over the years, changes in criminal justice policy and crime trends led to increases in the population at Rikers. In 1971, President Richard Nixon declared that "America's public enemy No. 1 in the United States is drug abuse. To fight and defeat this enemy, it is necessary to wage a new, all-out offensive."[29] New York State's Rockefeller Drug Laws, enacted in 1973, increased penalties for the sale and possession of "narcotic" drugs.[30] As a result, arrests and incarceration for heroin use and later crack cocaine use and sales led to dramatic increases in the number of people jailed at Rikers Island.

In 1979, in a first attempt to end the city's presence on the island, city officials proposed leasing the island to the state for $200 million a year; the plan was to use the money to build eight smaller jails in the boroughs. The state would also spend $100 million to upgrade Rikers. A city report called the *Rikers Island Project Working Document* observed that the jails on Rikers were "in a decrepit condition which creates a potentially dangerous environment for both staff and inmates."[31] While some city officials supported the plan, others, including community groups and the Correction Officers' Benevolent Association (the union representing correction officers), opposed the plan, the latter because they worried about its impact on public safety or their members' interests. By 1981, this opposition led Mayor Ed Koch to quietly drop the idea, leaving Rikers in place.[32]

More than twenty-five years later, Martin Horn, Mayor Michael Bloomberg's commissioner of the Department of Correction, again called for closing Rikers in 2006 because of the city's inability to improve conditions there or make the jail safe. He proposed a new 1,700-bed jail in Brooklyn. At first, some reformers supported the proposal, but then a fierce "not-in-my-backyard" grassroots opposition mobilized to defeat it, rejecting the idea of new jails in their neighborhoods. "I was buzz-sawed," Horn said. A decade later, reflecting on this experience, Horn told a *New York Times* reporter that closing Rikers "can be done physically, it can be done programmatically. But I don't think it's any more politically feasible today than it was then."[33]

Subsequent campaigns to close Rikers continued to face these challenges—community and correction-officer opposition and the reluctance of politicians to allocate the billions of dollars needed to build new jails and close existing facilities. New York City jails continued to serve as a national symbol of failed correctional policies. In her 2016 State of the City speech, City Council Speaker Melissa Mark-Viverito, one of the elected officials actively supporting the campaign to close Rikers, observed, "Rikers Island has come to represent our worst tendencies, and our biggest failures. . . . For too long, Rikers has stood not for more justice, but for revenge. We must explore how we can get the population of

Rikers to be so small that the dream of shutting it down becomes a reality."[34]

By the second decade of the twenty-first century, the political and institutional context that shaped jail policy had changed significantly, presenting new opportunities for rethinking the role of Rikers Island and New York City jails. What were some of these changes? In 1995, 121,412 people were admitted to city jails, mostly at Rikers Island, the highest number ever.[35] By 2019, annual admission had dropped to 34,389 people, a decline of 72 percent from 1995. Using the average daily census rather than annual admissions, this metric shows that at the peak in 1991, 21,674 people were locked up at Rikers; this average daily census had dropped by 80 percent to 4,541 in 2020, the lowest since 1949.[36]

Other trends and political developments set the stage for renewed activism focused on closing Rikers. In 2010, Michelle Alexander published *The New Jim Crow*, a book that both recognized and invigorated a mass movement against incarceration.[37] By tracing the origins of mass incarceration to the history of slavery, Alexander and the activists of Critical Resistance, the Campaign to End the New Jim Crow, All of Us or None, and other movement groups made the fight to end mass incarceration a critical civil rights and social justice battle of the early twenty-first century.

Black Lives Matter is a national movement that began in 2013 and defines its mission as working "inside and outside of the system to heal the past, reimagine the present, and invest in the future of Black lives through policy change, investment in our communities, and a commitment to arts and culture"; it also works to confront police violence against people of color.[38] When a New York City police officer choked Eric Garner to death in 2014, this movement erupted in New York City, highlighting the long history of police killings of Black and Brown people.[39]

Growing evidence and support for the idea that simply locking up more people did not improve public safety or reduce crime focused attention on another question. If jails and prisons are shut, what happens to the people leaving these institutions? As criminal justice reformer and scholar Jeremy Travis had noted, however many people are incarcerated, the vast majority return home, and if their lives and communities have not changed, the cycle of incarceration can begin again.[40]

Activists, politicians, and the public have thus asked, What policies and practices can rehabilitate those damaged by violence, drugs, and incarceration? What changes were needed in the communities to which incarcerated people returned to enable those returning from incarceration to live more stable lives, find housing and health care, rejoin their families and communities, and contribute to society? Their answers to these questions influenced their decisions to support or oppose closing Rikers.

IS CLOSE RIKERS ISLAND A HEALTH CAMPAIGN?

The campaigns to close Rikers are a social justice initiative that seeks to transform New York City's criminal justice system, make improvements in public safety, reduce mass incarceration, and recognize the human rights of those incarcerated. They are also health campaigns. For decades, Rikers Island in particular, the NYC criminal justice system, and jails more generally have been recognized as places that damage health in many ways. Research has shown that jails

- amplify transmission of infectious diseases like tuberculosis, HIV infection, hepatitis C, other sexually transmitted infections, and COVID-19;[41]
- concentrate and aggravate mental health conditions like depression, anxiety, post-traumatic stress, and other forms of serious mental illness;[42]
- perpetuate and aggravate interpersonal, gender-based, family, and correctional officer violence inside the jail and after release;[43] and
- fail to ameliorate the pervasive levels of drug and alcohol use and serious psychiatric illness among those incarcerated.[44]

Moreover, the adverse impact of the policies and practices at Rikers Island and other New York City jails harm most those populations in the worst health such as Blacks and Latinés, young people, drug users, LGBTQI individuals, and people with disabilities. In this way, conditions at Rikers

Island perpetuate and widen the health inequities that characterize New York City. Numerous reports showed that the New York City Department of Correction routinely violated the 1976 US Supreme Court decision in *Estelle v. Gamble*, which determined that ignoring a prisoner's serious medical needs can amount to cruel and unusual punishment. As a result, the department's routine practices amplified the threats to health faced by inmates, their families and communities, and correctional staff, and thus worsened several of New York City's most serious health problems.[45]

Too often, those released from jail encounter problems in finding the health care, drug treatment, mental health services, housing, work, education, or family support they need.[46] Thus, incarceration undermines the post-release health of those who pass through the jail gates—and their families.[47] Transforming the practices, policies, and systems that have made Rikers Island an incubator and amplifier of many of New York City's most serious health problems makes campaigns to achieve these changes a public health priority.

HOW THE CAMPAIGNS TO CLOSE RIKERS HAS INTERACTED WITH OTHER PLAYERS

Since 2010, activists and their organizations have launched a variety of campaigns to shut down the Rikers Island Detention Center. Their activities have used a wide range of strategies and tactics and interacted with the range of allies and opponents described in the first part of this chapter.

Over the years, advocates for closing Rikers organized several alliances, coalitions, and campaigns, listed in table 7.1, that mobilized a variety of partners in New York City and beyond. This plethora of partnerships demonstrates the appeal of closing what *The New York Times* in 2019 called "the most notorious jail in America."[48]

On the one hand, these campaigns show the diffuse energy and momentum cutting across the often siloed activist organizations and interest groups that wanted to make ending mass incarceration, reforming jails, and/or improving public safety political and policy priorities. Constituencies that supported these campaigns included legal defense and civil right groups, the families of those in jail, health professionals, labor unions, and several elected officials. This momentum was a remarkable asset for the campaigns to close Rikers. On the other hand, focusing and directing this energy in the face of powerful opposition proved to be an ongoing obstacle to success.

Within this changing cast of coalitions, supporters of closing Rikers had several differences in opinion, proposed strategies, and values. These differences included the following:

- What principal goal to pursue—to move forcefully and rapidly for the abolition of jails and incarceration as the best strategy for promoting social justice and improving public safety, or to focus on creating smaller, more humane jails for New York City?
- What timetable to follow—one that focuses on rapid closure to end the violence and abuse documented at Rikers, or a more gradual plan that gave time for enlisting community support and building new facilities?
- What mix of strategies to use—those that emphasized winning over the mayor and other elected officials, or more disruptive ones that employed litigation, civil disobedience, and mass demonstrations?

To better understand the interactions between the campaigns and their allies and opponents and the role these differences played, I examine the exchanges between the campaigns and five key players: Mayors Bill de Blasio and Eric Adams, city council leaders, the Correction Officers' Benevolent Association, several civil society groups, and the handful of researchers and academics involved on both sides of the campaign.

Mayors Bill de Blasio and Eric Adams. Multiple stakeholders must approve any big change in municipal policy, or at least not actively oppose it. For a decision as far-reaching as closing the city's main jail, the approval of the mayor was essential. The campaigners wanting to close Rikers made getting both a yes and the follow-up action to turn that yes into reality a top priority first from Mayor Bill de Blasio (2014–2021) and then from his successor, Eric Adams (2022–2025).

TABLE 7.1 Selected Organizations and Coalitions Supporting Closing Rikers Island

NAME OF ORGANIZATION	BRIEF DESCRIPTION	DATES
Campaign to Close Rikers	Led by survivors and family members who've been directly affected by the injustice and conditions at Rikers, and supported by faith leaders, service providers, community organizations, and other allies; sponsors include Freedom Agenda and Urban Justice Center and others.	2016–
Campaign to Shut Down Rikers	A grassroots collective of NYC activists dedicated to the immediate shutdown of Rikers and long-term abolition of jails in NYC.	2014–2016
#Close Rikers Campaign	Katal Center for Health, Equity, and Justice partnered with JustLeadershipUSA to campaign to close Rikers and enact city and state reforms to support this transition.	2015–2017
Freedom Agenda	A member-led project that organizes people and communities affected by incarceration. Seeks to defend the human rights of incarcerated people, divest from systems of punishment, and redistribute resources to people and communities most harmed by mass criminalization and systemic racism. Housed at Urban Justice Center.	2016–
Jails Action Coalition	A coalition of activists including the formerly and currently incarcerated, their family members, and other community members working to promote human rights, dignity, and safety for people in New York City jails.	2011–

TABLE 7.1 (*continued*)

NAME OF ORGANIZATION	BRIEF DESCRIPTION	DATES
JustLeadershipUSA	A national organization that provides training, resources, and access to activists and advocates in the movement to decarcerate the United States. Cofounder of #Close Rikers Campaign with Katal Center.	2014–
Katal Center for Health, Equity, and Justice	Develops intergenerational leadership and organizing capacity to build community-based power and win systemic change for equity, health, and justice. Cofounder of #Close Rikers Campaign with JustLeadershipUSA and later sponsor of ShutRikers Now.	2016–
Lippman Commission	An independent commission appointed by then City Council Speaker Melissa Mark-Viverito to make recommendations for closing Rikers Island. Chaired by former Chief State of New York Judge Jonathan Lippman, its 2021 report proposed strategies and a plan for closing Rikers. In 2023, City Council Speaker Adrienne Adams reappointed the commission to continue to advise the city.	2017–
No New Jails NYC	Formed after Mayor de Blasio launched the formal land-use approval process for the jail expansion plan to build power in communities throughout New York City and with incarcerated people. Envisioned abolition of incarceration in New York City through divesting from police and prisons and investing in community.	2018–2019

(*continued*)

TABLE 7.1 (*continued*)

NAME OF ORGANIZATION	BRIEF DESCRIPTION	DATES
Resist Rikers	Seeks to dismantle the system of mass incarceration, targeting solitary confinement, abuse, and corruption at Rikers Island. Organized a series of demonstrations at the gates of the Rikers jail complex.	2014–
#Shut Rikers	Katal Center's organizing and outreach to continue pressure to close Rikers after #Close Rikers Campaign ended.	2023–

In a 2019 report on the lessons they had learned from the campaign from 2015 to 2017, Katal Center staff observed that "campaign leaders knew that moving Mayor de Blasio and the broader political establishment to the position of closing Rikers would mean making that the only viable option."[49] To achieve that goal, Katal staff had organized a broad base of support, a cross-sectional organizational alliance, and an insider/outsider strategy that including working with officials within the system while simultaneously pressuring government from the outside through protests and media campaigns. The campaign sought to deliver the following messages to the mayor:

- Supporting closing Rikers was good policy and good politics.
- To maintain his base of support among communities of color and white progressives, he had to take a position on this issue.
- Winning reelection in 2017 depended on this base of support, which might go to other candidates if he failed to speak out on Rikers.

Critically, the campaign leaders decided to focus on the question of closing Rikers and to delay raising the question of what came next, which they believed was "largely hypothetical" at this stage.[50] They hoped this strategy would enlist the support of both the abolitionists who wanted to close all jails in the city and reformers who wanted to improve them, making it harder for the mayor to divide the supporters of closure.

In 2017, Mayor de Blasio released the city's *Roadmap to Closing Rikers Island* in ten years. His plan included proposals to reduce the jail population in New York City and make the new jails to replace Rikers safer and fairer.[51] Two years later, after the city council had revised and approved this plan, de Blasio said, "This is about valuing our people, no longer condemning people and sending them on a pathway that only made their lives worse and worse. Today we made history: The era of mass incarceration is over."[52] In their analysis of the campaign, Katal Center staff concluded that their success in getting the mayor to say, "Close Rikers" affirmed the basic organizing rule of focusing relentlessly on the primary target.[53]

While campaigners had succeeded in getting de Blasio to yes, he left office long before he could translate the words into practice. The campaign's interactions with his successor, Eric Adams, were more problematic. In an interview during his 2021 mayoral campaign, Adams told journalist Errol Lewis that he does believe the Rikers Island jail complex should close and be replaced with borough-based jails. "I believe we need to change the ecosystem of our incarceration system," he added.[54]

Three years later, Gabriel Sayegh, a leader of the campaign to close Rikers, wrote an op-ed for *Amsterdam News* titled "Mayors Adams Talks About Closing Rikers While Working to Keep It Open." Sayegh noted that since Adams took office, "he's failed to meet almost all of the closure plan's legal deadlines and process benchmarks."[55]

In 2025, as a candidate for mayor, Zohran Mamdani pledged he would do "everything in my power from the very beginning to follow that law [to close Rikers] and to ensure that we are reducing the jail population," thus ensuring that another mayor would be judged by his success or failure in realizing that commitment.[56]

City Council leaders. Three successive New York City Council Speakers, the leaders of the council, supported the plan to close Rikers and helped to persuade or pressure Mayors de Blasio and Adams to act.

In 2017, in her State of the City speech, Speaker Melissa Mark-Viverito (2014–2017) called for closing Rikers and announced that she was appointing an independent commission, chaired by the former chief judge for New York State, Jonathan Lippman, to advise the city on how to close Rikers.

In a *New York Times* op-ed coauthored with Judge Lippman, Mark-Viverito wrote, "The main obstacle [to closing Rikers] is political. We need to motivate our elected officials and the general public. We need to articulate a simple truth: We are better than this. Rikers Island is an affront to the civic values of New York City. Reforming our jail system and closing Rikers Island is not simply good public policy—it is a moral imperative."[57] In their assessment of the campaign, its activist planners credited the Lippman Commission appointed by the Speaker with their success in getting Mayor de Blasio to agree to support the closure of Rikers. It provided what they called an "insider vehicle" of respected public officials and community and foundation leaders to convince the mayor. Campaigners then used their resources to ensure that the commission used its formal and informal influence to make shutting Rikers a feasible, politically acceptable, and ethical decision for the mayor.[58]

After the city council passed a resolution in 2021 barring the New York City Department of Correction from using Rikers Island as a jail after 2026, another Speaker, Corey Johnson (2018–2022), observed that the resolution to close Rikers Island as a correctional facility by 2026 "shows our deep commitment to moving away from the failed policies of mass incarceration."

In a 2019 speech at John Jay College, Johnson observed, "Going forward, our default response to most arrests should be diversion, treatment, and rehabilitation—not incarceration. We need to increase our investment in alternatives to jail and prison. And importantly, we need to take the money we used to spend on our jails and invest those funds in the communities directly impacted by mass incarceration."[59]

In 2023, six years after Mark-Viverito had created the Lippman Commission, a new Speaker, Adrienne Adams (2023–2025), concerned about the lack of progress in closing Rikers under the new Mayor Eric Adams (no relation), reappointed the commission. She explained that she wanted its members to "bring stakeholders together towards getting the plan to close Rikers back on course and helping ensure it finally closes."[60]

By maintaining pressure on the mayor over many years, New York City Council Speakers helped to keep the issue of closing Rikers on the city's policy agenda. They also worked closely with the activist coalitions to pass a series of legislative acts that helped to advance the goal of reducing the number of people incarcerated at Rikers and initiating the reforms needed to transform the city's correctional system. Table 7.2 lists these laws and their objectives, evidence of the city council's deep engagement in the effort to close the jail—but also its failure to achieve the goal of shuttering Rikers.

Correction Officers' Benevolent Association (COBA). COBA represents twenty thousand active and retired correctional staff members within the New York City jails. After the police union, it is the second-largest trade union for law enforcement in New York City and the largest municipal jail union in the United States.[61] COBA has also been the most formidable opponent of closing the Rikers Island jail. Its priority has been "support without strings" to its members, "no matter their stage of their career or their individual needs."

Labeling correctional officers as "New York's boldest," COBA represents itself as an essential bulwark for public safety and reduced crime and violence. In a radio interview in 2017, COBA's newly elected president, Elias Husamudeen, explained his opposition to closing Rikers and building new community jails. "The guy that shot the 5-year-old, so now you want him next door to the mother, to the father? You want him in the community, the one who raped the old lady? You want him next door?"[62] With these emotional appeals, COBA reinforced community opposition to closing Rikers and served as a focal point for critics of the plan. Its opposition to closing Rikers stemmed in part from its concerns about public safety, but also its reluctance to disrupt a system in which it had long had a powerful voice.[63]

Under its previous president, Norman Seabrook, COBA had been a forceful advocate for protecting correction officers accused of excessive violence

TABLE 7.2 Selected Laws Supporting Closure of Rikers

LAW	SUMMARY
Local Law 192 (2019)	Requires Board of Correction to report on impact of closing Rikers on inmates and requires Mayor's Office of Criminal Justice to report on progress closing jails on Rikers Island.
Local Law 193 (2019)	Establishes a commission to make recommendations on reinvestment in communities impacted by Rikers Island.
Local Law 16 (2021)	Approves transfer of land, buildings, and facilities of Rikers Island to the Department of Citywide Administrative Services by 2027 or earlier for portions not used by Department of Correction.
Local Law 31 (2021)	Aims to transform Rikers Island by ending its use as a jail and replacing it with sustainable green infrastructure. Local Law 31 codified this plan, which was the result of years of community organizing and policy advocacy.
Local Law 42 (2023)	Restricts solitary confinement in city jails and limits use to four hours per day for emergency de-escalation; requires officers to check on inmates every fifteen minutes and write a report explaining why isolation was necessary.
Resolution 504 (2024)	Authorizes the Speaker to commence legal action on behalf of the New York City Council to oppose the Department of Correction's efforts to suspend Local Law 42 of 2024.

against inmates, opposing plans to reduce the size of the jail, as well as advancing the interests of its members, the basic responsibility of any union. Within the city jails, Seabrook often seemed more powerful than the commissioner. "I came to think that my wardens believed Norman was more important to advancing their careers than I was," Martin Horn, the city's correction commissioner from 2003 to 2009, told a *New York Times* reporter.[64]

Seabrook also had close relationships with the mayor. At a union charity fundraiser, Mayor de Blasio told the crowd of seven hundred correction officers and their families, "Norman is a friend. Norman has been a great leader in this town, [and] I want to thank him for all he does."[65] Under its new leadership, COBA continued to have a strong and positive relationship with Mayor Adams. Through these relationships, COBA leaders had private access to decision-makers and opportunities to contest the messages promoted by activist campaigners, a phenomenon that is long a reality in New York City politics.

Another reality was corruption. In 2019, Seabrook was sentenced to five years in prison for taking a $100,000 kickback from a hedge fund in return for investing $20 million of union funds, of which $19 million was ultimately lost. In 2023, a judge released Seabrook after he had served twenty-one months of his sentence, based on Seabrook's claim that he had received a harsher sentence than the businessman he had paid off.[66]

In sum, COBA's determined opposition to closing Rikers was both a real obstacle and a symbol to which elected officials who opposed closure could point when claiming that closing Rikes would threaten public safety.

Civil society groups. Civil society groups played a key role in advancing the campaign. By the time Mayor de Blasio announced his support for closing Rikers in 2017, almost 125 groups has signed on to support this demand.[67] While many were other activist groups, supporters also included legal defense groups (e.g., Legal Aid Society, Brooklyn Defenders Services, Association of Legal Aid Attorneys, Federal Defenders of New York), service providers (Fortune Society, Osborne Association, STEPS to End Family Violence), youth groups (Youth Represent, Brotherhood/Sisterhood Sol, Community Connections for Youth), and health-related groups (New York Academy of Medicine and the New York City chapter of the National Association of Social Workers). These groups demonstrated broad support for the campaign and their members testified before the city council and other bodies and sent letters of support to their elected officials.

The various close Rikers coalitions (shown in table 7.1) depended on these organizations and their members to exert their influence in the political arena, giving the campaign far more power than if it had acted only on behalf of its principal supporters. And for these civil society groups, supporting the campaign enabled the organizations and their members to advocate on behalf of a moral and political goal they strongly supported. They could do this without having to organize the events themselves or jeopardize their tax-exempt status by participating directly in legislative advocacy or lobbying, activities restricted for tax-exempt nonprofit organizations.

Researchers and academics. Criminal justice, public health, medical, and social science experts provided evidence to the campaigns on the legal, ethical, health, and economic consequences of Rikers, the feasibility of alternative plans, and the rationale for closing the jail.

While the campaigns to close Rikers emphasized the importance of having people who had themselves experienced incarceration in their leadership, organizers also recognized the value of having researchers and experts to support their work. At one of its early meetings in 2016, the campaign to close Rikers invited Michael Jacobson, who had served at various times as the commissioner of the city's Departments of Correction and Probation and deputy director of the city's Office of Management and Budget as well as the former president of the Vera Institute of Justice and the executive director of the Institute for State and Local Governance at the City University of New York. His presentation on the jail was data-driven and politically informed. As campaign organizers noted, "precisely because he is not an activist, his remarks had the effect of turning some skeptics in the room into believers that closing Rikers would be possible."[68] Over the following years, experts at the Vera Institute of Justice, the CUNY Institute for State and Local Governance, the Columbia University Justice Lab, the Brennan Center for Justice at New York University, and other research centers provided high-level and credible evidence on the costs and consequences of Rikers Island to the campaign, the Lippman Commission, the media, the public, and city officials.

ASSESSMENT OF SUCCESSES AND LIMITS OF THE CLOSE RIKERS CAMPAIGN

Like many of the city's activist campaigns, the multiple initiatives to close Rikers Island met with a mix of successes and failures, making any simple assessment of its record impossible. Through its interactions with a variety of external institutions and actors and its considered choices of strategies and tactics, the close Rikers campaigns achieved significant victories. As of 2025, however, activists had not succeeded in their goal of shutting down the detention center, nor did closure seem on the visible horizon. How can activists judge the success and limitations of these campaigns?

Putting the question of whether Rikers should be shut down directly on New York City's political and policy agenda was the most significant accomplishment of the campaigns. While the city's political establishment has not yet definitively answered that question, the campaigns' ongoing mobilizations, media coverage, and supportive public officials have kept the issue in the public eye for more than a decade. By linking a specific policy question to the broader national debates on mass incarceration, effective strategies for protecting public safety, and ending racial inequities in applying criminal justice policies, campaigners have maintained public and media attention on Rikers.

Second, the campaigns organized several powerful coalitions and alliances that helped to keep policymakers' attention on the issue. The experienced activists who led these coalitions, including individuals who had themselves experienced incarceration, brought together activists, families of the incarcerated, civil society groups, sympathetic politicians, and others to focus their attention on the issue and mobilize their support at critical moments. By assisting a variety of civil society groups to provide ongoing support for shutting Rikers, the campaigns augmented their own limited power.

The May 2025 decision by a federal judge to put the jail temporarily in federal receivership is another indicator of the campaign's success in forcing action (but not achieving resolution). In her ruling on the takeover, Laura Taylor Swain, a judge in the Southern District of New York, wrote,

> Nine years have passed since the parties first agreed that the perilous conditions in the Rikers Island jails were unconstitutional; that the level of unconstitutional danger has not improved for the people who live and

> work in the jails is both alarming and unacceptable. . . . The city has demonstrated in virtually every court area that neither court orders nor the monitors interventions are sufficient to push the Department of Correction towards compliance.[69]

Third, the campaigns enlisted and maintained the support of a wide variety of city and state elected officials and agency staff. This success prevented the government from speaking in a unified voice in favor of keeping Rikers open. In other campaigns, the unified opposition of government (e.g., to defunding the police) often limited the capacity of activists to maintain public attention on issues or to achieve significant victories.

Closing a major public institution is always a challenge since most have multiple constituencies who benefit from the status quo. In the case of Rikers, the intense national and local political debate on criminal justice further complicated any effort to begin transformative changes in New York City's approach to public safety. Moreover, the backlash against reform, symbolized and stoked by the reelection of Donald Trump in 2024, created a much more hostile national climate for any justice-oriented transformation of criminal justice policies.

Of concern here, however, is how the decisions that campaigners made (or failed to make) influenced the outcome. Three shortcomings seem important. First, campaigners were unable to achieve consensus on what comes after they succeed in closing Rikers. One bloc proposed moving as quickly as possible to the abolition of jails and incarceration in New York City, believing that the nation's incarceration policies were so tainted by their origins in slavery and their continuing practice of racism that no reforms, only transformation, could solve that problem. Another bloc, more pragmatic but in the view of their opponents less principled, believed that building replacement jails was a reasonable interim step to getting to yes on closing Rikers, a view supported by some residents of over-policed communities of color.

Th #CLOSErikers campaign proposed focusing first on closing Rikers, deferring the question of what comes next until after that decision had been made. In practice, this seemingly reasonable approach did not quell the debates. Whether some other resolution was possible is unknown, of course, but the failure to have a unified plan for what comes next handicapped the campaign's ability to move forward.

Communities understandably want assurances that any new criminal justice policies will protect their safety. Their concerns on this issue, motivated both by prior experiences and reasonable fears and fanned by racist, right-wing propaganda, made it easier for elected officials to oppose closing Rikers and harder for activists to win unified community support.

Second, while the activist campaigns succeeded in putting closing Rikers on the city's policy agenda, they were unable to muster sufficient power to overcome the opposition of entrenched interests, players in what Newfield and Du Brul in 1981 called "the permanent government," which they said really ruled New York.[70] The reluctance of mayors beholden to powerful law enforcement unions and politicians who represented conservative neighborhoods, the concealed power of COBA, and the political influence of civil society and political groups from communities where residents insisted that no jail would be built in their backyards blocked continued progress on closing Rikers.

In sum, close Rikers campaigners succeed neither in constructing a detailed, compelling picture of viable effective alternatives, nor in communicating that vision to the broader public. These limitations contributed to their inability to achieve their primary goal as of 2025. Whether future changes in the national or political environment will enable the city to close Rikers and further reduce its reliance on mass incarceration remains to be seen.

What does seem clear is that even modest changes in jail policy and practices can save lives, shrink the number of incarcerated people, and reduce the harm of the status quo. By monitoring the impact of these incremental changes and identifying windows of opportunity for accelerating them, activists can leverage their limited victories to support more transformative changes.

SOME PRINCIPLES FOR INTERACTING WITH ALLIES AND FOES

The various iterations of activist campaigns to close Rikers interacted with dozens of external organizations, compiling a sprawling body of evidence on what kinds of interactions work or do not work to move toward campaign goals. The previous campaign profiles in this book provide additional insights into interactions with other key policy actors. My assessment of these cumulative experiences leads me to suggest five basic lessons for more effective transactions between activist health campaigns and external organizations.

EFFECTIVE CAMPAIGNS DEFINE SHORT- AND LONG-TERM GOALS FOR EACH OF THEIR EXTERNAL ALLIES OR OPPONENTS AS THEY PLAN THEIR STRATEGIES AND TACTICS

The priority of the campaigns to close Rikers, for example, was to persuade the mayor to announce that he supported closing Rikers Island jails. Campaigners used their interactions with successive New York City Council Speakers and with civil society groups to achieve that goal. Their next goal was to develop an implementation plan and timetable for the closure. They achieved these objectives (but not yet their ultimate aim of shutting the jail) by focusing their activities on these outcomes.

Most campaigns have dynamic interactions with a changing set of actors. Thus, articulating in advance the relationships among the key actors and the sequence of steps needed in New York City's political and governance processes to move this plan forward can help activist organizations move from a reactive to a more intentional mode. Of course, circumstances may change, and their plan may need to be modified, but with no road map, as the cliché goes, any road seems to take you where you are going.

EFFECTIVE CAMPAIGNS ENGAGE WITH ENDURING GOVERNMENT PARTNERS WHO CAN SERVE AS RELIABLE ALLIES

Long-term legislative partners can assist campaigns to advance their legislative priorities, anticipate political changes, and frame their proposals to adapt to changing circumstances. Richard Gottfried, the chair of the New York State Assembly's Health Committee from 1987 until he retired in 2022, played this role for campaigns to enact universal health care in New York State.[71] During his long tenure, *The New York Times* observed, New York "lurched to the left and embraced many of the policies [Gottfried] had long supported."[72]

Between 1992, when Gottfried first introduced a single-payer health-care bill to the New York State Assembly, and 2018, when that body (but not the Senate) first passed the bill, national campaigns for universal health care and the Affordable Care Act changed the opportunities for activism around universal health care. Gottfried's commitment to universal care, his deep understanding of the issue, and his ongoing relationships with other legislators helped campaigners to move their cause forward.

Similarly, the campaigns to close Rikers, and its predecessor campaigns in the area of criminal justice reform, worked closely with New York State Assembly Member Jeffrion Aubry, who represented Black and immigrant communities in Queens. In 1997, Aubry introduced legislation to repeal the Rockefeller Drug Laws, a goal he pursued until partial success was achieved in 2009. Subsequently, Aubry championed ending the practice of treating juveniles as adults, expanding alternatives to incarceration, and developing stronger and better-funded reentry programs, all measures designed to reduce the number of people incarcerated on Rikers Island and thus to make it easier to close the facilities.

As Gabriel Sayegh, a close Rikers campaign leader observed, Aubry "emerged from [and] remained rooted in the community, and stayed in the fight for justice for the long haul, even against daunting odds and when his party wasn't with him. New York is better—and the national movement to end mass incarceration stronger—because of his work."[73] Long-term advocates like Gottfried, Aubry, and others have helped activists negotiate the legislative maze, plan strategy, and seize emerging opportunities. Finding such an ally adds an invaluable asset to a campaign's toolbox.

EFFECTIVE CAMPAIGNS SEIZE WINDOWS OF OPPORTUNITY TO ESTABLISH NEW PARTNERSHIPS OR CONFRONT NEW OPPONENTS

The political scientist John Kingdon hypothesized that when policy ideas, public opinion, and political leadership align, windows of opportunity for meaningful policy change open. He wrote that when "a problem is recognized, a solution is available, and the political climate happens to be right, all at the same moment," those seeking change can make significant advances.[74] By establishing processes to identify such openings, campaign planners can find opportunities to promote existing policy goals more forcefully, escalate their activities, find new partners, or challenge opponents more vigorously.

After David Dinkins lost his 1993 mayoral reelection bid to Rudy Giuliani, the leaders of WE ACT for Environmental Justice recognized they had a narrow window to reach a settlement of the lawsuit they and the Natural Resources Defense Council had filed against a mayor who had often been an ally of their efforts to close the sewage treatment plant in Harlem or make it safer. Just hours before the inauguration of a mayor anticipated to be an opponent, Rudy Giuliani, WE ACT and NRDC reached a settlement with the city. The two plaintiff groups were designated to enforce the consent decree, giving WE ACT an ongoing voice in decisions about the plant. The agreement also provided $1.1 million to establish the North River Fund, with the public funds to be used to tackle environmental and health issues in West Harlem.[75] By being ready to take advantage of the political calendar, WE ACT won an important victory.

In 2015, Kalief Browder, a young man who had spent almost three years at Rikers and eight hundred days in solitary confinement for allegedly stealing a backpack, a crime the city later admitted he did not commit, killed himself after several bouts of depression. "Before I went to jail, I didn't know about a lot of stuff, and, now that I'm aware, I'm paranoid. I feel like I was robbed of my happiness," Browder told a reporter.[76]

His suicide presented the campaign to close Rikers with a grim opportunity to use this tragedy to make a more compelling case for closing the jail. The campaign planners later wrote that "Kalief's story and his death laid bare the absolute scandal of Rikers Island and a broken justice system. Shortly after his death, activists in New York City, including Akeem Browder, Kalief's brother, launched a new effort, the Campaign to Shut Down Rikers, using direct action and protest to call for the facility's closure."[77] By being ready to publicize the inevitable calamities that activists confront, campaign planners can enlist new allies and further shame their opponents (see figure 7.2).

EFFECTIVE CAMPAIGNS CREATE ALLIANCES TO MOBILIZE CONSTITUENCIES THAT CAN BUILD THE POWER TO ACHIEVE THEIR GOALS

Each of the profiled campaigns created alliances or coalitions that could bring together diverse constituencies that supported their work. The Young Lords worked closely with the Health Revolutionary Unity Movement (HRUM), an organization of health workers, and a variety of community organizations to make Lincoln Hospital more responsive to the South Bronx communities it served. HRUM and the Young Lords also worked at Gouverneur, Morrisania, Fordham, and Greenpoint Hospitals, each a part of New York City's public hospital system. By bringing together the voices of health-care workers and patients, the Young Lords built a more powerful force for change. For the next twenty years, these alliances, sometimes working with more established unions, sometimes not, resisted the budget cuts, layoffs, and threats to close the city's public hospitals triggered by the city's 1975 fiscal crisis. This political force has continued to play a key role in defending and maintaining public support for the city's public hospitals.

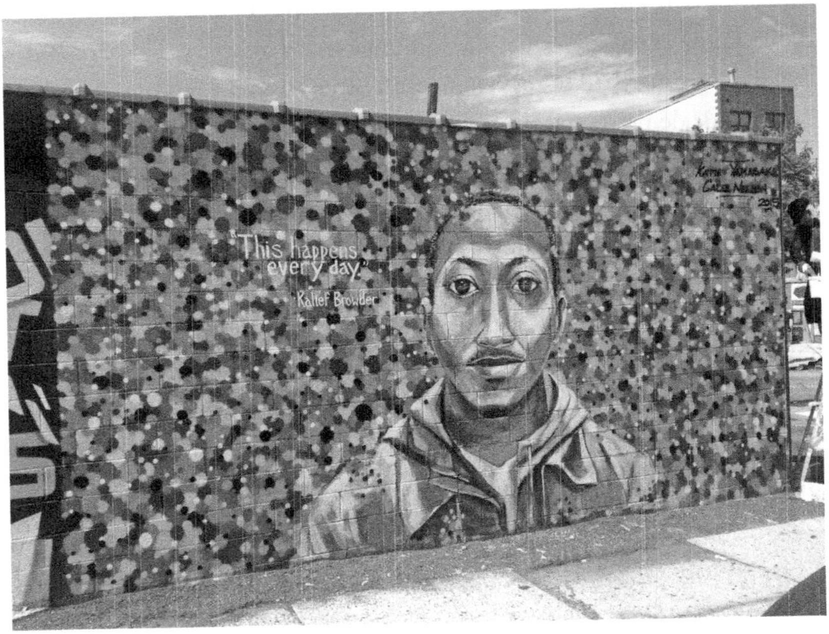

FIGURE 7.2 A mural by Caleb Neelon and Katie Yamasaki commemorates Kalief Browder, an African American youth from the Bronx who was held at the Rikers Island jail complex, without trial, between 2010 and 2013 for allegedly stealing a backpack containing valuables. During his time in jail, Browder was kept in solitary confinement for eight hundred days. He committed suicide in 2015 at the age of twenty-two. His story and the advocacy of his brother contributed to the movement to close Rikers.

Source: Caleb Neelon and Katie Yamasaki. https://www.calebneelon.com/world

MRNY allied with New York Communities for Change, Service Employees International Union, and others to support Fight for $15, a campaign profiled in the next chapter that advocated for increased wages for fast-food and other low-wage workers. ACT UP created numerous coalitions with the Women's Health Action and Mobilization and other feminists to challenge the Catholic Church's efforts to defeat health policies that supported the sexual and reproductive health rights of women and the human rights of LGBTQI individuals. In each of these cases, the lead organization's ongoing relationship with one or more external organizations served to advance the campaign's policy goals.

EFFECTIVE CAMPAIGNS CREATE SPACES WHERE THEY CAN SAFELY NEGOTIATE OR DEBATE WITH POTENTIAL ALLIES AND OPPONENTS

Developing relationships with outside organizations, especially when the activist group and the partner are in different systems and respond to different political forces, can facilitate ongoing negotiations and the ability to compromise. Several of the profiled campaigns created such spaces: The private meetings between ACT UP's Treatment Committee, themselves experts in the science of clinical trials, and the scientists at Burroughs Welcome or the FDA became places to have those discussions. For the campaigns to close Rikers, the deliberations of the Lippman Commission, where both activists, community leaders, and city officials were active participants, also served that purpose. By making the creation of such spaces an explicit goal, and creating them before significant conflicts arise, activists and their partners can be ready to work out the conflicts that will inevitably arise—or agree to disagree while continuing to talk about other issues of mutual interest.

* * *

Organizing effective activist campaigns is both an art and a science. No playbook can tell activists what to do when in a specific situation; that requires the application of their wisdom and experience to the circumstances in which their campaign is unfolding. But the cumulative evidence of many campaigns suggests that groups that follow these principles are more likely to achieve a greater share of their goals than those that do not.

Each suggestion requires longer-term planning than most campaigns have been able to carry out. Activist campaigns in New York City and elsewhere usually make their priority reacting to the unfolding events and political circumstances that seem relevant to their immediate policy goals, an understandable response to often rapidly changing political landscapes. But by designating time, people, and spaces for this planning process, activist organizations can move from reacting to these events to anticipating them and responding in ways that maximize their chances of achieving their political objectives.

8

HOW ACTIVIST CAMPAIGNS INTERACT WITH LOCAL, NATIONAL, AND GLOBAL MOVEMENTS

Fight for $15, the local, national, and global campaign to raise the pay of low-wage workers, was launched in New York in 2012. Sponsored by community organizations and the Service Employees International Union (SEIU), the national union representing low-wage workers in service industries such as health care, home care, cleaning, and public service, Fight for $15 organized fast-food workers in a variety of corporate chains. By 2015, Fight for $15 had mobilized what its organizers called "the largest low-wage protest in U.S. history," attended by more than 60,000 people in 200 cities.[1] Six years later, according to a study by the National Employment Law Project, Fight for $15 and its offshoots had won $150 billion in raises for a total of 26 million workers across the United States, including nearly 12 million workers of color and 18 million women.[2]

This chapter describes how the Fight for $15 campaign linked with other local, national, and global activist campaigns and social movements. These organized mobilizations constitute another constituency that organizers rely on, like their core supporters, activist allies, government partners, and external organizations considered in previous chapters. The questions I look to answer include the following:

1. Why and how have New York City health activist campaigns interacted with local, national, and global activist campaigns and social movements?
2. What are the risks and benefits of such interactions?
3. What steps can activist campaigns take to maximize these benefits and minimize the perils?

PROFILE: FIGHT FOR $15

The Fight for $15 campaign, which became a national and international movement to improve the lives of low-wage workers, got off the ground in September 2012 at a meeting at the United Federation of Teachers office in Downtown Manhattan.[3] That evening, forty fast-food workers met with an organizer for SEIU, one of the largest, most active unions in New York City. For the past several months, New York Communities for Change (NYCC) had been sending organizers door-to-door to identify issues that could mobilize political action in the city's low-income communities. NYCC is a membership organization that works to build community power to improve the lives of its members and their communities. Through their canvassing, the organizers learned that many residents in these neighborhoods worked in the fast-food industry and that the $7.25 hourly minimum wage made it impossible for them to earn enough to support their families.[4]

At the meeting, the fast-food workers described not only low wages, irregular work hours, and wage theft, but also pervasive disrespect from their employers. Almost every worker displayed a burn or scar they had suffered in their workplaces. From this and other such discussions came the plan for Fight for $15, a group that helped to instigate the national movement across industries and states to raise the minimum wage to $15 an hour.

Participants at the first New York City meeting recruited coworkers and friends for a second meeting in October, which attracted 80 people. In

November 2012, two hundred fast-food workers from various New York City fast-food chains, including Burger King, Wendy's, Taco Bell, Kentucky Fried Chicken, Domino's Pizza, and McDonald's, walked off their jobs to attend a demonstration. Chanting "$15 and a union," they called for better working conditions and more respect in their workplaces. The demonstration attracted coverage in *The New York Times* and won support from several candidates in the upcoming 2013 New York City mayoral election. Mary Kay Henry, the president of SEIU, observed that the fast-food companies could afford to pay their employees more. "People who work for the richest corporations in America," she said, "should be able to afford at least the basic necessities to support their families."[5]

How did the organizers decide on $15 an hour? They debated between $10 and $15, Alvin Major, a Fight for $15 organizer and a father of four who worked three part-time jobs at different KFC restaurants, explained to Steven Greenhouse, a labor journalist. "Some people at the meeting said $15, and some believed that was crazy, you would never get $15. Some people were even saying $20, some $25. Then people said $10, but that was too little. It came back to $15. That's enough to survive on. Fifteen is a great number."[6]

The workers recognized that $15 an hour would more than double their pay and help them to afford basic necessities. They also believed that the hugely ambitious goal would inspire and excite many fast-food workers, enabling them to win new support.

Over the years, many have debated what constitutes a living wage. Generally, it is defined as a wage that enables a worker's household to afford adequate shelter, food, and other necessities and to earn enough income to avoid falling into poverty.[7] In recent years, activists and scholars have noted that while $15 an hour is much better than $7.25, by 2020, it was no longer a wage that enabled people to escape poverty or adequately support their families,[8] leading some campaigners to call for setting $20, $25, or more as the minimum hourly standard.

Over the next dozen years, Fight for $15 and several other established and newly formed New York groups achieved an impressive list of legislative and policy accomplishments. How did these groups extend the victories of Fight for $15, and what accounts for this list of successes? The surge in national union organizing that began after the fiscal crisis of 2008, growing attention among policymakers, the media, and the public about persistent and increasing income inequality, and the successful mobilization of thousands of fast-food workers in communities throughout New York City and beyond contributed to these successes. In New York, both the city and state legislatures and the mayor and governor passed laws and issued executive orders that raised the minimum wage for various groups of low-wage workers.

SELECTED ACCOMPLISHMENTS OF FIGHT FOR $15 AND ITS ALLIES AND SUCCESSORS IN NEW YORK, 2013–2025

- 2013: Based on a study by Fast Food Forward (a national organization supported by SEIU that later changed its name to Fight for $15), the New York State attorney general began an investigation of wage theft by fast-food chains, an investigation that eventually led to stiff fines and a jail sentence for one Papa John's franchise owner.[9]
- 2014: New York City Mayor Bill de Blasio signed an executive order requiring employers receiving financial assistance of more than $1 million a year from the city to pay no less than the minimum wage.
- 2015: New York City and State Wage Boards approved a $15 minimum wage for fast-food workers.
- 2015: Governor Andrew Cuomo extended the $15 hourly wage to other sectors of the economy.
- 2017: The New York City Council approved and the mayor signed the Fair Workweek Law, which required employers to provide workers with at least two weeks' advance notice of work schedules and extra compensation if workers were required to stay beyond regular hours to open and close the store. It also provided workers with the option of making voluntary paycheck-deduction contributions to a not-for-profit nonunion

organization of their choice. The National Restaurant Association challenged this requirement in court but lost in 2019.[10] The law recognized the long-term complaints of fast-food workers that unpredictable scheduling and last-minutes changes in shifts make it impossible for many workers to arrange for childcare, attend college, schedule second or third jobs, or pay their monthly bills.[11]

- 2021: New York City Council approved and the mayor signed the Just Cause Termination law that prohibits firing workers or reducing hours by 15 percent or more absent just cause, defined as unsatisfactory job performance or misconduct—or a "bona fide economic reason."
- 2023: Seeking to extend minimum-wage laws to food-delivery workers employed at DoorDash, Uber Eats, and Grubhub, the city's Department of Consumer and Worker Protection set a wage of $17.96 per hour, a significant increase from the average $7.09 per hour that these workers were making at the time. In response to a lawsuit challenging the rule, a federal judge temporarily stayed implementation, leaving the ultimate outcome in doubt.[12] Later in 2023, the New York State Supreme Court lifted the stay, leading to implementation of the higher wage.

FIGHT FOR $15 ALLIES WITH MOVEMENTS TO GO NATIONAL

Another cause of Fight for $15's success was its capacity to join or inspire similar efforts in cities and states around the country, making the campaign a national phenomenon rather than only a local one. Contributing to the campaign's national spread were its connections to several nationwide social movements. These linkages to the early work of Fast Food Forward highlighted the moral and social justice dimensions of the struggle, helped to promote big ideas that challenged the market-oriented status quo, and offered key constituencies—low-wage workers, Black, Latiné, and other immigrant workers, women, and young people—a choice of identity-based routes into activism.

Trump's 2024 presidential election win and the right-wing agenda of curtailing labor rights threatened this progress in raising the minimum wage. Even in 2024, however, voters in two states that Trump won voted to approve raises in the minimum wage, joining the thirty states and sixty-three localities that had previously approved such measures.[13] A 2024 national opinion poll showed that 86 percent of likely voters (89 percent of Democrats, 86 percent of independents, and 84 percent of Republicans) agreed that $7.25 was too low a minimum wage, and 64 percent (85 percent of Democrats, 65 percent of independents, and 45 percent of Republicans) favored a minimum wage of $17 an hour.[14] Most voters, it seemed, still supported higher pay for low-wage workers.

Labor Movement. Several movements interacted with the Fight for $15 campaigns that were springing up around the country, each opening distinct pathways for expanding the struggle. The labor movement provided strong support for Fight for $15. SEIU paid the salaries of the New York Communities for Change staff who organized the first campaign activities in Brooklyn and later helped to support Fight for $15 organizing in other cities. Over the next decade, low-wage workers in other companies and sectors in New York City and elsewhere also organized to raise their wages to $15 an hour or more. This included workers at Starbucks,[15] Chipotle, a national restaurant chain with a record of anti-union activity,[16] warehouse workers at Amazon, supported by the Teamsters Union,[17] and graduate students at several New York universities, also demanding at least $15 an hour.[18] This surge of labor organizing publicized and normalized the fast-food workers' campaign and helped to make their demands a national social justice issue.

Another labor movement contribution came from the worker centers that had sprung up around the country. By 2019, 220 such centers operated around the country, with 26 in New York City alone.[19] They represented a new generation of institutions that seek to integrate low-wage workers into the labor movement by offering these workers new opportunities to express their collective voice and take collective action.[20] Some focused on a particular job category—day laborers, for example—while others organized in a particular geographic community, such as Flushing, Queens.

Many worker centers reached out to immigrant workers and to sectors often ignored by traditional unions such as domestic workers or fast-food workers. Their support for Fight for $15 enabled the campaign to reach workers and communities less served by traditional labor unions, including the women and immigrant communities where worker centers often organized, places that were also home to many fast-food workers.[21]

While Fight for $15's name signaled their primary demand, their affiliations with the many strands of the wider labor movement showed their commitment to historic union values: the insistence that all workers deserved to be treated with dignity and respect and that all workers should have safe working conditions, decent benefits, and health and safety protections. And through their day-to-day battles, Fight for $15 activists communicated these values to their coworkers. "Some people are too scared to say anything," Arisleyda Tapia, a McDonald's worker in Upper Manhattan who had been fired for participating in a protest on her own time and then reinstated, told a reporter in 2014. "It's not that everybody working there supports the union," she said. "But they all want us to keep fighting. They're afraid to fight themselves, but they know they'll benefit when we win."[22]

For Lizett Aguilar, a Los Angeles McDonald's worker, the biggest impact of the campaign was not her pay increase, but the fact that "Fight for $15 has helped me lose my fear about speaking out against injustice."[23] Aguilar later led marches and lobbied legislators to win passage of California's Assembly Bill 257, which created sectoral bargaining for more than 550,000 California fast-food workers to help them win pay increases and reduce wage theft and sexual harassment. In another example of victories in one place inspiring similar efforts elsewhere, New York and several other cities and states passed similar bills.

Black Lives Matter. The Black Lives Matter (BLM) movement also helped to reinforce and build support for the Fight for $15 campaign. By integrating the fight against racism with the fight for improved pay and working conditions for low-wage workers—most fast-food workers in New York are Black or Latiné—BLM emphasized the shared values and goals of the movements for labor rights and racial justice. In 2017, on the forty-ninth anniversary of Martin Luther King Jr.'s assassination, BLM and Fight for $15 sponsored "Fight Racism, Raise Pay" protests in two dozen cities, including Atlanta, Milwaukee, Memphis, Chicago, Boston, Denver, and Las Vegas. A Fight for $15 organizer of these actions explained, "What we both realize is we're stronger when we operate together. . . . When MLK was assassinated, he was talking to workers who were dealing with union-busting, unfair wages. The bottom line is that every day, workers of color across the country face deep-seated racism that would seem to be out of Dr. King's era, but sadly it's still happening today."[24]

Occupy Wall Street. Another multilevel movement, Occupy Wall Street, played an important role in setting the stage for the subsequent Fight for $15 campaigns. Occupy Wall Street had attracted global attention when protestors against growing income inequality in the United States exacerbated by the 2008 Great Recession occupied Zuccotti Park in New York City's Financial District.[25] In the fifty-nine days the occupiers stayed in the park before their arrest, they and their supporters used social media, mass media, and street demonstrations to promote their message—"We are the 99 percent," in contrast to the wealthiest 1 percent, who claimed the right to make decisions for everyone else. That slogan soon spread around the world: Occupy organizers claimed that on October 15, 2011, demonstrations were planned in 951 cities across 82 countries in Europe, North America, Latin America, Asia, and Africa.[26]

Some critics on the left and right claimed that Occupy Wall Street disappeared without a trace, but in its 2021 assessment of the tenth anniversary of the initial action, *Time* magazine observed,

> There's a big problem with that conclusion, however: Occupy's messaging just won't go away. It permeates political discourse about the global economy. It has cemented notions of economic inequality squarely in D.C. policy debates. Ideas that were thought to be too socialist since the demise of the Eastern Bloc—class struggle, wealth distribution across social strata, or even flaws in the capitalist system—were suddenly aired loudly and frequently for the first time since the Great Depression.[27]

Fight for $15 benefited from the legacy of Occupy Wall Street in several ways. The campaign insisted that it was not fair that minimum wages did not allow workers to support themselves and their families while fast-food executives earned millions, a message that resonated with not only fast-food workers but also a growing proportion of the public. Occupy demonstrated that peaceful but disruptive protests could spread rapidly and change public opinion, thus reinforcing fast-food workers' determination to use similar tactics.

In some ways, Fight for $15 managed to turn Occupy's abstract call to end inequality into a specific demand that could change the lives of low-income workers and mobilize them for political action.[28] In this way, the campaign offered Occupy activists a new path to pursue.

#MeToo. The national and international movement fighting to end sexual harassment and sexual abuse, known by its online handle #MeToo, offered another way to align several battles. Like other low-wage workers, especially those in the service sector, food-service workers reported high levels of sexual harassment from both customers and managers.[29] A study found that 42 percent of women in the fast-food industry who reported experiencing sexual harassment put up with it over fears of losing their jobs.[30]

In a 2018 Fight for $15 strike in ten cities, many strikers carried banners that read, "#MeToo McDonald's!" In Chicago and elsewhere, women wore tape over their mouths with the words "#Me Too."[31] By emphasizing the connections among the fights for respectful treatment of women with the struggles for fair pay, safe working conditions, and recognition of workers' family responsibilities, #MeToo and Fight for $15 acknowledged that the campaigns recognized that fast-food workers joined as workers and as women, two intersecting identities that shaped their experience on and off the job.

Through these movements and additional support from the immigrant rights, food justice, faith-based, and antipoverty movements,[32] Fight for $15 campaigns in New York City and elsewhere won media coverage, widespread public support, and ongoing connections to networks of activists, activist organizations, and supportive public officials around the country. Fight for $15 also showed that organizing campaigns could start in one or two communities, spread to others, then become a national political force. The national movements that supported higher wages became the megaphones that enabled local campaigns to amplify their impact.

FIGHT FOR $15 SUCCESSES

How did the Fight for $15 campaign differ from previous efforts to organize low-wage workers? Several characteristics distinguish it from more traditional labor activism. First, the group did not focus its organizing at a single workplace or brand. The 2012 demonstration in New York City included workers from multiple fast-food chains. This sectoral or industry-wide approach to organizing recognized the challenges of organizing shop by shop in small workplaces, especially when the parent multinational dedicated significant resources to resisting unionization, as did McDonald's, Chipotle, Starbucks, and other chains. Organizers also used neighborhood-based outreach, recognizing that fast-food workers knew neighbors and family members who also worked in the sector, providing networks and connections for education and support outside the specific workplace. These approaches demonstrated the impact and power of organizing workers to demand policy changes at the city, state, and national levels as well as organizing at specific workplaces.

Second, Fight for $15 encompassed both unions and other organizations. SEIU provided crucial financial, logistical, and media support, but so did groups like New York Communities for Change, the community partner for the first Brooklyn campaign. Make the Road New York, profiled in chapter 2, organized immigrant workers and communities to support the $15 wage, as did numerous churches and faith-based groups (see figure 8.1).

New York's Catholic Cardinal Timothy Dolan, for example, gave his support to the campaign, saying, "the status quo is not working," and in 2016 calling the then state minimum hourly wage of $9 per hour "too low." Dolan wrote in *The New York Daily News* that "we can all agree that a minimum wage is valuable protection for laborers, and that the current level is too low. We can also find common ground in recalling that our

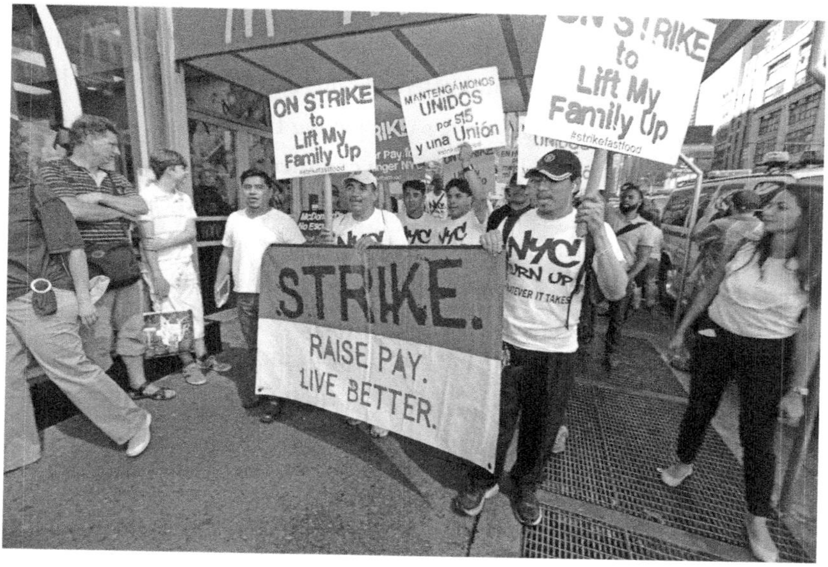

FIGURE 8.1 In 2014, fast-food workers and their supporters march along Eighth Avenue calling for an increase to the minimum wage. Some blocked traffic on the street, leading to several arrests by NYPD.

Source: Shutterstock. https://www.shutterstock.com/image-photo/new-york-city-september-4-2014-215115700

workers not only deserve a living wage, but also benefits to help with health insurance, pensions, sick leave, and vacation."[33]

Each partner brought specific skills and networks, expanding the campaign's breadth and depth. New groups emerged, like Fast Food Justice, which sought to enroll individual fast-food workers and become their public voice across chains. The New York chapter of the Restaurant Opportunity Center (ROC), founded in 2001 by restaurant workers employed in the World Trade Center who had survived 9/11, strived to improve working conditions across the restaurant industry. ROC campaigned for higher minimum wages and better benefits for food-service workers in New York, nationally, and across its nine chapters in other parts of the country. ROC also offers training to food-sector workers, conducts research, and files complaints and lawsuits, illustrating the breadth of services some of these new groups provided.[34] In San Francisco and New York, ROC organized and promoted "high road employers," food establishments that willingly paid living or better wages and offered more adequate benefits.[35] These restaurants showed other businesses that paying living wages and treating workers with respect could contribute to commercial success by retaining skilled workers and attracting customers who supported these values.

Third, Fight for $15 illustrated and advanced the idea of worker centers, the entities that sprang up around New York and elsewhere that made organizing women, people of color, low-wage workers, and others often overlooked by traditional unions their priority. For some union activists and scholars, worker centers represented the best hope for the future of the labor movement and for organizing low-wage, immigrant, women, and people-of-color workers.[36]

In other ways, Fight for $15 used the familiar strategies of the earlier labor movement, especially the traditions of "social unionism," which focus on improving the conditions for all workers, compared to business unionism, which focus on those already members.[37] Like these predecessors, Fight for $15 emphasized dignity and respect, powerful draws to workers and communities so often treated disrespectfully by their employers and managers. By tapping into fast-food workers' desire for respect, Fight for $15 was able to empower participants to become organizers. As Shantel Walker, a Papa John's worker and then a Fight or $15 organizer, explained, "Discrimination happens a lot in the workplace, but customers . . . don't have any idea what's happening behind that counter. They don't see the retaliatory measures. They don't see your hours getting cut and cut. They don't see your boss talking to you like you're worthless. That's why I'm so vocal and adamant with what I do."[38] In this way, Fight for $15 put a face and a story about fast-food workers in front of millions of Americans.

Like previous campaigns, Fight for $15 also enlisted politicians to support their demands for improved pay and working conditions. In 2012, New York City mayoral candidates and other elected officials and candidates for office supported their November demonstration. In 2014, Governor Andrew Cuomo, once a staunch opponent of increased minimum wages, did an about-face and acted to increase the pay of fast-food

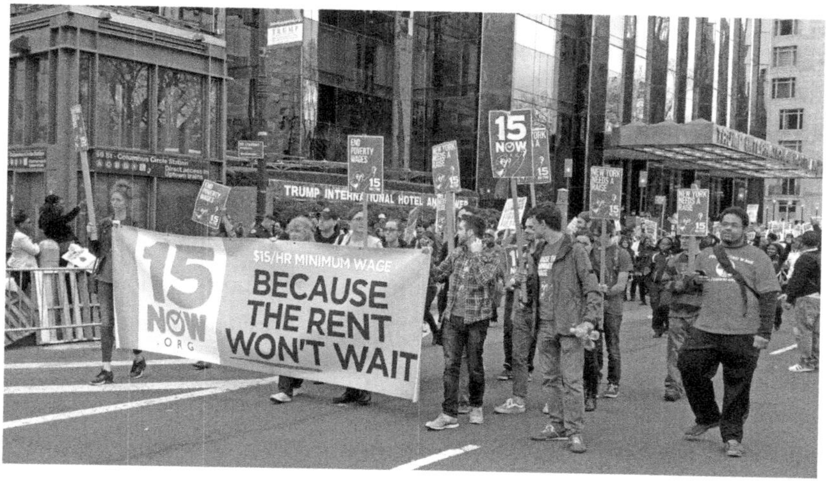
15 NOW
.ORG
$15/HR MINIMUM WAGE
BECAUSE
THE RENT
WON'T WAIT

FIGURE 8.2 A Fight for $15 rally and march in front of Trump International Hotel in New York City to support raising the minimum wage, April 15, 2015.

Source: All-Nite Images, commons.wikimedia.org. https://commons.wikimedia.org/wiki/File:Fight_for_$15_on_4-15_%2816954296607%29.jpg

workers.[39] In 2015, Fight for $15 demonstrated in front of Trump Tower in Midtown Manhattan, showing the contrast between their positions and that of the man who would openly declare his 2016 candidacy at the site two months later (see figure 8.2).

FIGHT FOR $15 LIMITATIONS

Of course, Fight for $15 campaigns also have their limitations. For the most part, these and similar campaigns have failed to organize workers into unions in specific workplaces or companies, a significant defeat and one that failed to reverse the long decline in union membership in New York and the nation. Some activists have come to believe that organizing workers shop by shop in industries like fast food is a Sisyphean task, doomed to failure. Some union leaders believe that only when the number of workers belonging to unions returns to previous levels will workers have the power to win significant concessions. SEIU's Mary Kay Henry told a reporter that minimum wage legislation is great, but only "collective bargaining can set a standard that obviates legislation."[40] However, as Henry also observed in 2014, "the fight for $15 is growing way beyond fast food. It's getting to be what the eight-hour day was in the twentieth century."[41]

By the end of 2025, although millions of workers across the United States had won billions of dollars in higher salaries, no progress had been made at raising the national minimum wage, the most efficient path for improving the pay of all workers. In 2013, President Barack Obama announced support for a $9-an-hour minimum wage, and a year later he called for a raise to $10.10 an hour, still lower than the inflation-adjusted minimum wage of $10.95 needed to avoid poverty in 1968, almost fifty years earlier.[42] In the subsequent twelve years, however, Congress has been unable to reach agreement on raising the minimum wage.

Like other activist campaigns, those organized by fast-food workers and their allies encountered intense opposition from business groups that favored lower wages. In 2025, twenty-one states raised their minimum wage, increases set to help more than 9.2 million workers, many of whom fall below the poverty line.[43] The National Restaurant Association—sometimes called the "other NRA"—opposed every proposal from Fight for $15 and its allies, lobbied vigorously to defeat them at the city, state, and federal levels, and often went to court to seek to overturn them. The NRA also opposed the Affordable Care Act, worker-safety regulations, restrictions on marketing junk food to children, and a variety of public health measures, making it a target for alliances of activists working in other struggles.

In March 2025, President Donald Trump issued an executive order undoing a Biden-era regulation that raised the minimum wage for private-sector workers on federal contracts to $17.75 per hour. That rule had raised the wages of hundreds of thousands of workers and helped ensure government contractors paid workers a decent wage.[44] This action followed the recommendations of Project 2025, the blueprint for the Trump presidency published by the Heritage Foundation and other right-wing groups before the 2024 election.[45]

As part of the 2025 federal budget bill, President Trump—with the support of the NRA—eliminated taxes on tips but opposed any effort to raise the base pay of tipped workers. This led some low-wage workers to support the end of taxes on tips but oppose a raise in base pay in the belief that both changes were not possible. By deploying the classic divide-and-conquer strategy, Republicans and the NRA hoped to defeat any further increases in the minimum wage.[46] At the national level, Project 2025 proposed allowing states to opt out of federal overtime and minimum-wage laws, a move that could jeopardize progress to date.[47]

Other business groups took a slightly different approach. Katherine Wylde, then CEO for the business group Partnership for New York City, emphasized that fast-food franchise owners were small businesses deserving protection from burdensome laws. Speaking of the proposed city law to terminate the licenses of businesses that were repeat offenders of wage laws, she noted, "This is an impact on franchise owners who are mostly small businesspeople and many minorities. Imposing more fines and requirements on them seems to go in the opposite direction of the supposed desire to help recovery [from the pandemic]. It's not the big corporations that get stuck with these fines."[48] While it is true that some fast-food businesses are franchises operated by struggling owners, the national fast-food chains use franchising to shift risk to smaller businesses, hardly a practice to be rewarded.

Many elected officials supported the policy changes proposed by Fight for $15 campaigners, but others depended on the New York National Restaurant Association and other food industry trade associations for campaign contributions and were reluctant to disagree with reliable patrons. Between 2007 and 2021, as overall national NRA spending on politics and lobbying more than doubled, a significant portion went to state associations for their lobbying expenses.[49]

THE ROLE OF MOVEMENTS IN HEALTH CAMPAIGNS

The critical role that other social movements played in advancing the Fight for $15 is not unique to that campaign. Social movements offer activist health campaigns resources, publicity, access to experienced organizers, and the moral appeal of a social justice vision, as illustrated by the following stories.

UNIVERSAL HEALTH CARE

Another example comes from the campaign for universal health care in New York, led by Metro New York Health Care for All (Metro NY), a coalition organized in the early 1990s to advocate for universal health care, and the New York State Nurses Association (NYSNA), the largest union and professional association for registered nurses in New York State, representing more than 42,000 members. Both these organizations had deep roots in other social movements, including the civil rights, AIDS, labor, and women's movements. As an organization founded and staffed by former ACT UP members and as a labor group that represented primarily female workers, Metro New York and NYSNA shared values and goals with the AIDS, labor, and women's movements.

After the defeat of Bill and Hilary Clinton's national health care plan in 1994,[50] Metro NY was created to campaign for universal health care in New York State. Over the years it has participated in and supported several coalitions, including Health Care for All New York, the Campaign for New York Health, Coverage for All, Community Voices for Health System Accountability, Medicaid Matters New York, and New Yorkers for Accessible Health Coverage. Its longtime director, Mark Hannay, had started as an HIV activist with ACT UP New York and Gay Men's Health Crisis, experiences that informed his strategic and tactical thinking and his understanding of the needs of New Yorkers without adequate health care.

While universal health care became its advocacy priority, Metro NY also led or supported campaigns to enact a Consumers Bill of Rights for Medicare Patients; created New York Family Health Plus, a program that expanded access to health care coverage for low-income families; opposed cuts in the New York State Medicaid budget; and supported President Obama's Affordable Care Act.[51] As Hannay explained,

> These efforts include the defense, improvement, and expansion of existing public health and health care programs, strengthened regulation and oversight of the health care industry, advancing health equity, and supporting unionized workers as they seek to maintain and improve with their negotiated health care benefits. Our member-partners support the broad range of policy goals from incremental reforms to Medicare-for-All, and so we understand our work to be not either-or but rather both-and, to advance toward health care for all across New York and the U.S.[52]

By taking on these multiple advocacy efforts, Metro NY shows its members and the public that it is possible to support both incremental and transformative changes, to ameliorate some of the health-care problems patients and community residents face on a daily basis while still advancing solutions based on a commitment to health care for all as a human right. Some health-care activists believe they cannot work on the two levels simultaneously, a belief that Metro NY's actions refuted in practice.

The fights for universal health care also demonstrated both the potential and risks of moving between city, state, and national campaigns and of forging alliances with the coalitions operating at each level. On the one hand, working across levels gave Metro NY and NYSNA more opportunities to keep organizing, even when one level encountered obstacles that stopped progress. It also gave these groups and their leaders a more nuanced understanding of the potential for new partners or new settings for their universal care advocacy.

On the other hand, jumping back and forth across levels forced campaigns to perform a tightrope act that risked confusing their supporters, diverting energy from a promising campaign at one level, and dissipating their impact on key actors. The fragmented US health-care system, the wide variation in care across state and cities, and the separation of health care, mental health, and social service systems compound these difficulties.

At best, success at one level could reinforce accomplishments at other levels. "Passing the New York Health Act, which NYSNA has helped popularize through consistent organizing," explained Judy Gonzalez, a NYSNA leader and an emergency room nurse at Montefiore Hospital, "would be beneficial to all New Yorkers and help propel the movement nationally, along with the other states engaged in the same process."[53]

Health-care activists also worked closely with immigrants' rights groups. In 2023, Metro NY together with Make the Road New York and several other groups supported the Coverage for All Coalition's effort to expand health-care coverage to low-income New Yorkers regardless of their immigration status. When the state assembly failed to vote on the bill, Coverage for All wrote that "It is deeply shameful that Speaker Heastie and his leadership colleagues refused to lead on this issue and gave in to Governor Hochul's antiimmigrant exaggerations about the Coverage for All bill."[54] While some advocacy organizations avoid shaming language, Metro New York did not, perhaps hoping that moral appeals would reach some people more effectively than political ones. "Every day undocumented New Yorkers without health insurance are forced to forego the health care they need and continue to suffer in silence," the coalition's staff wrote. "Speaker Heastie and the Assembly's inaction will continue to put the health and lives of these New Yorkers at risk." By 2025, New York State had not yet passed its universal health care act.

STRATEGIES TO ENLIST MOVEMENTS IN HEALTH CAMPAIGNS

How have local campaigns enlisted other movements in their campaigns? Many planners of activist drives are tempted to invest the bulk of their intelligence and energy in responding to the day-to-day developments in the hurly-burly world of their campaigns. While pragmatically understandable, in my view, this tendency handicaps their success and advantages their opponents. Compared to activists, protectors of the status quo usually have more resources and deeper roots in the political system that enable them to plan and implement long-term strategies for winning. By forging partnerships with social movements, organizers of local health campaigns can benefit from their resources, experience, political power, and wide tactical repertoire. In return, movements gain new supporters, deeper local roots, and the potential for more power—a win-win relationship.

Based on experiences of Fight for $15 and other profiled campaigns, I describe several approaches that organizers have used to enlist other movements in their campaigns.

IDENTIFY MOVEMENTS THAT SHARE VALUES AND GOALS TO IDENTIFY STARTING POINTS FOR COLLABORATION

Strategic planning provides the opportunity for activists to set priorities based on a comprehensive assessment of their current and emerging political landscape. By making the time for this exercise, identifying its members and allies who can complete this mapping, and debating the options identified, activist groups can compensate for the greater resources of their adversaries. Activist groups whose leaders or members are already immersed in social movements have an advantage over organizations with less experienced participants. ACT UP, the Coalition for Abortion Rights and Against Sterilization Abuse, and Make the Road New York are groups whose members synthesized available intelligence on opportunities for partnering with other movements. Less experienced groups may need to find movement elders or leaders of sister groups who can provide similar insights.

Fight for $15 used its shared memberships, ongoing dialogues, and previous partnerships with labor unions and worker centers, Black Lives Matter, #Me Too, and other campaigns to highlight common values and specific policy goals. Their shared activities—planning a demonstration, lobbying in support of a bill, or testifying at legislative hearings—helped to transform organizational relationships into personal friendships, common social networks, and shared values. Together these activities created the foundation for their evolving alliances with these movements.

SEQUENCE OVERTURES TO OTHER MOVEMENTS TO KEEP CAMPAIGNS FOCUSED AND WORKLOADS MANAGEABLE

As activists wander through the candy store of other campaigns, movements, and struggles in their effort to build the power needed to win, it can be tempting to taste every treat, to seek every possible partnership simultaneously. But few activist organizations have the capacity to initiate or pursue more than a few such relationships at a time. Using the results of their strategic assessment, organizers can choose which alliances to pursue first and which to defer to later stages of their campaigns.

However, activist choices that open one door may close another. The first goal of the campaigns to close Rikers (chapter 7) was to get the support of the mayor, so their priority was to make alliances that would convince the mayor to say yes. Their initial success in this goal validated this emphasis. But as noted in that profile, their decision to defer proposing what should follow Rikers' closure, part of an effort to avoid the debate between jail reformers and abolitionists, made the next stage more difficult, an obstacle yet to be resolved. What does seem clear is that activists who make informed choices about priorities after considering their options are more likely to be successful than those who skip this step.

IDENTIFY SPECIFIC ACTIONS THAT TWO OR MORE MOVEMENTS COULD SUPPORT TO BUILD MOMENTUM FOR FURTHER ALLIANCES

The coalitions between Fight for $15 and other movements, or between Metro Care for All and national universal health-care advocates, were forged based on concrete joint actions. Examples include the "#MeToo McDonald's!" banners that Fight for $15 strikers carried in ten cities; the Black Lives Matter and Fight for $15 slogan "Fight Racism, Raise Pay"; union leaders like SEIU's Mary Kay Henry, who made forceful statements in support of Fight for $15 at their rallies; and Metro NY's support for nurses' strikes at various New York hospitals.

Collaborative campaigns such as those between Fight for $15, Make the Road New York, #MeToo, Black Lives Matter, and others provide a very visible manifestation of solidarity. These human and physical representations of shared goals and actions strengthen alliances more than do ideological statements divorced from participants' experiences. Stories, actions, and human relationships build human and emotional connections between supporters of local campaigns and national movements.

CREATE SPACES WHERE ACTIVISTS FROM DIFFERENT MOVEMENTS CAN EXCHANGE IDEAS, DEBATE STRATEGY, AND ANALYZE THEIR EXPERIENCES

Many campaigns operate in silos and rarely have the opportunity to learn from activists from other campaigns. In the mid-twentieth century, movement organizers created schools or institutes to train and educate activists from different parts of the country. The Highlander Research and Education Center, founded in 1932 in Tennessee, trained labor activists from Appalachia and later civil rights activists from throughout the southern United States.[55] In the 1940s, Saul Alinsky's Industrial Areas Foundation trained organizers from around the country to lead campaigns in their neighborhoods, a tradition other groups have since emulated.[56] The Midwest Academy, founded in Chicago in 1972 by Chicago organizer Heather Booth, trains people "in the skills and strategies needed to build powerful organizations and governing majorities that win important victories for their communities and drive forward the movement for justice for all."[57] These centers provide useful models for today's activists to find common ground and forge alliances with other movements and campaigns.

Since the mid-1960s, similar organizations have taken on this task in New York City. Three of these, created at different times to serve different constituencies, shared the goals of creating spaces where activists engaged in different campaigns and movements exchanged ideas and plans.

Founded in 1968 at the peak of the 1960s movements, the Health Policy Advisory Center (Health/PAC), brought together activists, organizers, and academics working in campaigns to prevent hospital closures, support the Young Lords and Black Panthers health initiatives, and document the rise of medical empires in New York City. Participants exchanged ideas, published their work, and sparked cross-cutting strategy discussions. Its contributors came from the New Left, anti–Vietnam War, civil rights, community control, women's, and labor movements; Health/PAC provided the physical and intellectual space for organizers, mainly based in New York City, to analyze their work and chart future directions.

Its journal, *Health/PAC Bulletin*, and its books, including the *American Health Empire: Power, Profits, and Politics* (1970) and *Prognosis Negative: Crisis in the Health Care System* (1976),[58] brought its messages to health professionals, students, and activists in New York and around the country. At its offshoot, the East Coast Health Discussion Group, more than two dozen activists from the East Coast gathered regularly to analyze changes in the health-care system, the role of the women's movement in transforming health care, and the potential of community control of health care. They then brought these insights to the campaigns they were organizing, providing more unified messages and goals than would have been possible had each group operated in isolation. For example, in the 1970s and 1980s, activists' growing understanding that austerity politics and the rise of neoliberalism was driving health-care transformation facilitated a more integrated response across local and national levels.

In a 2011 history of Health/PAC, the public health historian Merlin Chowkwanyun concludes that

> Health/PAC's crowning achievement was situating health care politics in a wider political-economic context and bringing intellectual rigor to activism. It struggled constantly with identifying the most promising methods for change in the health sector, but it must be credited, too, with revisiting that question, often in a ruthlessly self-critical way. . . . We would all do well to recall Health/PAC's political spirit and analytic totality and to revive the ambitious parameters of debate that it set.[59]

A second example, the Center for Popular Democracy (now simply Popular Democracy), founded in 2014 by activists including three leaders of

Make the Road New York, promotes equity, opportunity, and a dynamic democracy in partnership with innovative, community-based organizations, and local, state, and national progressive networks across the country.[60] Based in Brooklyn, New York and Washington, DC, Popular Democracy develops cutting-edge state and local policies that seek to deliver tangible benefits to communities and help build stronger infrastructure and capacity to drive local fights for positive change. The group works on education, housing, the role of the Federal Reserve, immigrants' rights, electoral politics, and other issues.

Popular Democracy now includes fifty grassroots organizations across thirty-four states and DC that demand transformational change for Black, Brown, and low-income communities. By providing economic analyses, policy reports, and messaging guidance to community organizations around the country, the organization helps to break down the local/national divide and to enable cross-cutting learning across issues and places. By listening to community activists and helping to elevate their concerns, the group helps to balance the sometimes unequal voices of local and national groups.

The third example, Equity Advocates, differs from the two previously described, more comprehensive New York–based groups in that it works solely on food policy and has its roots in the food justice movement. But by including activists working on school food, urban agriculture, hunger and food insecurity, municipal food policy, and food workers' rights, the group also brings together organizers and leaders from multiple movements, enabling them to exchange experiences, identify common grounds, and plan strategies at the city, state, and federal levels. Its commitment to equity helps to align equity-focused work across the food movement, while its training programs assist the members of its partners to operate more effectively in city, state, and national food politics.

Equity Advocates sponsors the NYC Food Policy Alliance, a multi-sector group of more than sixty food organizations from across New York that work together to identify and advocate for public policies and funding that respond to current economic and hunger crises, while also addressing the ongoing vulnerabilities and injustices of the food system.[61] The NYC

Food Policy Alliance and the advocacy-training programs sponsored by Equity Advocates provide activists working on food issues across New York communities with the space to learn from each other, develop new partnerships, build capacity, and identify common policy messages and goals.

These organizations illustrate the valuable role that similar organizations can play in making it easier for activists to overcome the siloization and isolation that block the creation of more powerful and unified social movements that can advance a common agenda. By strengthening these cross-cutting, unifying groups, and creating new ones to meet emerging needs, activist organizations can build their power and create more effective movements for change.

Activist campaigns arise at different levels. Some begin in one neighborhood, others in a city or county, and still others emerge from state and national political currents. Wherever they start, campaigns that link their messages, goals, and activities to the work of other campaigns and take on related problems at different levels create the potential for amplifying their work, building more power, and therefore achieving more success.

In summary, by (1) connecting to other movements that share values and goals, (2) choosing partners that will help to achieve specific short-term campaign objectives, (3) launching specific activities that build momentum for expanding alliances, and (4) creating spaces where activists from different movements can exchange ideas and debate strategy, organizers of activist campaigns can reap the benefits of working with other movements.

9

HOW ACTIVISTS EVALUATE THEIR WORK

At some point, the planners and participants in every activist campaign ask, "Is what we are doing working?," "Are we achieving our goals?," or "What should we be doing differently?" To answer these questions, activists have devised various ways to monitor, assess, and improve their activities. They use their responses to modify their strategies as needed, document their impact on policy and health, or share their lessons with others. In this chapter, I review some of the ways that health campaigns and social movements in New York City have evaluated their work. My focus is on evaluations that measure the health impact of the changes and the effect of their campaigns on the capacity of activist organizations to achieve their goals.

In the evaluations of campaigns reviewed here, activists have sought to answer some mix of the following questions:

- Did our work raise awareness and concern about the problem we tackled?
- Did our activities lead to changes in policies, institutional practices, or the health of our populations of interest?

- Did our activities reduce the problem we had identified? By how much?
- Did our endeavors strengthen the capacity of our organizations and allies or build the power of our organization or movement to win, or monitor, defend, and expand on our successes?
- Did our work suggest approaches that could be used successfully in other circumstances?
- What could we have done differently to better achieve our goals?

No single evaluation can answer all these questions, but by determining its evaluation priorities and calibrating methods to its priority concerns, every activist campaign can learn from a thoughtful assessment of its work. More broadly, by analyzing the longer-term trajectory of successes and failures of a social movement, its leaders can make changes in strategy, tactics, and goals based on the assessment of its accomplishments and the changing context of the work. In this chapter, I illustrate this process by presenting brief profiles of five activist campaigns launched in New York City from the late 1960s to 2025, each designed to expand or protect what is now called sexual and reproductive health and justice.

PROFILES: ASSESSING ACTIVISM THAT ADVANCES SEXUAL AND REPRODUCTIVE JUSTICE

Feminists, scholars, and activists from women-of-color and health movements have defined and refined their definition of sexual and reproductive health and justice over the years.[1] First defined by women of color in 1994 to inform the development of the 1993 Clinton health care plan, Women of African Descent for Reproductive Justice published a statement signed by more than eight hundred women insisting that any national health care plan must address the unmet reproductive health needs of Black women.[2]

In 2025, the New York City Department of Health wrote that "Sexual and reproductive justice exists when all people have the power and resources to make healthy decisions about their bodies, sexuality and reproduction." The definition includes the rights of all people to choose whether to have or not have children; the conditions under which to give birth or create a family; care for their children with the necessary social support in a safe and healthy environment; and control of their own body and self-expression, free from any form of sexual or reproductive oppression.[3]

By examining the changing ways that New York City and national groups mobilized to protect and expand sexual and reproductive health and justice over the last several decades, how these groups assessed the impact of their campaigns, and what changes they made based on those evaluations, I extract lessons that can inform a deeper understanding of the potential and limits of the evaluation of activist campaigns and movements.

LEGALIZING ABORTION IN NEW YORK STATE, 1970

On February 13, 1969, demonstrators interrupted the staid meeting of New York State's Joint Legislative Committee on the Problems of Public Health, convened to discuss whether to liberalize the state's eighty-six-year-old criminal abortion statute. The proposed changes would make abortion legal in cases where a woman's physical or mental health was at risk, or when she was a victim of rape or incest.[4]

A nun, the only woman among the fifteen experts asked to testify, told the legislators that abortion was a mortal sin. A former judge—a man—testified that abortion might be allowable only after a woman had already had four children. Members of a new radical feminist group called Redstockings also attended the hearing. After hearing from the judge, a Redstockings member shouted, "All right, now let's hear from some real experts—the women." Other women stood up to demand that people who had had abortions needed to speak. The hearing moved into an executive session behind closed doors, while activists protested outside, insisting that they were the authorities to whom the legislators needed to listen.[5]

A month later, Redstockings organized its own hearing in which twelve women described their experiences with illegal abortion. "We are the true experts, the only experts, we who have had abortions," one witness said.[6] At this meeting, New Yorkers for Abortion Law Repeal, an alliance of groups working to repeal New York State's ban on abortion, distributed their proposal for a model bill that would establish public abortion and contraception clinics. "This is the abortion law that every state will have when present abortion laws are repealed," they proclaimed.[7]

In 1970, after intense debate, the New York State Legislature passed a bill to decriminalize abortion in the state. In the Senate, the law passed by one vote after a Catholic senator from upstate New York changed his mind to support legalization. "I don't think I have the right to force my morality on anyone else," he said. Governor Nelson Rockefeller signed the law. He acknowledged the role of activists in passing the law, telling reporters that "Women's liberation played an important part in the passage of this bill" and that "the wives of the Senate and the Assembly put this bill through."[8]

The legalization of abortion in New York State provided public health professionals and abortion-rights activists with an opportunity to assess the impact of the change for the health of women and babies. Prior to the passage of the new law, John Lindsay, then mayor of New York City, and Dr. Jean Pakter, the director of the Bureau of Maternity Services for the New York City Department of Health, had decided to support advocates' calls for the state decriminalization of abortion. The mayor used Pakter's data on maternal illnesses and deaths associated with illegal abortion to persuade state legislators that decriminalization could reduce the number of illegal abortion–related deaths, an argument that legislators accepted.[9]

Pakter and her colleagues then had the task of proposing regulations for implementing legalization in New York City in consultation with an Advisory Committee on Obstetrics and Gynecology. The proposed rules, intended to ensure that abortion was both legal and safe, specified the settings in which abortion could take place, the procedures to be followed, and mandated public education so that New Yorkers would know how to obtain a legal abortion. Some activists objected, claiming these rules restricted access for low-income women and "created a two-tier system that unfairly restricted the options of poor women," but the new rules were adopted and implemented.[10] The city's Department of Health was also required to monitor abortion services and make public reports on the results, evidence activists could use for their own monitoring and advocacy.

In 1971, using these monitoring reports, Pakter and Frieda Nelson, the Health Department's principal statistician, published an article summarizing the results of the first nine months of legalization. Their report provided data on the number of abortions performed, the type of hospitals in which they were performed, the methods of termination, the types of complications reported, and the fees paid. Significantly, the study showed that the ratio of maternal deaths due to abortion fell from 17 per 100,000 live births in the first four months of 1969 to 7 per 100,000 live births in the first four months of 1971, after the new law went into effect, a decline of almost 60 percent. The authors concluded that after the new law, "women have sought and obtained abortions earlier in pregnancy, complication rates are declining . . . and abortion mortality rates have decreased markedly."[11]

A second study by the Health Department staff provided updated results for the first two years of the new law. Pakter and her colleagues reported that nonresidents of New York State accounted for almost two-thirds of all abortions performed during the two-year period, and that complication rates for early termination declined while rates rose for terminations after sixteen weeks, a more complicated procedure. During this two-year period, the report showed unprecedented lows were recorded for maternal and infant mortality in New York City.[12]

In 1973, the US Supreme Court used data from Pakter's and other studies to reach its landmark *Roe v. Wade* decision on abortion. In their decision, the justices wrote that "mortality rates for women undergoing early abortions, where the procedure is legal, appear to be as low as or lower than the rates for normal childbirth. Consequently, any interest of the State in protecting the woman from an inherently hazardous procedure, except when it would be equally dangerous for her to forgo it, has largely disappeared."[13]

Pakter and her colleagues were public health professionals, not activists, but they were committed to documenting and publishing their assessment of the impact of a new law designed to improve women's health.

Their monitoring reports and journal articles provided health professionals, public officials, and women's health activists with the evidence they needed to identify problems, improve implementation, demonstrate the law's success in achieving key health outcomes, and expand its reach to other states and, in 1973, to the nation.

CESA and CARASA: Linking Sterilization Abuse and Abortion Rights, 1975–1980

In the mid-1970s, two organizations, the Committee to End Sterilization Abuse (CESA) and the Committee for Abortion Rights and Against Sterilization Abuse (CARASA), campaigned to end sterilization abuse, first in New York City and then nationally. Their political goal was to develop a shared policy agenda that combined the fights against sterilization abuse and for abortion rights. Sterilization abuse describes sterilizing women without obtaining their informed consent, misleading them about the reversibility of the procedure, or obtaining consent while a woman is giving birth or having an abortion. According to a 1975 lawsuit filed by the Center for Constitutional Rights, prior to the establishment of the guidelines that CESA convinced public hospitals in the city to adopt, sterilization abuse was each year leading thousands of New York City women, disproportionately Black and Latiné, to be sterilized without their informed consent, because they had been misinformed about the irreversibility of the operation or coerced into consenting.[14]

CESA started first, and later evolved into CARASA, sharing some members and goals, but also differing in focus and composition. Like other sexual and reproductive justice activists that followed these two groups, CESA and CARASA strived to expand public understanding of reproductive justice and to speak to the needs of and engage Black, Latiné, working-class, and other women in this movement.

The story of the evolution of CESA into CARASA and their successes and limitations in creating a multiracial, equity-focused movement for sexual and reproductive health and justice highlights the early challenges these activists faced. The ways that each group gathered evidence on the context and impact of their work adds to the repertoire of approaches that those evaluating activism have used.

Committee to End Sterilization Abuse. In 1974, ten women from Puerto Rican, reproductive health, health-care, and legal activist groups in New York City formed CESA to fight sterilization abuse in Puerto Rico and New York City. Catalyzed by a legal case challenging the forced sterilization of two teenage Black girls in Alabama in 1973 and the federal Department of Health, Education and Welfare's (HEW) failure to implement its own sterilization guidelines, the founders of CESA wanted to end forced sterilization in New York City.[15] Their first target was the New York City Health and Hospital Corporation (HHC, now named NYC Health + Hospitals), the city's network of public hospitals. CESA organized an Advisory Committee on Sterilization to assist the hospital system to create regulations that would protect women from sterilization abuse.

By 1975, CESA had made impressive steps toward this goal. HHC had approved new guidelines that required hospitals to institute a thirty-day waiting period after women had given consent, used a detailed and explicit consent form, and provided counseling to those considering sterilization in the women's own language. The Center for Constitutional Rights successfully defended these rules against a lawsuit filed by several directors of obstetrics and gynecology from the public hospitals.

CESA then helped to win approval for a city council law that required private New York City hospitals to follow the public hospitals' sterilization rules; to defeat a New York State law that would have weakened the rules across all hospitals in the state; and to implement new federal HEW regulations on sterilization abuse in all hospitals in the United States that received federal funding.[16]

How did CESA and its supporters succeed in expanding its success in one city hospital system to secure new state and national rules protecting against sterilization abuse? Proponents of the guidelines deployed a mix of strategies that contributed to their ultimate success. First, they mastered and embedded themselves in the internal institutional practices and processes of the institutions that needed to act to end the abuses. At HHC,

CESA helped to create an HHC Advisory Committee on Sterilization. It was cochaired by Esta Armstrong, a veteran HHC administrator, longtime activist, and CESA member, and other HHC physicians, including Dr. Helen Rodríguez-Trias, a pediatrician at Lincoln Hospital, and Karen Stamm, a CESA cofounder and spokesperson. Representatives of other health centers, community organizations, and Puerto Rican, women's, and legal advocacy groups also served on the advisory committee. The guidelines proposed by this group won unanimous approval from HHC's Board of Directors.[17] In their subsequent interactions with the New York City Council, the New York State Legislature, and HEW, CESA members similarly identified allies among elected officials and their staff and used these relationships to advance their goals.

Second, CESA members used their insider knowledge to cultivate elected officials who could serve as public spokespeople for the sterilization abuse rules and forged relationship with politicians who could help to win passage of the guidelines at each political level. By having public champions who could bring their case to other legislators and the media, CESA amplified its influence.

Third, CESA members launched an educational, organizing, and communications blitz to encourage public support for the guidelines. Stamm described how CESA organized community meetings to discuss the issue, encouraged "thousands of people" to write "hundreds of letters," testified at public hearings, won endorsements from medical, faith-based, and community groups, and developed alliances with women's, civil rights, Black, and other groups. These activists helped to strengthen the backbones of elected officials and institutional staff members, reinforcing their prior efforts to encourage these individuals to resist conservative and religious opposition to the guidelines.

This public support also enabled CESA to overcome significant opposition from some physicians and medical societies who viewed regulation as an intrusion on physician autonomy. Among major physician groups, only the National Medical Association, a membership organization of Black doctors, supported the HEW guidelines on sterilization abuse.[18] Planned Parenthood and the Association for Voluntary Sterilization opposed the guidelines, arguing that the waiting period limited women's freedom to choose.

Some women also challenged the waiting period. At a public meeting, an angry woman asked how activists could justify abortion on demand, but not sterilization on demand. "It's my body, and no one else's," she said. Rodríguez, the pediatrician who helped to found CESA, responded, "It's the slight inconveniences of [a] 30-day waiting period versus the danger of many instances of abuse. Frankly, I would choose to inconvenience the few."[19]

Rodríguez serves as an example of the many influential leaders in New York City's activist movements. She played prominent roles in the Young Lords, CESA, CARASA, and several other activist and health organizations. For thirty years, she brought together the diverse constituencies that she represented both in New York City and nationally. She served as a credible and charismatic spokesperson, using her skills in eliciting the differences among groups and then bringing these people together to find common ground.

During her medical internship in Puerto Rico, Rodríguez saw a mother of five die from a botched abortion, an important influence on her subsequent political development. She later explained, "What brought me to the women's movement was the women's health movement. The cultural elements of feminism didn't resonate with me, but abortion resonated with me. I became part of the women's movement in October 1970 at an international meeting on abortion rights attended by several thousand women and held at Barnard College in New York City."[20]

Rodríguez was a cofounder of CESA and helped to bring other physicians, health providers, and health professionals' associations to support the proposed changes in the public hospital system's guidelines on sterilization abuse, then the New York City Council law, and finally to the US Health, Education and Welfare hearing in Washington, DC, that led to making the New York City's guidelines the national standard. By providing an authoritative physician's voice as well as acknowledging the importance of the sterilization and birthing experiences of Puerto Rican women and the patients in city hospitals like Lincoln, Rodríguez became a recognized leader of local and national campaigns to end sterilization abuse.

At a conference on the health of women of color held at Stanford University in the 1990s, Rodríguez described her formative years in the movements for abortion rights and against sterilization abuse:

> Women activists in the women's movement, who were primarily concerned with removing all legal obstacles to abortion, opposed the notions of guidelines, regulations, or legislation that in any way restricts access to sterilization. As we thrashed out the differences, we . . . began to listen to each other and to understand our personal experiences were different because our race, class or ethnicity exposed us to different institutions or practices. A basis for working together was solidly laid [for] identifying and understanding our commonalities.[21]

Rodríguez went on to beseech her listeners "to consolidate our ranks and focus our strength that we may create a universal equitable system fully consonant with our values of compassion and freedom." This task of finding the commonalities that can accelerate its successes while acknowledging the differences among its constituencies has remained a continuing goal of the movement for sexual and reproductive justice.

<u>Committee for Abortion Rights and Against Sterilization Abuse.</u> After its New York City and national successes, CESA slowly dissolved. As Karen Stamm later noted, "There seemed to be no particular need for [CESA] anymore, which was too bad."[22] But CARASA, an organization founded in 1977, absorbed several CESA members, including Stamm and Rodríguez, and continued the battles for sexual and reproductive justice.

On July 13, 1977, a lightning storm caused a major blackout in New York City. CESA members were meeting at Rodríguez's Upper West Side home at the time. Rather than sending people into the dark night, Rodríguez, as always "cool as a cucumber," in Stamm's words, "invited us to stay on the couches, floors, bathtubs, where we could fit."[23] At that all-nighter emerged the idea of an organization that espoused a new politics of reproductive rights that both embraced abortion access and opposed sterilization abuse. Its founders were white feminists, Latina activists from CESA, and feminist scholars, diverse in terms of class, but not including many from other racial/ethnic groups.

CARASA was formed in response to the increasing backlash against the gains women had won in the 1960s and early 1970s. These included the Supreme Court decision allowing states to cut off Medicaid funding for abortion and the legislative Hyde Amendment, which cut off all Medicaid funding for abortions except in cases of rape, incest, or physical danger to the women, and the persistence of sterilization abuse. CARASA's principles of unity proposed an expansive vision of "reproductive freedom for all women" that included the following:

- Abortion rights; guarantees against sterilization abuse; safe birth control; sex education in schools; and the "right to conduct one's sex life as one wishes, regardless of marital status or sexual preferences."
- Equal wages for women, enough to support a family, alone or with others; welfare benefits for an adequate standard of living; decent housing to provide a comfortable, secure place to live and rest; reliable and skilled childcare and schools to enable our children to become healthy adults; and safe and affordable health care for everyone.[24]

Reflecting its roots in the women's, civil rights, Latina, lesbian, and gay, socialist, and other movements, CARASA sought to integrate feminist, class, and racial/ethnic perspectives. Unlike the more nationally focused reproductive justice movement founded a few years later, CARASA did not center racism and African American women in its early statements, nor did it use the word "justice" in its definition. It did, however, highlight its commitment to community organizing, building broad coalitions, and creating a large mass movement. "Only in this way," its principles of unity asserted, "will we be strong enough to successfully pressure the government, win against the political power of the Catholic Church and other antichoice religious groups, and defeat the right wing's general offensive against the rights of all oppressed people."[25]

To achieve these lofty goals, CARASA pursued several activities. First, its members spent hours meeting to formulate ideas about how to integrate the goals of the diverse strands of its constituent movements into a coherent agenda, followed by more hours to discuss how best to communicate these ideas to potential supporters. In 1979, CARASA's scholar-activist members published a manifesto, *Women Under Attack*, to define and explain the concept of "reproductive freedom." "When we say women must have reproductive freedom," they wrote, "we mean the possibility of controlling for themselves in a real and practical way—that is free from economic, social or legal coercion—whether and under what conditions, they will have children."[26] In community meetings, op-eds, its newspaper, and testimony before legislative bodies, CARASA members promoted and debated these ideas with activists from other organizations and movements, helping to broaden their call beyond abortion access (see figure 9.1). By carefully defining reproductive freedom, the group also made it possible to track the movement's success in advancing this concept.

Second, to make progress on achieving specific policy aims, CARASA forged alliances with the diverse constituencies with experience and a stake in these issues. It joined a coalition with students from City University of New York to promote subsidized childcare so that working-class women raising children could attend college. Following the lead of the Coalition for the Reproductive Rights of Workers and several labor unions, CARASA joined in challenging corporate policies that required women exposed to toxic chemicals to undergo sterilization, rather than require the companies to eliminate the exposures. The organization supported welfare rights and advocated for better access to birth control and sex education. Several lesbian women created the CARASA Lesbian Action Committee to urge other members to add lesbian rights to the reproductive freedom agenda and form alliances with outside lesbian and gay rights groups.[27]

In some ways, however, by 1985, CARASA's ambitious goals contributed to its demise. Its effort to integrate and reconcile multiple issues led to conflicts. Members disagreed about key questions such as how best to incorporate lesbian rights, how best to engage with and support Black women, what role disruptive tactics should play, and how to integrate calls for both reproductive and sexual freedom. The endless meetings that had previously led to resolution of issues now often ended in conflict. Stamm

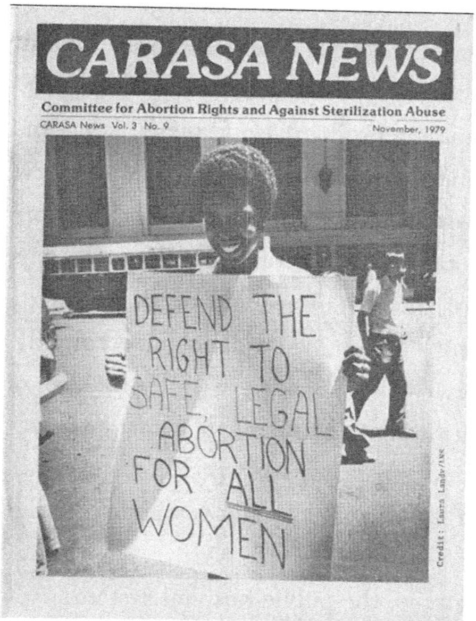

FIGURE 9.1 1979 newspaper of the Committee for Abortion Rights and Against Sterilization Abuse (CARASA).

Source: CARASA. https://www.zinnedproject.org/materials/peoples-history-of-abortion-care-in-the-us/

recalled a year of meetings that left members "demoralized and disheartened," leading many to drop out.[28] By the early 1980s, CARASA had disappeared as an organizational presence.

Nevertheless, its ideas, insights, and members lived on. CARASA activists continued to join and lead reproductive justice campaigns. Its broader view of reproductive freedom still influences national and New York City activism related to reproductive health. In 1978, several CARASA members helped to form the Reproductive Rights National Network, which eventually included about fifty feminist organizations seeking to make reproductive choices available for all women in the United States. A key priority of the network was to create a national infrastructure to fight the strengthening alliance of conservative political groups and antiabortion religious groups. It also ended after a few years, but its efforts, albeit unsuccessful, to create an organization that Black women would join set the stage for the emergence over the following decade of a reproductive justice movement focused on the intersecting roles of racism and sexism in shaping reproductive and sexual freedom.

Both CESA and CARASA, in different ways, developed innovative methods of assessing their work. CESA's sterilization guidelines at the public hospital, city, and national levels each required monitoring implementation of the guidelines and producing regular reports. Each hospital community board, as well as city council committees and HEW staff, reviewed these reports. While the level of monitoring varied across institutions, the mandate to report created data, an accountability mechanism, and an opportunity for activists, elected officials, and agency staff to identify and investigate problems and celebrate successes.

In 1975, for example, the public hospital system's Advisory Committee on Sterilization prepared a report concluding that some doctors were ordering hysterectomies as sterilization rather than the less risky tubal ligation to give trainees experience in surgical techniques. "These factors . . . create an atmosphere for concern," the committee noted, leading it to strengthen its recommendations for medical training and patient education.[29]

In CARASA's report *Women Under Attack*, first published in 1979, a collective of feminist activist-scholars assessed the state of the movement for abortion rights and against sterilization abuse. By analyzing the context and consequences of the last decade of activism for reproductive rights and health, the authors sought to answer these questions:

- Why has abortion become such a fiercely contested political issue?
- What is its current legal status in the United States and how is that changing?
- What forces are behind the recent attacks and what do they want?
- What do people, but especially women, of differing ethnic, economic, and religious backgrounds stand to lose from this attack?
- How can women join to defend their reproductive freedom?[30]

Several characteristics of *Women Under Attack* make it a useful model for deeper analyses of activists' problems and accomplishments than those asked in other, more superficial accounts. First, it asks profound political questions, seeking to understand the backlash to the movement for reproductive freedom, the political dimensions of the fights on abortion, and the potential for framing messages that will bring in new supporters. This distinguishes it from other activist assessments that avoid political questions.

Second, it grounds its analysis in extracting lessons from previous battles of women's health activists, providing the historical context that activists caught up in their day-to-day battles sometimes miss. Third, because the authors are scholars and activists, they are willing to use theoretical frameworks to inform their assessment and to make policy and practice recommendations, a task that more traditional academics sometimes avoid for fear of compromising their scholarly detachment.

The report concludes with a call to action:

> The imminent threat to our reproductive freedom has necessitated much stronger actions of unity and protest. In 1977 and 1978, CARASA and other groups mobilized many people to demonstrate against anti-abortion politicians and officials, and on several occasions we have picketed "Right-to Life" headquarters and conferences. We have also organized groups of women to defend abortion clinics against harassment and invasion by "Right-to-Life" groups and are working closely with the clinics to develop long-range strategies to maintain their integrity and security in the face of these attacks. These actions are an important beginning; but we must mount a campaign that is national in its scope and decisive in its impact. From firebombers to population controllers, from the "Right-to-Lifers" to the Church hierarchy, the forces against women's control over their bodies and reproductive processes are everywhere. They are organized, well-funded and prepared for a long political fight. To defeat them, we must build a national network that includes masses of women and men of all racial, economic, religious, and age groups. We believe that the fight for reproductive

> freedom for women shares important goals with the struggles of minority groups, working people, welfare recipients, the handicapped, and all those affected by unemployment and the decline in social services. We want to unite everyone to fight against the attacks on reproductive freedom and for a radical change in existing social conditions.[31]

By using its assessment of the state of the reproductive freedom movement to make recommendations about what this movement should do next, the CARASA report fulfills the ultimate reason activists need to evaluate their work: to inform future strategies, tactics, and goals.

PREVENTING DISCRIMINATION AGAINST PREGNANT WORKERS: A BETTER BALANCE'S CAMPAIGN FOR THE NEW YORK CITY PREGNANT WORKERS FAIRNESS ACT, 2014

The successful passage of New York City, State, and federal laws to prevent workplace discrimination against pregnant workers illustrates another approach to expanding reproductive rights, one that builds on the work of the labor movement, takes a human rights approach, uses courts and litigation to win new rights, and, in the case described here, addresses the specific needs of the 47 percent of New York State's labor force who are women.

Lenora Lapidus, the director of the ACLU's Women's Right Project (founded by Ruth Bader Ginsburg), made a succinct case for why pregnancy discrimination needs to be high on the agendas of the labor and feminist movements: "The twenty-first century reality is, the majority of women work. Most women who have children work. Workplaces need to change so that pregnancy is just a normal condition of the workplace."[32]

The story of activism to end pregnancy discrimination in New York also spotlights another type of activist group, A Better Balance (ABB). Created in 2005, ABB provides direct legal and advocacy services to individuals as well as promoting local, state, and national legislation that bans pregnancy discrimination and litigating to ensure enforcement. In the words of Dina Bakst, cofounder and former copresident of the organization, and Sarah Brafman, staff attorney, ABB was founded to ensure "that all workers can care for themselves and their families without compromising their health or economic security."[33]

In 1978, Congress passed and President Jimmy Carter signed the federal Pregnancy Discrimination Act (PDA), an amendment to the Civil Rights Act of 1964. The legislation resulted from more than a decade of women's and human rights activism. It also had limitations: PDA only covered workplaces with fifteen or more employees, thus excluding the millions of women who worked for smaller employers, and it required employers to accommodate pregnant workers only if they covered other employees who are "similar in their ability or inability to work." Consequently, an employer was not obligated to provide paid sick leave to an employee simply because she is pregnant so long as the employer denies paid sick leave to employees who are not pregnant.

Under the 1978 PDA, an employer may deny a reasonable accommodation to an employee only if those accommodations would impose an "undue hardship" on the employer, defined as a significant difficulty or expense incurred by the employer in making the accommodation. These exclusions, added to the bill at the behest of employer groups to win majority support in Congress, illustrate the compromises activists make to get a bill passed. However, in this and other cases, the shortcoming also set the stage for the next round of advocacy.

To complicate matters, as legal historian Deborah Dinner noted, while feminists put pregnancy discrimination on the national political agenda, various antiabortion and pro-family groups also supported the bill, setting the stage for ongoing battles about the rationale for ending pregnancy discrimination.[34] At the heart of the debate was whether pregnancy was a private decision with private costs, as businesses and conservatives claimed, even those who supported ending pregnancy discrimination, or a social good, a public need, and a basic human right, as feminists and labor advocates asserted. Some supporters believed that guaranteeing the rights of pregnant workers could reduce the needs for abortion.

Through the 1970s and 1980s, a variety of organizations used litigation in the federal courts to clarify and expand the protection of reproductive rights. In the view of sociologist Mark Evan Edwards, this litigation—with its limitations—raised issues that created the opening for and necessity of the state and local legislative efforts of the following decades.[35]

In New York City, ABB played a leading role in winning approval for the city's 2014 Pregnant Workers Fairness Act, first drafting the legislation and then helping to get the city council to pass it. ABB's work on the act began in the early 2000s, when, as Bakst and Brafman explained, "we began to hear from pregnant women across New York City and beyond who faced the impossible choice of maintaining a healthy pregnancy or earning a paycheck."[36] For example, a pregnant retail worker told ABB staff that she had to be rushed to the emergency room when she fainted on the job because her employer would not let her take a drink of water.[37] A supermarket worker who could not lift heavy boxes during her pregnancy was sent home and forced to take disability insurance, which expired a month before she gave birth, causing her to lose her health insurance.[38]

As the city council took up the bill in 2012, ABB invited the women who told these stories as well as medical experts to testify at legislative hearings. They also invited experts. Wendy Chavkin, a public health ob-gyn at Columbia University, for example, informed the council members that "physically demanding work—including prolonged standing, long work hours, irregular work schedules, heavy lifting and high physical activity—has consistently been shown to be associated with a statistically significant increased risk of preterm delivery and low birth weight."[39] By bringing scientific evidence and multiple voices and points of view to the city council, ABB and its allies convinced the council to pass and Mayor Bloomberg to sign the Pregnant Workers Fairness Act, which went into effect in January 2014.

Both before and after the law was enacted, ABB also operated a free legal hotline, where workers encountering discrimination could get immediate help. It also educated workers and distributed flyers and brochures at workplaces and to unions. A particular focus of this outreach was to inform low-wage workers about the law, especially women working in male-dominated industries such as construction, where they may be less likely to learn about their rights, and to inform young workers and disabled workers.[40] This hotline also provided ABB with ongoing evidence on the implementation of the law and the problems various groups of women encountered in having their new rights recognized. The analysis of these records enabled ABB to evaluate the law's success and identify unsolved problems, an important goal for the assessment of policy advocacy.

In another evaluation strategy, in 2019, five years after the law had been passed, ABB analyzed its implementation and enforcement and made recommendations for improvement to the New York City Commission on Human Rights, the city agency charged with enforcing local human rights laws and educating the public about their rights. Based on this assessment, ABB staff made three recommendations. First, they encouraged the city to fast-track pregnancy accommodation complaints, especially when the worker's health is at risk. This was based on ABB's experience that it often took months to investigate and resolve complaints, delays that endangered pregnant workers and their future babies. Second, they encouraged more active investigation of pregnancy discrimination complaints in male-dominated (e.g., construction) and low-wage (e.g., fast-food and domestic work) industries, sectors where ABB regularly found problems and limited enforcement. Finally, ABB encouraged the commission to increase public education and outreach on pregnancy discrimination to ensure that all pregnant and potentially pregnant workers know about their rights and how to resolve problems before they arose. ABB also called on the city council to increase funding for enforcement of the law and to reverse recent cuts in the budget for the Commission on Human Rights.[41]

By educating workers about their rights, providing legal services to those who experienced problems, and monitoring the city's funding, implementation, and enforcement of the Pregnant Workers Fairness Act, ABB filled some gaps that other activist organizations miss. These efforts helped to ensure that their legislative victory had an ongoing impact, and it helped set the stage for subsequent campaigns to pass a New York State and then a national act to prevent pregnancy discrimination (see figure 9.2). By including labor unions, immigrants' rights groups, and civil liberties organizations in its advocacy campaigns, ABB showed the diverse support

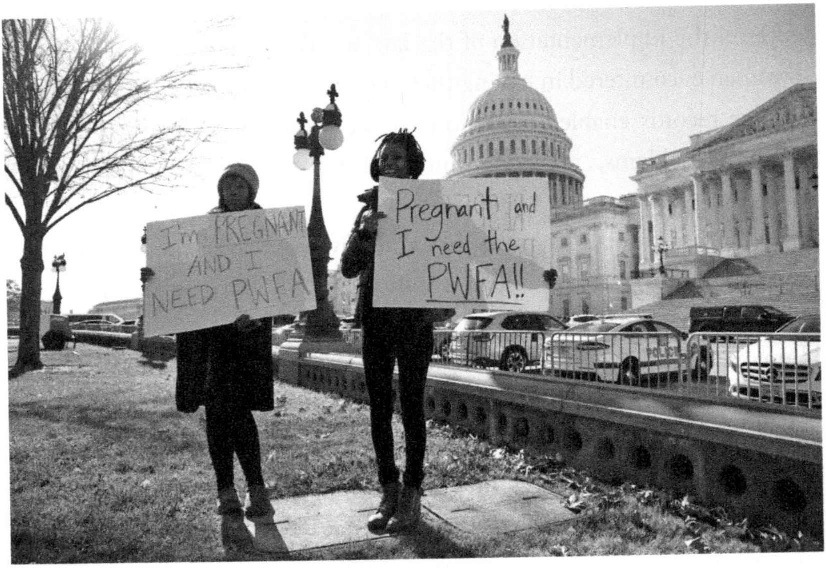
I'm PREGNANT AND I NEED PWFA
Pregnant and I need the PWFA!!

FIGURE 9.2 In December 2022, participants in a campaign to persuade the US Senate to pass the Pregnant Workers Fairness Act led by the New York City-based group A Better Balance, which rallied supporters at Capitol Hill to call on Senate Majority Leader Chuck Schumer to bring the bill to a Senate floor vote.

Source: A Better Balance. https://www.abetterbalance.org/pregnant-workers-advocates-and-legislators-rally-together-on-capitol-hill-to-demand-a-pregnant-workers-fairness-act-vote/

for ending pregnancy discrimination and the potential of the law to reduce gender, racial/ethnic, and other forms of inequity.

New York's changing politics contributed to the momentum to take on pregnancy discrimination. The day after Alexandria Ocasio-Cortez won her primary election against the Democratic machine–endorsed candidate for Congress, Governor Andrew Cuomo, facing growing challenges from progressive and feminist groups, announced a state investigation of pregnancy discrimination, a phenomenon one observer called the "AOC effect" to describe mainstream politicians' fear of progressive insurgents that sometimes led them to support activist demands.[42] By focusing public attention on the need for stronger action to end pregnancy discrimination,

ABB's activism put indirect pressure on other politicians to show their support.

By 2023, thirty states and five localities had passed pregnancy accommodation laws, providing confirmation that these laws worked and that there was popular support for a national law to protect all pregnant workers and their families. As ABB's Bakst explained, these successes "helped show members of Congress that these laws were working, because we brought many examples of workers to members of Congress to show that the state laws were helping keep pregnant women healthy and attached to the workforce."[43] ABB played a vital role in providing national, state, and local legislators with the evidence they needed and the access to experts to approve new laws.

In 2023, Congress passed and President Joe Biden signed a federal Pregnant Workers Fairness Act to close a gap in coverage for pregnant and postpartum workers and applicants. Passage of the act culminated an effort that had started in 2012 when Bakst, Copresident Sherry Leiwant, and other ABB staffers first met with New York Congressman Jerry Nadler, who invited them to meet with him in the wake of a *New York Times* op-ed Bakst had written on pregnancy discrimination.[44] Nadler wanted their advice on how to craft a national version of an act to prevent pregnancy discrimination.[45]

The campaigns to pass New York City, State, and federal laws to eliminate pregnancy discrimination took place over more than a dozen years. Their successes showed it was possible to change laws at all three levels. Activists successfully moved a topic from the back burner to the front burner of policymakers' agendas. They combined public education, litigation, direct services, and advocacy to achieve a cumulative impact far greater than any of these strategies alone could have achieved. The multilevel pregnancy and discrimination acts also demonstrated how adept advocates can move from the local to the state and national levels and back, creating synergies and openings for policy change. In addition, as public policy experts and activists, the leaders and staff of ABB provided evidence to policymakers and activists around the country that could be used to advance legal protections for pregnant workers. Finally, the campaigns showed the value of an intersectional approach, one that integrated, rather than pitting against each other, the concerns of women workers with those of Black and Latiné workers, immigrant workers, workers with disabilities, and young workers.

Laws alone, of course, cannot end pregnancy discrimination, a practice deeply rooted in the structures of sexism, racism, and gender stereotypes. But by combining a health and human rights approach, ABB and other activists fighting to end pregnancy discrimination contributed specific victories that improved the well-being and working conditions for pregnant workers and opened the doors for additional reforms to realize ABB's vision of a society where all workers can care for themselves and their families without compromising their health or economic security.

ACTIVISM TO REDUCE BLACK MATERNAL MORTALITY AND MORBIDITY, 2020–2025

In the early 2020s, Black women giving birth in New York City were more than nine times more likely to die in pregnancy or childbirth than white women,[46] an appalling disparity more than three times higher than the national Black-white ratio (2.6:1) of deaths.[47] US Centers for Disease Control researchers estimated that more than 80 percent of pregnancy-related deaths in the United States are preventable,[48] suggesting that the persistence of this inequity reflects more than the lack of medical knowledge.

Black women also experience serious pregnancy-related health problems at higher rates than other women. Severe maternal morbidity (SMM) describes significant health problems experienced by pregnant women. In 2018, 3,311 deliveries in New York City were associated with SMM, and Black women were more than twice as likely to experience SMM as white women.[49]

Not only were Black women experiencing higher rates of pregnancy-related health problems, but they also reported difficulty getting care or receiving poor quality or unsatisfactory care. Studies in the United States and New York showed that a few hospitals, mostly nonteaching ones in Black communities, had much higher maternity mortality and severe morbidity rates than other hospitals.[50] Echoing the earlier complaints of Black and Latiné women protesting sterilization abuse, Black women criticized the inadequate information and disrespectful treatment they experienced, a practice some activist-scholars label "obstetric racism."[51]

As in previous community mobilizations on health and policing in New York, it was the deaths of Black people that got the attention of birth justice activists. Several maternal deaths in 2020 and 2021 show that this tragedy strikes Black women from different socioeconomic backgrounds, medical conditions, and sources of hospital care. Cordielle Street, who came to New York from Trinidad to work as a journalist, died a week after giving birth to her second daughter.[52] That same year, Amber Isaac, a graduate student, died at Montefiore Hospital shortly after delivering her son.[53] Less than three months later, Sha-asia Washington, twenty-six years old, died shortly after delivering her daughter in an emergency C-section at Woodhull Hospital in Brooklyn. Denise Williams, a twenty-nine-year-old mother of two, went to Queens Hospital Center seeking treatment for postpartum depression. Two days later, Williams's family learned she had died.

These deaths led to protests. At Queens Hospital, for example, protestors gathered to demand an explanation of Williams's death. "We don't want condolences, we want answers," said Charlene Magee, Williams's maternal aunt. "It's been three weeks, and [my sister] has no idea what happened to her child." Later, the medical examiner attributed the hospital death to a pulmonary embolism that had gone undetected.[54] Bruce McIntyre, the partner of Amber Rose Isaac, who had died after an emergency C-section at Montefiore Medical Center, attended the protest and spoke out in solidarity with Williams's family.

The deaths of Black pregnant women were not new, but the combination of Black Lives Matter's visible public focus on preventable deaths of Black people, new media attention to maternal mortality,[55] and the emergence of a birthing justice movement with ties to (and differences from) the reproductive justice movement contributed to new birth justice activism in New York City.

Brief profiles of a few organizations involved show the diversity of participants and strategies. The New York Coalition for Doula Access, for example, aims to increase access to doula care for Black maternal health patients and low-income Medicaid patients in New York State. Doulas are women, usually without formal obstetric training, who are employed to provide guidance and support to a pregnant woman during labor.

Reproductive justice advocates, women's health activists, and some research evidence shows that increasing access to doulas can reduce SMM and improve the birthing experience, especially for Black women and others experiencing high rates of adverse birth outcomes. A study comparing demographically matched pairs of women who had and had not received doula care in three states found that those with doula care had lower odds of having a C-section and of experiencing postpartum depression or anxiety.[56]

Another group, the Coalition for Doula Access, sought to increase the availability of this care by advocating for changes in the Medicaid reimbursement rate for doula care. In a 2023 appearance at the New York State Senate Committees on Health, Mental Health, and Medicaid Reimbursement, Michelle Zambrano, the coalition's colead, testified as follows: "To improve maternal and child health outcomes, doulas need to be compensated through a statewide Medicaid reimbursement program that meets a standard for living wages. . . . I am here today to talk about ensuring financial sustainability for the doula workforce. . . . [This change] will also make New York a leader in addressing the maternal health crisis and a safer and more equitable place to give birth."[57] After eleven years of advocacy, the coalition convinced the New York State government to include funding for doula care in its 2024 budget for Medicaid, but advocates continued to believe that the funding proposed was lower than needed to address the doula shortages. A year earlier, New York City Mayor Eric Adams signed a bill that required the Department of Health and Mental Hygiene to provide no-cost doula services to neighborhoods with high rates of adverse pregnancy outcomes and establish a doula training program, one component of a package of new laws designed to reduce maternal mortality in the city.[58]

Bx (Re)Birth is a reproductive and birth justice collective comprising experienced doulas, midwives, and lactation counselors founded after the death of Amber Rose Isaac. Its members provide care to support healthy births by seeking to meet the range of needs of pregnant women by "fostering pro-Black, inclusive, and trauma-informed initiatives." Its doulas and midwives also educate women in the Bronx about alternatives to hospital-based birth, "collaborate with people and programs that are committed to revolutionizing the way we birth in our communities," and "strive to return universal dignity and care to the sacred ceremony that is birth."[59]

Finally, the Movement to Birth Liberation is a "network of birth workers, birthing and birthed peoples working together to" imagine and work toward birth liberation. Many of its members are health professionals who cared for women who died in childbirth. Its founder, Katy Cecen, is a nurse-midwife who became a whistleblower, activist, and community organizer. In 2017, she testified before the New York State Senate and Assembly Health Committees on her views on preventable deaths of Black mothers she witnessed at Downstate Medical Center. She described unsafe patient care caused by understaffing and charged that "Governor Cuomo chose to unlawfully withhold [a] disproportionate share [of] hospital payments, huge sums of federal financing to reimburse hospitals for services they had already provided, which sends public hospitals into hiring freezes." These freezes, Cecen argued, led to the staffing shortages that contributed to the deaths she witnessed.[60]

The Movement to Birth Liberation also organized to win passage of New York State's Universal Health Care Act, which it believed would reduce the wide inequalities in access to quality maternity (and other types of) health care. It also supports families of those who have died of pregnancy-related causes in New York City hospitals.

While activism to reduce Black maternal mortality and morbidity in New York City is still in a formative stage, it has the potential to make important contributions to the reproductive justice movement and health activism more broadly. First, reducing maternal morbidity and mortality (MMM) requires tackling systemic racism, a fundamental obstacle to more equitable health. The high burden that MMM imposes on Black women and the multiple pathways by which it exerts its impact—from obstetric racism to the implicit bias of health professionals to segregated housing and health care—requires activists to develop and implement strategies to change the systems and practices of racism, a formidable but vital challenge.

Second, MMM puts a spotlight on several other health problems that Black and other women of color face—inadequate or inaccessible health care; family, community, and police violence; drug use; inadequate management of chronic diseases; and other types of inadequate sexual and reproductive health services, including infant mortality. By educating their communities about the common causes of intersecting health concerns, activists can build the foundation for multi-issue coalitions that increase community power.

Finally, reducing MMM requires integrating upstream and downstream solutions, offering the wider movement the opportunity to gain experience in taking on this critical task. Yes, obstetric care must be improved, and obstetric racism confronted. Yes, doulas and midwives can provide more culturally appropriate, humane, and patient-centered care. But to bring about meaningful reductions in MMM, activists will also need to create more equitable access to high-quality hospital care, more affordable housing, stronger protection against pregnancy discrimination, better pay and more decent jobs for women, and the other life opportunities that contribute to safe birthing, healthy parenting, and equitable communities.[61]

Most profoundly, the birth justice movement has the potential to take on the most fundamental causes of MMM and other health problems facing women of color: the pervasive influences of racism and sexism that continue to compromise the ability of health care, public health, social service, and other systems to deliver on the promise of health for all.

To realize this potential, the green shoots of the birth justice movement will need to find common ground with other streams of sexual and reproductive rights activism, forge alliances with intersecting movements of women, people of color, and health-care reformers, and define specific short- and longer-term policy objectives.

Like other activists, those fighting for birth justice have used various approaches to document and evaluate their work and thus to learn from their successes and failures. In 2022, the New York City Council passed a package of ten birth equity laws and resolutions, the result of years of activism, media attention, and the support of several progressive legislators. City Council Speaker Adrienne Adams noted that "Black women and birthing people have faced a maternal health, mortality, and morbidity crisis. The lived experiences that far too many people have endured are striking and the disparities for Black, Latino, and Indigenous people are horrifying. This package of legislation is an important step designed to eliminate the inequities so that all women and birthing people are safe and protected."[62]

Activists and health professionals contributed two bodies of evidence to inform passage and implementation of the birth equity package. First, several testified at city council hearings on the legislative package, bringing their experiences as clinicians, advocates, and birthing women to the legislators' attention. Paige Bellenbaum, the founding director of the Motherhood Center, testified on the importance of addressing the mental health needs of pregnant and postpartum mothers. "As a survivor of severe postpartum depression and anxiety that nearly ended my life 18 years ago," she said, "I strive to ensure that other new mothers and birthing people do not have to suffer silently as I did."[63]

Lorena Kurousias, the executive director of Mixteca, a community organization serving the growing Mexican and Latin American immigrant population in Sunset Park, Brooklyn, testified about the difficulties their clients confronted in getting help for the problems they faced from sexual violence and the process of immigration. She reported that women even had trouble getting pregnancy tests in shelters or social service agencies to find out whether they were pregnant.[64] Each of these and other witnesses helped educate council members about the unmet needs of various populations and the value of creating laws and programs that addressed the real needs their clients were experiencing.

Second, the activists and legislators insisted that the new laws include mandates for systematic documentation of problems, monitoring their implementation, and reporting the results to the city council, activists, and the public. The assessment measures included in the birth equity legislative package included the following:

- A requirement for the New York City Department of Health to post its annual *Maternal Mortality and Morbidity Report* on its website, a requirement previously missing.
- A mandate to post online the methods the city used to educate various populations on maternal health services to select populations.
- An obligation for regular Health Department reports on sexual and reproductive health disparities across New York City neighborhoods, enabling community residents, activists, and the city to assess progress and identify unmet needs.

These and other requirements ensured that the new laws would provide relevant actors with the readily accessible, understandable information they needed to assess the progress of their implementation, identify emerging needs, and hold public agencies accountable. By themselves, these requirements did not reduce the problems of concern, but they provided key constituencies with the evidence they needed to identify successes and failures and chart future actions, a key purpose for the evaluation of activism.

To assess the new programs and policies designed to reduce Black MMM, activists, evaluators, and policymakers will need to create more comprehensive and systematic evaluation studies that can attribute changes to specific strategies—for example, improved access to doulas, higher-quality obstetric care in hospitals serving low-income communities, better health care for women of all ages, and improvements in housing and working conditions for low-income women in their child-bearing years. Such evidence can guide the choice of priorities that will lead to measurable progress in closing Black-white gaps in maternal mortality and morbidity.

EVALUATING REPRODUCTIVE HEALTH AND JUSTICE ACTIVISM SINCE THE 1970S

Over the last sixty years, reproductive and sexual health and justice activists in New York decided how to modify their goals, strategies, and activities in response to changes in city, state, and federal policies, laws, and institutional practices that emerged over this period. Changes in local and national politics and beliefs during this era also influenced the course of sexual and reproductive justice activism.

A third influence, the focus here, was activists' own formal and informal assessments of their work and its accomplishments. Several sources of evidence informed these assessments: public health data on changing rates of births, abortions, maternal and infant deaths, and other public health outcomes; studies by researchers, health professionals, and activists of the impact of changing policies and laws; and reports by activists, sometimes in partnership with scholars, analyzing the impact, potential, and limitations of their work.

Examples of how assessments using these sources influenced policy or practice come from the profiles in this chapter. The assessment of the impact of New York State's decision to legalize abortion in the 1970s showed that the change in the law was associated with a decline in maternal and infant deaths, a finding that contributed to the 1973 *Roe v. Wade* Supreme Court decision to legalize abortion nationally. CESA's 1975 mandate for city government to monitor and report on compliance with the city's sterilization guidelines showed a reduction in sterilization abuse. This evidence influenced the subsequent adoption of national guidelines to monitor sterilization abuse in all hospitals receiving federal funds. Activists used New York City Health Department reports on racial inequities in Black maternal morbidity and mortality to convince city and state governments to pass new measures to close this gap.

Another kind of evidence came from policy analyses of the changing political context for advancing sexual and reproductive health and justice. CARASA's *Women Under Attack* report, written by a collective of activist-scholars, made the case for the movement to shift from a narrow focus on abortion access to a broader one on what is now called reproductive justice, emphasizing the importance of addressing women's and families' needs for childcare, accessible health care, contraception, and the other pillars of reproductive choice. The report also emphasized the importance of tackling the influence of racism and class in shaping the choices of different populations of women. The 1994 statement by the Women of African

Descent for Reproductive Justice in *The Washington Post* provided a political and moral framework for the next decade of Black women's sexual and reproductive justice activism.[65]

More recently, an analysis of the opportunities for post-*Dobbs* reproductive justice activism by Suzanne Staggenborg, a sociologist who studies social movements and abortion politics, compared opportunities for activism in the *Roe v. Wade* and post-*Dobbs* periods. She concluded that the *Dobbs* decision created opportunities for the reproductive justice movement to switch from defending *Roe* to developing strategies to attract new supporters and build broader coalitions to oppose the constellation of attacks on women's rights.[66] These deeper assessments of changing political circumstances can help activists take a step back from the day-to-day struggles to reconsider and modify their long-term strategies and goals, a crucial task for an effective movement. More research evidence on the impact of health-enhancing and health-harming influences of current policies could guide this search for emerging windows of opportunity in the policy realm.

The *Dobbs* decision crystallized threats to reproductive justice that had been gathering over the years. On the one hand, it provided activists with both the opportunity and necessity of looking at the years since *Roe v. Wade* to ask what had and had not worked to expand access to quality abortion and other reproductive health services over the years. On the other hand, it required those committed to expanding reproductive justice to take a step back and ask, What do we need to do differently in this era? What new strategies, message frames, alliances, and goals will be needed in the coming years to protect and expand sexual and reproductive health and justice for all people?

INTEGRATING EVALUATION INTO ACTIVIST CAMPAIGNS

While activists frequently think about and discuss the impact of their work, most do not use formal evaluation methods to assess their activities or the impact of their campaigns. Evaluation is not an end but a means to more effective work. So how can organizers and leaders of activist campaigns better integrate an evaluation perspective into their ongoing work?

A starting point might be in the planning stages to identify all the possible outcomes of a campaign or a series of campaigns. Such a list would enable campaign planners to discuss which outcomes were their highest priority, what resources would be needed to make progress on each, and how the group could determine the level of success on each.

Based on her review of activism on reproductive health justice in South Africa, reproductive rights researcher and evaluator Barbara Klugman concluded that "failure to maintain strong organizations and continually rethink strategies contributed to the loss of government accountability and focus on implementation of new policies."[67] In other words, by focusing only on whether they got the policy they wanted, activists missed opportunities for ongoing learning to improve the success of their efforts and to plan the ongoing pressure that could ensure that the policy was fully enacted. To remedy this problem, Klugman proposed a broader approach to evaluation and identified seven outcomes that evaluators of activism can assess to gain practical insights into strengthening their work.[68] Using Klugman's suggested outcomes for assessing progress,[69] I list the types of questions health activists in New York have asked about their campaigns for each outcome.

SEVEN OUTCOMES THAT ACTIVISTS CAN ASSESS TO STRENGTHEN THEIR WORK

1. Strengthened organizational capacity

- Did the campaign leave our organization better able to take on the next issue?
- Did our organization develop new ways to find financial support or manage our resources?

- Did we increase our capacity to identify and nurture new leaders?

2. Strengthened base of support and alliances

- Did we forge new alliances and coalitions with new constituencies?
- Did we win institutional support for our goals?
- Did we expand our membership?

3. Increased data and analysis from a social justice perspective

- Did we gather and analyze different kinds of evidence from a variety of sources to make our case to decision-makers?
- Did we use diverse sources of evidence to assess our campaign's successes in improving health and social justice?
- Did our campaign lead government agencies or businesses to make useful new data available to the public?
- Did we create ongoing alliances with researchers who could help collect and analyze data?

4. Increased support for a specific problem definition and policy options

- Did we change the way key actors defined the problem we were taking on?
- Did we add new policy options to the remedies policymakers were considering?
- Did our proposed solutions win media and public attention?
- Did we gain public support for our goals?

5. Increased visibility of the issue in policy processes resulting in positive policy outcomes

- Was our group successful in identifying and using "windows of opportunity" to advance our policy goals?
- Did our activities put our issue higher on policymakers' agenda?

- Did community residents and neighborhood organizations win new rights to participate in making decisions on our problem of interest?

6. Shift in social norms

- Which public beliefs need to change for our campaign to achieve longer-term successes?
- Did public understanding and support for our values and the changes our group proposed increase?
- Did our campaign "de-normalize" the beliefs or institutional practices of our opponents?[70]

7. Changes in impact

- Did the health of our population of concern improve?
- Were inequalities in health reduced?
- Did our campaign lead to meaningful reductions in specific social injustices?

This expanded list of evaluation questions informed by Klugman's framework provides those wanting to assess their campaigns with several benefits. To start, it converts the yes/no binary of "Was our campaign effective?" into more than twenty questions, giving campaign planners an array of choices for evaluation that can match their interests, resources, and capacities.

Evaluators often seek to answer another question. After ascertaining whether or not any of the outcomes of interest have changed, evaluators also want to ask whether the observed change can be attributed to the activities under study, in this case activist campaigns and the policy changes it won. Being able to attribute desired changes to planned activities gives the leaders and evaluators of traditional or activist health interventions confidence that their efforts made a difference.[71]

To give an example, the Lunch for Learning campaign found that after the implementation of free universal lunches, the number of children eating lunch in school, the desired behavioral change, increased. But can this increase be attributed to the new policy rather than some other factor? Two studies provide relevant evidence. One, using school records of lunches served, found that an additional 26,000 New York City students were eating lunch at school—4.5 million additional meals per year—after the new policy compared to before, a bigger increase than had been observed in previous year-to-year data before the expansion.[72] A second study from researchers at Syracuse University determined that making free lunch available to all students boosted academic performance among New York City middle school students, again using before-and-after comparisons.[73] These two studies suggest that the campaign was effective in bringing about behavioral and educational changes and that it is likely that these changes can be attributed to the policy changes activists pursued.

By considering the questions proposed to assess Klugman's suggested outcomes and selecting those that are most relevant to their goals, resources, and evaluation capacity, organizers of health activist campaigns can create realistic and fit-for-purpose evaluation plans. From the campaign profiles in this book, coupled with the larger body of evidence on the evaluation of health activism,[74] I suggest some best practices for the evaluation of this activism. As organizers plan their campaigns, they should also plan their evaluation. The goal is to evaluate activities as they are launched.

STRATEGIES FOR EVALUATING ACTIVISM

By starting to think about evaluation as they begin to plan their campaigns, activists can gather the appropriate indicators of success, articulate the narrative of their campaign that they hope to document, and elicit suggestions from relevant actors such as participants, leaders, funders, and policymakers. The following recommendations, again based on the goals Klugman proposed, are listed in suggested sequential order of implementation.

BEFORE IMPLEMENTING CAMPAIGNS, ACTIVISTS SHOULD IDENTIFY OPTIONS FOR EVALUATION STRATEGIES AND POSSIBLE SOURCES OF SCIENTIFIC AND FINANCIAL SUPPORT

The scope of an evaluation is determined by the resources available. Some activists view evaluation as a diversion of resources from campaign activities. While understandable, this short-sighted view limits the capacity of activists to learn from their successes and failures or win new funding or political support for their policy goals. Many campaigns will not have the resources needed for a systematic or rigorous evaluation of their work. But every activist initiative can do something to assess impact, identify obstacles and facilitators, and gather evidence to inform next steps.

By creating a repertoire of evaluation strategies and methods and a checklist of possible sources of support, campaign organizers can consider their options. WE ACT for Environmental Justice, the Harlem-based environmental group, for example, has researchers on staff, partners with academic institutions, offers field placements for graduate students, and recruits local young people to help collect and analyze data. Depending on the resources available for any project, WE ACT can choose an affordable but appropriate mix of partners to assist with its evaluation activities.

ACTIVISTS AND THEIR RESEARCH PARTNERS SHOULD IDENTIFY PUBLIC EVIDENCE TO ASSESS THEIR CAMPAIGNS

Using public evidence (e.g., Health Department statistics on births, deaths, or illnesses) is an effective way to reduce the demand for organizational resources for evaluation and to institutionalize monitoring. Campaigns can work to convince government agencies that they should collect, analyze, and report to the public data that monitors the implementation and impact of the policies that activists seek to win. Requiring the city's public hospitals to monitor implementation of sterilization guidelines, the Department of Education to report levels of participation in school breakfast and lunch programs, and the Department of Health to analyze racial/

ethnic disparities in maternal morbidity and mortality and make their findings publicly available and accessible illustrate this approach.

ACTIVISTS SHOULD ENGAGE COMMUNITIES EXPERIENCING PROBLEMS TO EVALUATE CAMPAIGN IMPACT

In recent decades, both activist groups and researchers have promoted the benefits of community-based participatory research, also called participatory action research. This approach uses community members as well as researchers to design the evaluation, collect and analyze data, and prepare and present the results. Its proponents argue that it can provide additional insights into a given problem and its perception among the affected populations, new ideas for solutions and communications campaigns, and another way to engage residents in activist campaigns.[75]

For groups such as ACT UP, Make the Road New York, or the Young Lords, whose participants are themselves from the communities they seek to organize, participatory research can include these members, although ensuring representation of all sectors of the community can be difficult. Groups with professional staff may need to enlist their constituencies' members in recruiting community researchers and to create opportunities for participation that diminishes power differentials. United Bronx Parents, the educational reform group in the South Bronx, WE ACT, UPROSE (an environmental justice group in Sunset Park, Brooklyn), and other activist campaigns have hired and trained young people from the community and created youth councils where young community residents can forge their opinions on their own, then discuss them with the group's staff and leaders.[76]

In their interactions with legislators and policymakers, many activist organizations recognize that their members can use their own experiences to educate key decision-makers. "We are the true experts, the only experts, we who have had abortions," said the Redstockings member who testified at the 1969 forum organized by New Yorkers for Abortion Law Repeal to write the bill that served as a model for New York State's legalization of abortion. Like researchers and scholars, those who have experienced a problem can contribute their insights into the policy process, another form of evidence to guide practice.

EVALUATORS SHOULD CHOOSE SOURCES AND METHODS FOR THEIR EVALUATION THAT ARE COMPELLING FOR THEIR PRIMARY AUDIENCES

Like a communications strategy or a political plan, an evaluation plan should choose the variety of sources and methods that will be most compelling for the various audiences the campaign planners want to reach. Politicians and journalists like stories, often told by their own constituents; health professionals want scientific data, collected using rigorous methods they understand; and citizens want to know how the proposed changes will improve their health or lives. By using the variety of methods that will engage key constituencies, evaluators can produce narratives that will build support for the campaigns they assess. Consulting experts in health communications, evaluation research, and of course community residents will enable activists and their evaluators to make more informed choices.

ACTIVISTS AND RESEARCHERS SHOULD ENCOURAGE RESPECT FOR SCIENCE AND EVIDENCE TO COUNTER DISINFORMATION AND CONSPIRACY THEORIES

In the last two decades, corporate leaders from fossil fuel, food, and pharmaceutical industries have led aggressive disinformation campaigns to counter the evidence that their products and practices harm health.[77] Right-wing political groups have promoted conspiracy theories about the harms of vaccinations, the origins of the COVID-19 pandemic, and the role of immigrants in crime and violence.[78] The Trump administration has used misinformation and disinformation campaigns to discredit the science that supports taking action on global warming, regulation of harmful corporate practices, and support for reducing health inequities.[79] These activities have contributed to a growing distrust of science and evidence, a trend that can also complicate the work of health activists and their supporters.

By creating a culture of respect for science and evidence, activists can counter disinformation campaigns and conspiracy theories. By assisting their supporters to analyze information, distinguish scientific claims from political opinions, and counter disinformation, activist organizations and their science and research supporters can mitigate the harmful impact of disinformation. And by insisting they will not succumb to the temptation to distort or make up evidence to support their case, even if it seems that everyone else does this, activists can maintain the trust of their constituents as well as honest policymakers.

CAMPAIGN LEADERS SHOULD MODIFY AND CHANGE THEIR APPROACHES TO EVALUATION AS CIRCUMSTANCES CHANGE

Finally, organizers benefit from taking a step back from the implementation of their campaign and its evaluation to ask certain key questions: "What should we be doing differently?" "How have politics or public perceptions changed such that what we planned a year or two ago needs to be reconsidered and perhaps modified?" And "What new questions has our work illuminated that we now need to include in our evaluation?" The CARASA report *Women Under Attack* illustrates this approach.[80]

A key goal of *Fighting for New York*, considered in the next chapter, is to understand how activists can use assessments of their campaigns conducted since 1965 to improve the effectiveness of future health activism in New York City and beyond. Synthesizing their own experiences, the documented practice-based evidence on the impact and outcomes of activism, and the relevant research studies provides activists, health professionals, and scholars with a powerful resource. Activists can use this eclectic body of knowledge to make their future work more effective and more successful.

10

WHAT NEXT?

Translating Lessons from Sixty Years of Health Activism in New York City Into Practice

For more than sixty years, health activists and social movements in New York City have battled to win new public resources for improving health and living conditions. They have mobilized to end health-harming business and government policies and practices, win improved access to vital services, and get more dignified and respectful treatment from New York's institutions for all sectors of the population.

A few examples of these movements' successes illustrate their contributions. More than a million New Yorkers get free or subsidized health care at the city's public hospitals and community health centers every year, services that community activists and health-care workers' unions have consistently defended against closure and budget cuts since before the city's 1975 fiscal crisis. Every school day almost a million New York City schoolchildren eat lunches and breakfasts that are tastier, healthier, and more culturally tailored than in the past. This food helps many children avoid hunger and food insecurity and saves overburdened parents from the daily time and expense of preparing meals to send to school. These improved meals are now free thanks to decades of activism by students, parents, teachers, and others.

In 2024, 795,000 New York City low-wage workers had their pay lifted to $16 an hour, thanks to an increase in the minimum wage, achieved after years of activism by Fight for $15 and other labor and community groups.[1] This increase earned these workers an additional $2.3 billion a year in income, an average raise of almost $3,000 per year. And since the COVID-19 pandemic, housing activists have persuaded legislators to pass new laws ensuring the right to counsel in housing court, a moratorium on evictions during the pandemic, and added pressure on the court system to enforce these new rights. As a result of these changes, thousands of families have avoided the heartache, stress, or descent into homelessness resulting from evictions. Between 2016 and 2024, evictions in the city dropped by nearly 26 percent.[2]

These examples illustrate some of the concrete improvements in living conditions that health activists have contributed over the years, making New York City a healthier and fairer place to live.

Activist campaigns have failed too, of course, as described in previous chapters. Despite broad public support for universal health care, no such law for New York State has yet been approved since the first such bill was introduced in 1991. Immigrant New Yorkers, long targeted by city, state, and federal politicians who see them as convenient scapegoats, face greater legal and health perils than ever. There are still 1.2 million city residents who face food insecurity or hunger. In 2024, more than 140,000 people experienced homelessness on any given night, an increase of 127 percent since 2022.[3] In the 2024–2025 school year, more than 154,000 public school students experienced homelessness—a record high.

NEW THREATS TO HEALTH, NEW OPPORTUNITIES FOR ACTIVISM

At the start of the second quarter of the twenty-first century, New York City faces a cascade of new and recurrent threats to health, social justice, and democracy. But, as in the past, every threat also presents new opportunities for activism, resistance, and political mobilization. By looking across the health campaigns profiled in *Fighting for New York*, I hope to identify some approaches that activists, health professionals, and scholars can use to overcome threats to the well-being of the people of New York and other cities.

EMERGING AND RECURRENT THREATS

In the first quarter of the twenty-first century, a cascade of medical, environmental, political, and social threats bombarded New York City, adding new perils to health and social justice. These include a rising burden of chronic diseases such as diabetes, cardiovascular diseases, and psychiatric illnesses; the persistence of infectious diseases such as tuberculosis, syphilis, and HIV infection; and acute epidemics of COVID-19, mpox, measles (in 2018–2019), pneumonia, and influenza.

Recurrent environmental and climate threats including hurricanes, heat waves, floods, droughts, smoke, and pollutants from fires (both local and from as far as Canada and California) have sickened or killed tens of thousands of New Yorkers. As always, these have disproportionately burdened those exposed because of their age, low incomes, poor health, racial and ethnic characteristics, or social isolation.

High and growing levels of income and wealth inequality, exacerbated by tax cuts for the wealthy, leave a tiny fraction of New Yorkers living in luxury while forcing millions of middle- and working-class residents to struggle for adequate and affordable housing, food, health care, childcare, and employment. At the same time, new right-wing authoritarian movements and political leaders have espoused austerity budgets that cut safety-net programs, enacted policies to demonize recent immigrants, LGTBQI residents, and homeless people, and strived to undermine democratic reforms on voting, public participation, and campaign contributions.

A defining characteristic of the current period are the persistent efforts to roll back the advances of the 1960s movements and to return to what supporters of this path view as traditional American values of the past. An effective movement for the future must confront this nostalgia for an often imaginary past, frequently spiced with racism, misogyny, and homophobia. Health might serve as one focal point for this alternative vision, a unifying common ground for all those concerned about their own well-being, as well as that of their families and their communities.

The Make America Healthy Again (MAHA) movement instigated by Donald Trump and his secretary of health and human services, Robert F. Kennedy Jr., similarly claims nostalgia for a healthier past.[4] But both public health experts and the real-life experience of many ordinary Americans confirm that closing the gap between actual population well-being and the potential given the nation's wealth and scientific knowledge is a future project still to be realized, not a past accomplishment.[5]

OBSTACLES TO A REVITALIZED HEALTH MOVEMENT

To mobilize a successful movement for health in the coming years, activists will need to overcome three major obstacles—backlash, distrust of science, and growing feelings of hopelessness. Backlash, defined as the negative reaction of significant sectors of a population to a social or political development, emerged in response to the civil rights, labor, women's, and environmental movements of the 1960s. In the health arena, fights to legalize abortion, defund the police, close the Rikers Island Detention Center, improve care for people with mental illness, and pass universal health care also triggered opposing constituencies.[6] Backlash forces activists to consider how they can effectively anticipate, prevent, or mitigate this threat.

Second, distrust of science and evidence has grown, encouraged by false or exaggerated claims by Big Pharma, Big Oil, the food industry, government health agencies, and activists from both the right and the left.[7] In the last few years, the MAHA movement led by Robert F. Kennedy Jr. has co-opted some of the left-wing critiques of corporations and government and blended them with its own dark conspiratorial theories on vaccinations, autism, food, and other health issues.[8] In the future, activists committed to health and social justice must find ways to confront the frequent misuse of science and demand that government, scientists, corporations—and activists—use evidence appropriately.

Finally, a growing epidemic of hopelessness makes it more difficult for activists to mobilize, organize, and maintain their own optimism about a better, healthier, more just future.[9] This pessimism about the future, transmitted by person-to-person contact as well as by mass and social media, infects activists across age, class, and population groups. In recent years, hopelessness has served as a powerful deterrent to activism and organizing, a fact recognized by those who deliberately promote the view that the current political reality is inevitable and unavoidable.

In the coming decades, effective activism will need to confront both the political, social, and economic threats to health and the psychological and cultural forces that discourage people from fighting for their health. Fortunately, the current era also opens some new doors for activists.

NEW OPPORTUNITIES

Despite—or sometimes because of—these threats, activists and social movements also have new opportunities to confront the obstacles that can undermine their success. First, it is clear that business as usual is not working. The worsening environmental, health, and economic impact of global warming threatens the survival of humans and the planet's other life while public policy on health, strong safety nets, and democracy in the United States is moving backward. Despite public and scholarly recognition that rising inequality endangers the economy and health of New York and the nation,[10] the 2008 fiscal crisis, the COVID pandemic, and the budget and policy priorities of the Trump administration separately and together have widened inequalities. As the status quo becomes more problematic for more people, more people are open to seeking alternatives.

Second, in the past two decades, waves of activism have swept New York City and the nation. Occupy Wall Street, Black Lives Matter, #MeToo, the Sunrise Movement (young climate activists who emerged to promote the Green New Deal), Fight for $15, the 2017 Women's March on Washington and the national mobilizations against Trump's Muslim ban, as well as the 2025 No Kings days supporting immigrant rights, federal funding for research, and support for democracy, and continuing widespread opposition to the Russian invasion of Ukraine and Israel's decimation of Gaza and the West Bank, show that protest and activism are alive and energetic. Together they provide evidence that, as always, a desire for a better, fairer, healthier world moves people to act. The policy successes of these activists have been mixed, but their impact on the national discourse has been profound.

Despite the national rightward drift of the last few years, local activist groups continue to mobilize New Yorkers and their communities. In 2024 and 2025 alone, the North Star Fund, a longtime philanthropic supporter of the city's grassroots activism, has funded more than sixty-five activist groups to organize, educate, and take action to address dozens of social justice issues, another indicator that the history of the people of New York fighting for a more just city continues.[11]

Third, public opinion polls show that many New Yorkers—and many in other parts of the United States—support some of the more transformative ideas of activists and social movements.

- A 2022 poll of New York State residents by the Community Service Society found that 58 percent of New Yorkers favored big, fundamental changes to the health system to make health care more affordable, with only 27 percent supporting smaller, more modest changes.[12] A 2024 Gallup national survey found almost two-thirds of Americans believe that the federal government should ensure that all Americans have health insurance coverage, and just one-third disagree.[13]
- In 2024, a survey of crime victims in New York City found that 80 percent think incarceration generally worsens mental illness and increases the safety risk when people leave incarceration. Nearly 90 percent of New York City crime victims support moving people who have mental illness and addiction issues from jails into secure treatment facilities.[14]
- More young people have negative views of capitalism and favorable views of socialism than in the past. A 2021 Gallup poll found that just under half of young Americans aged eighteen to thirty-four had a positive view of capitalism—down nearly twenty points from a decade earlier. Meanwhile, a 2025 survey by the Cato Institute and YouGov found that

62 percent of Americans aged eighteen to twenty-nine say they hold a "favorable view" of "socialism."[15]

These surveys show that even when public officials and business interests oppose progressive reforms, the broader public often supports such change. This suggests that activists may not need to spend so much time convincing people to alter their views and can instead work harder to build the political power to convert majority views into public policy.

Fourth, as this book and its more than six hundred references show, activists and scholars have created an extensive body of evidence documenting which strategies usually work and which often fail. Organizers and activist leaders can leverage this practice-based evidence into pragmatic guides to action.

Fifth, the emergence of the MAHA movement provides health activists with an opportunity to engage many Americans who share concerns about the health status of the American people and disagree with the often weird and dangerous solutions proposed by President Trump and HHS Secretary Robert F. Kennedy Jr. The "again" in the MAHA slogan also enables those opposing Trump and his Make America Great Again (MAGA) movement to question the nostalgic reverence for a past characterized by ill-health and poverty for many. It thus offers health activists the opportunity to propose an alternative vision for future well-being.

National public opinion polls in 2025 showed that large majorities of American voters agree with some MAHA positions—95 percent want fresh fruits and vegetables with every school lunch, 96 percent support warning labels on foods with high levels of chemicals, and 93 percent say bureaucrats should disclose ties with drug and food companies.[16] Another poll found that 63 percent of voters support banning artificial dyes, 66 percent favor stricter FDA review of food additives, and 51 percent endorse restricting ultra-processed foods in federal programs.[17] However, this poll also found that 55 percent oppose the decision to cut twenty thousand federal health agency jobs and 44 percent worry that Kennedy's policies overall may endanger public health (compared to the 33 percent who feel his policies will result in a healthier population).

Moreover, as Erin McAleer, a food advocate in Massachusetts, observed, "We Can't 'Make America Healthy Again' Without SNAP and Medicaid."[18] The cuts in the federal budget for public benefits, scientific research, and the support of local and state public health agencies will endanger the health of many people. By looking for principled common ground with MAHA followers and articulating the differences, health activists may find they can attract new supporters.

The polarized debate about the country's response to the COVID-19 pandemic has left the American people confused and upset, which presents an opportunity for public discussion about what policies will best protect the American people.[19] To this end, activists must consider certain key questions: How can our country find the right balance between individual and collective responsibility for protecting health? What roles should the evidence produced by scientists play in setting policy? How can the public assess evidence without falling into unquestioning trust or paranoid conspiracy theories? And what role should tobacco, food, pharmaceutical, fossil fuel, and health-care corporations play in setting public policy? A movement that creates spaces for these conversations has the potential to gain new trust and win new supporters. Community activists may be better positioned to convene these forums and engage new supporters than academics or scientists.

Finally, in the last several years, a new progressive movement has emerged in New York City, a movement that is willing to combine electoral politics with street protests, lead community struggles while also joining citywide, regional, national, and global movements, and work across issues, populations, and identities. This nascent, diffuse, heterogeneous movement has contributed to the congressional election of Alexandria Ocasio-Cortes in 2019, the defeat of the Democratic state senators who voted with Republicans from 2011 until they were swept from office in 2018 (Independent Democratic Conference) by candidates supported by the Working Families Party (WFP), and the election of progressives like Jumaane Williams and Brad Lander to citywide offices.

The mayoral election victory of Zohran Mamdani in November 2025 expanded this trend. Mamdani's campaign recruited and trained tens of thousands of young people, made affordability for average New Yorkers the central issue, and offered an alternative to the business-as-usual mainstream candidates. Mamdani, a member of the New York Democratic Socialists of America (NYDSA), won more than 50 percent of the vote in the ranked-choice voting, defeating two mainstream but unpopular former Democrats, New York State Governor Andrew Cuomo and the incumbent Mayor Eric Adams, who also ran on an independent line.

While in his campaign Mamdani emphasized affordability, expanded housing, and inclusion rather than explicitly health and health care, his administration provides health and social justice activists with remarkable opportunities. In the coming years, the city's health movements and the mayor could advance a shared agenda that would seek to do the following:

- Align activist campaigns and legislative initiatives for health, social justice, and democracy.
- Create new avenues for democratic participation in community boards and public health agencies as well as sponsor popular assemblies to elicit community voices on key health issues.
- Begin to implement Mamdani's campaign proposals for free and fast public busses, public supermarkets, affordable housing, new mental health and community safety services, and free universal childcare. Progress on these measures would demonstrate both the potential for expanding the public sector to meet people's needs and more effective ways for city government to tackle the social determinants of health.
- Forge new and effective alliances among activists, community organizations, and political parties, including progressive Democrats, NYDSA, and WFP.

Long-standing opponents of a more just city and nation—the 1 percent and their billionaire leaders, the finance, insurance, and real estate business sectors, MAGA sponsors, and the wealthy and middle-class communities who have long insisted that desegregated, undesirable, or unsafe facilities should not be located in their backyards—will of course oppose such an agenda. But the emerging coalition that elected Mamdani, the rising costs of food, health care, and housing, and the growing bipartisan support for affordability provide grounds for cautious optimism.

How this budding movement can survive and thrive in New York in the age of Trump and his MAGA and MAHA movements remains to be seen. But growing ties among groups like Make the Road New York, the close Rikers campaigns, Housing Justice for All, and Fight for $15 show the potential for an alliance that includes local health and social justice campaigns, political activists from more progressive political parties, and representatives of the national social movements active in the city.

In sum, despite threats to the health of New York City, the opportunities for building a stronger movement to fight for health and social justice have never been greater—nor has the need been more urgent. The burning question, of course, is what activists and their supporters can do tomorrow, next year, and in the coming decade to realize these opportunities.

TOWARD A HEALTH JUSTICE ALLIANCE FOR NEW YORK—AND OTHER CITIES

What kind of activism can create a movement that can effectively fight for health in New York City in the coming decade? A New York City health justice alliance, the name I suggest, could build on the accomplishments, and overcome the weaknesses, of health activism in New York City of the last sixty years.[20] Such an alliance in New York and other cities could do a mixture of the following:

- Coordinate and align the work of a city's health campaigns, activist organizations, social movements, civil society groups, and sympathetic elected officials to build their collective power.
- Promote the ideas that all city residents have the right to health and that the role of government is to ensure that its policies, programs, processes, and practices make meaningful progress toward achieving that right.

- Create forums and social spaces where movement participants across sometimes siloed constituencies can identify shared goals and a common vision, but also debate differences in an environment of respect and collegiality.
- Develop communications and political strategies that welcome constituencies of diverse identities and experiences to jointly build political power to advance a shared agenda.
- Mobilize and organize both within and outside established political structures and processes, using both conventional and disruptive—good trouble—strategies and tactics to advance their policy and other goals.
- Build ongoing and sustainable alliances to advance shared goals with social movements and activists in other sectors, other cities, and other movements.

The activists, community leaders, health professionals, concerned residents, and committed political representatives who create the New York City health justice alliance will need to translate these broad goals into a specific platform and strategies attuned to current circumstances.

Is the development of a cross-cutting health movement for New York and other cities an ambitious, idealistic, and possibly extravagant and naive aspiration? Of course it is, especially in the current political climate. But given the dark plans that right-wing and corporate actors put before the American people, isn't a more hopeful plan a welcome relief for those urgently seeking alternatives? At a time when progressive people struggle to move beyond defensive reactions to each new assault on health, democracy, and fairness, citywide health justice movements can begin to create a coherent and comprehensive alternative vision for the future.

Other ideas—democracy, equity, human rights, or a sustainable planet—can also serve to unify and build the power of disparate movements and campaigns, but health has the potential to engage people across physical and social borders; connect emotions, politics, and everyday lives; and highlight the gap between what is and what could be.

I propose a health justice alliance for New York and other cities to encourage activists and their supporters to develop longer-term plans for the coming years, to move from reactive to visionary strategies, and to inspire others to propose additional long-term strategies for health movements.

ORIGINS OF CROSS-CUTTING HEALTH MOVEMENTS

The idea for a more comprehensive health movement is not new. In 1978, the World Health Organization issued the Declaration of Alma-Ata, which proclaimed the universal goal of "Health for All," stating that health is a fundamental human right and the aim of social and economic development.[21] Twelve years later, recognizing that an activist force was needed to make progress on the health-for-all goal, a People's Health Assembly brought together 1,450 grassroots activists and health professionals from ninety-two countries in Savar, Bangladesh, to produce a People's Health Campaign for Health for All Now!, a People's Charter for Health, and eventually an organization called the People's Health Movement (PHM).[22]

In 2025, PHM celebrated its twenty-fifth anniversary and reiterated its founding premise that the World Health Organization had failed to make progress toward its ambitious goal of health for all, and that more forceful activist movements were needed to restore that vision. At the celebration, Roman Vega, PHM's global coordinator, acknowledged that "We continue to face many of the same challenges. . . . We won't achieve Health for All unless we confront capitalism."[23] A successful movement will need to find accessible, compelling ways to talk about capitalism and its impact on the city and the planet.

Today, the PHM organization is a global network of grassroots health activists, civil society organizations, and academic institutions concentrated in the Global South. PHM currently has chapters in more than seventy countries,[24] including a few groups working in the United States. PHM seeks to connect activists from around the world to focus their efforts and amplify their voices. The proposal for a New York City health justice alliance borrows and modifies the PHM concept and gives it an urban focus.

For the most part, PHM activists work at the national and global levels.[25] However, some activists have attempted to organize at the city or regional level, as has happened in, for example, Bologna, Italy, Cape Town, South Africa, and Edinburgh, Scotland.[26] Synthesizing the lessons from these local endeavors can help to inform urban people's health movements in other cities.

This idea for a city-based health movement also draws on other national and global urban health initiatives, such as WHO's Healthy Cities program. WHO calls Healthy Cities "a strategic vehicle for health development and well-being in urban settings" and a force for implementing the urban-focused Sustainable Development Goals of the United Nations.[27] Additional initiatives seek to improve the health of urban populations in both the Global South and Global North.[28] In the later nineteenth and first half of the twentieth centuries, New York City was home to several cross-cutting reform movements that mobilized residents to improve housing, sanitation, access to healthy food, health care, and other necessities of life, a history that can inform and inspire future rounds of activism.[29]

The distinguishing features of PHM's transformative approach are its focus on partnerships with activists and social movements, rather than solely with health departments and city governments; on addressing the social, political, and commercial determinants of health, rather than mainly the behavioral and medical ones (such as tobacco, diet, physical activity, and health-care utilization); and its willingness to confront governments and businesses as needed, rather than concentrate on achieving consensus among these parties.

The accounts of activist campaigns and their lessons from US cities such as Los Angeles, Chicago, Detroit, and San Francisco provide further evidence to inform the creation of a health justice alliance for New York City.[30] A separate useful body of scholarship provides activists and academics with detailed descriptions of health movements and their interactions with other actors in other cities, often extracting cross-cutting lessons from comparisons across places.[31]

Another source for guidance on building a cross-cutting health movement for New York City comes from analyses of activism in cities in the Global South where social movements, often in partnership with labor unions and political parties, have long played a leading role in fighting for health. Princeton sociologist Benjamin Bradlow's comparison of the relationships between social movements and municipal governments in São Paulo, Brazil, and Johannesburg, South Africa, for example, offers insights that can inform the development of a health justice movement in New York City.[32]

Based on interviews with 225 activists and city officials in São Paulo and Johannesburg, Bradlow identified several movement practices in these cities that shaped how the interactions between city governments and social movements influenced policy and politics. His focus was on movements working in housing and land use in those cities, two sectors that influence health.

First, Bradlow concluded that movements more successfully influence government policy and practice when they emphasize citywide demands, rather than those of specific neighborhoods or communities. In Johannesburg, he found that powerful businesses and elite institutions had a stronger voice in city government than in São Paulo, leading South African activists to focus on the community or neighborhood level, where they believed they could make more progress. However, Bradlow noted that the campaigns of these groups often focused narrowly on demanding more effective administration of government programs in their community, rather than on changing policy or redistributing resources. In São Paulo, labor unions and social movement organizations have created a stronger presence in city government, making it possible for activists to advance their agendas for redistribution and policy change at that level.

Bradlow noted the greater success of citywide action in São Paulo compared to Johannesburg; in South Africa, wealthy powerful actors were often able to block citywide campaigns, forcing these movements to focus instead on local campaigns. The implication is that urban social movements should make limiting the power of those elite actors who support an unjust status quo a strategic priority, a goal easier said than done.

Second, Bradlow found that when activists worked closely with progressive political parties, they won a greater voice in city government than when they ignored or opposed all political parties. Having progressive political parties and officials within city government facilitated that process. In Johannesburg, sectarian conflicts and government and business corruption made it more difficult for social movements to work inside city government.

Third, in São Paulo, activists moved back and forth between city government and social movement organizations, creating channels of communication and cooperative interpersonal networks. In Johannesburg, social movement organizations were less integrated with political parties. Their memberships were place- and community-based rather than oriented to a wider agenda, and this limited their participation in the shaping of government policy.

Bradlow determined that the housing movements he studied had complex reciprocal relationships with political parties and municipal governments, and the nature of their interactions influenced their effectiveness. He concluded that "housing movements make local states and local states make housing movements," and "movements shape parties and parties shape movements."[33] His findings reinforced similar conclusions by social movement scholar Sidney Tarrow, who has looked at these issues in the United States.[34]

In the final analysis, activists' skills in building on the successes and overcoming the limitations of the last sixty years of activism depend not on what they say or think but on what they do in the real world. From the accomplishments of the activist campaigns profiled in previous chapters, the analysis of other historical and scholarly accounts of social movements and health activism, and my own observations of New York City's popular mobilizations on health in recent decades, I suggest six approaches that activists can deploy in the coming decades to create a powerful, effective health justice movement in New York City.

ACTIONS TO BUILD A MOVEMENT THAT CAN FIGHT FOR HEALTH IN THE NEXT DECADE

How can activists in New York City accelerate the transition from siloed alliances of activist campaigns, organizations, and movements to a more coordinated, aligned, and successful movement? How can they win more campaigns, build stronger coalitions and networks, and become a more influential force in enabling New York City to become a global showcase for healthier and more just cities? I suggest six approaches.

MAKE BUILDING POWER AND INFLUENCE THE LONG-TERM PRIORITY

Educating, mobilizing, and organizing are each important movement activities. But they are not ends in themselves. Their ultimate goal is to build a movement that has the political power to win changes that will lead to improvements in people's health and more equitable access to the necessities of life.

In an 1857 speech at Canandaigua, New York, the abolitionist leader Frederick Douglass famously said, "Power concedes nothing without a demand. It never did and it never will. . . . The whole history of the progress of human liberty shows that all concessions yet made to her august claims have been born of earnest struggle."[35]

One hundred sixty years later, Kimberlé Crenshaw, the Black feminist activist and scholar, elaborated on Douglass's idea: "It's not about supplication, it's about power. It's not about asking, it's about demanding. It's not about convincing those who are currently in power, it's about changing the very face of power itself."[36]

Through their actions, New York City activists have shown their understanding of the importance of power. When the close Rikers campaigns demanded that the detention center be shut, when Lunch for Learning insisted that all school lunches be free, and when feminist activists called for access to safe and legal abortion for all, they knew they were forcing powerful actors to relinquish something they wanted because more people wanted something else.

The work of developing a strategy to build power needs to be tailored to the specific circumstances and the demands that activists make. But the goal of building power can be a tool for focusing campaigns. As author-activist Jane McAlevey wrote, using the language of Occupy Wall Street, "In the organizing approach, specific injustice and outrage are the immediate motivation, but the primary goal is to transfer power from the elite to the majority, from the 1 percent to the 99 percent."[37] By keeping that goal front and center, activists can make informed decisions on what to do first, next, and thereafter, a process McAlevey describes in her portrait of Make the Road New York.[38]

ORGANIZE COALITIONS AND CAMPAIGNS THAT BRING TOGETHER DIVERSE CONSTITUENCIES

Another way to build power is to organize coalitions and campaigns that recognize the value of bringing together activists with different social identities (intersectional), those fighting in different sectors such as housing, health care, and labor (intersectoral), and those looking to bring benefits to all members of society (the sum-of-us universalists). Such alliances have broader appeal and the potential for winning more power than those that include only one group. The profiles of Make the Road New York, ACT UP, Lunch for Learning, Fight for $15, Housing Justice for All, and the various close Rikers Island campaigns show some of the ways that organizers of activist campaigns built such coalitions.

New York City activists have found many ways to use their coalitions to advance cross-cutting health issues and to link their campaigns to national and global initiatives. In 2023, for example, Metro NY, the group supporting New York State's universal health care bill, joined with Make the Road New York, the New York City Immigration Coalition, and several other groups to support the Coverage for All Coalition's effort to expand health-care coverage to low-income New Yorkers, regardless of their immigration status. Their proposal aligned the interests of low-wage workers and immigrants, two populations too often pitted against each other. At a rally in 2023 urging New York's governor to sign the bill, demonstrators dropped off empty medicine bottles to the governor's office to emphasize the importance of ensuring prescription drug coverage to everyone, including undocumented immigrants.[39]

Well-crafted coalitions facilitate bringing together constituencies harmed by a health or social problem, even when they differ in class, race/ethnicity, geography, gender, or other social characteristics. Coalitions can also unite groups working on different but related problems, such as advocates wanting to improve school food and those seeking better education for their children.

Successful coalitions create the potential for building sufficient power to initiate changes in policies and structures long opposed by entrenched political and business interests. Alliances can birth and nurture learning communities that bring people together across identities and sectors to analyze a campaign's successes, limitations, and changing political opportunities. This is especially important since many activist campaigns take years, even decades, to achieve their goals. Thus, developing effective mechanisms for assessing progress and responding to changing political and social contexts becomes vital.

Since the organizations participating in a New York City health justice alliance would be even more diverse and heterogeneous than the problem- or population-based coalitions described in the profiles, reaching agreement on a plan of action will be difficult. There is no alternative, I believe, to an incremental, trial-and-error approach. Activists will have to learn from their experiences, correct mistakes, and, over time, create decision-making processes and organizational cultures that can help New York City more fully realize its potential for better, more equitable health.

A city health justice alliance could also become the space where coalitions are formed to achieve a specific purpose. Organizers with years of experience negotiating coalitions in different settings on multiple issues could become the facilitators in this coalition incubator, saving groups the years of strenuous effort now often devoted to building such alliances.

EXPAND FROM SEEKING ONLY INCREMENTAL CHANGE TO ALSO PURSUING TRANSFORMATIVE CHANGE

The campaigns of Metro New York Health Care for All (described in chapter 8) to pass a universal health care act in New York State showed the tension between concentrating on incremental changes or transformative changes. With time, the group identified opportunities for aligning the two goals. As Mark Hannay, its director, explained, "Our member-partners support the broad range of policy goals from incremental reforms to Medicare-for-All, and so we understand our work to be not either-or but rather both-and, to advance toward health care for all across New York and the U.S."[40]

Health activists have found several ways to make the transition. Selecting incremental changes that set the stage for more profound transformations is one way. ACT UP used its success in lowering the price for one drug, Azidothymidine (AZT), to raise the larger question of what should be the government's role in setting drug prices to limit predatory pricing and ensure equitable access to all essential medicines. This question remains on the global and national health policy agenda today with some progress since ACT UP's partial victory.

Another approach, discussed in the profile of the campaigns to close Rikers, focuses first on an attainable win—the shutting of the jails on Rikers Island—and then moving on to the larger goal of implementing criminal justice policies that create alternatives to incarceration. Activists should anticipate how to order their demands from modest to more ambitious to transformative to build momentum and win converts along the way.

The trajectory of New York's sexual and reproductive health and justice movement illustrates this process. Activists went from making abortion legal in New York in 1970 to ending sterilization abuse first in city hospitals, then in all medical centers in New York, and, by 1978, in federally funded hospitals. Between 1978 and 2022, each level of government passed and then expanded laws to protect pregnant workers from workplace discrimination, an obstacle to women's full participation in the workforce as well as a threat to their health. In 2019, in the face of threats to the Supreme Court's *Roe v. Wade* decision, the state-level New York Reproductive Health Act codified and expanded previously federally protected abortion rights, shielding providers and facilities from legal challenges and ensuring insurance coverage for abortion.

This sixty-year-long march has strived to create a city and state that fully recognize the rights to reproductive justice for all people, as defined by Women of African Descent for Reproductive Justice in 1994,[41] and then modified by Sister Song a few years later.[42] Each new law or policy that activists won moved the needle in the right direction, set the stage for the next battle, and built support for the transformative vision of a still distant world where full reproductive justice was the norm rather than an aspiration.

Another dilemma for those balancing incremental and transformative change is when to compromise to achieve a partial win, and when to hold out for a more substantive victory. At the behest of employers and conservatives, proponents of the 1978 federal Pregnancy Discrimination Act agreed to exclude employers who had fewer than fifteen workers. They accepted this measure not because they believed these women were less in need of protection from discrimination, but because activists recognized that support from the small businesses who said they could not afford to pay leave would help achieve legislative approval. Although small employers were again excluded in the 2023 federal Pregnant Workers Fairness Act, in New York City and State, A Better Balance and its supporters were able to reduce the minimum number of employees to four, offering protection to a higher proportion of women.

Compromise always has costs and benefits. It can win new rights or protections for some while leaving other populations vulnerable, as the pregnancy discrimination example shows. It can also undermine the momentum of a growing movement. "The dilemma for a movement organization is that the very reforms it wins may defuse the crisis and lessen the incentives for people to continue to engage in protest," observed social movement scholars Frances Fox Piven and Richard Cloward.[43] In their book *Poor People's Movements: Why They Succeed, How They Fail* (1977), they contend that to achieve their social justice goals, activists should maximize the disruption they cause during periods of heightened social and economic crisis.

Table 10.1 compares the short-term goals with the more transformative longer-term aims of various New York City health activist movements. Every campaign and movement has a mix of both, and no litmus test can easily determine the best choice for a given time and struggle. Activists can make more informed decisions by mapping their options on this spectrum in advance and by plotting a trajectory from incremental to transformative informed by an assessment of the likely consequences of their choices. By resisting the temptation to put all their organizational resources into either the quest for short-term victories or the pursuit of societal transformation, activists can find the balance that has the potential to optimize both types of change.

To move from the short-term, incremental changes partially implemented in recent years to the more transformative changes needed to achieve our society's full potential for well-being will also require changing ideas, cultures, values as well as policies. Activists who seek to build power and change policy need to introduce new ideas and challenge cultures, beliefs, and values that harm health or justify inequality.

A few examples from the campaign profiles show how activists have done this:

- By popularizing the concept of environmental justice in New York City, WE ACT, the Harlem environmental group, promoted the idea that public policy should not disproportionately expose any community to pollution and toxins.
- Through the Stop the Church action, ACT UP and WHAM! challenged the Catholic Church's right to impose its religious beliefs on abortion, AIDS education in the schools, and gay marriage on all New Yorkers. ACT UP members argued the church should not be able to benefit both from its nonpartisan tax-exempt status and the First Amendment right to practice one's religion freely while also using its power and influence to violate the other part of the First Amendment, which prohibits the government from establishing or endorsing a specific religion.

TABLE 10.1 A Comparison of Short- and Long-Term Changes in Health and Social Justice in New York City

SECTOR/ DOMAIN	SHORT-TERM CHANGES	LONG-TERM CHANGES
Housing	Rent control; eviction moratorium; repairs to public housing; stronger and enforceable mandates for developers to include affordable housing in new projects	Social housing; expansion and improvement of public housing; stronger limits on rights of landlords vs. tenants; commitment and specific plan to end homelessness by a specified date
Health care	Expanded Medicaid; subsidized health care for the uninsured; legal protections of patients' rights; consistent support for public hospitals and health centers; parity for mental health and reproductive health services	Universal free health and mental health care for all residents, including primary and preventive care, medications, mental health services, and sexual and reproductive health care
Labor	Increased minimum wage; mandated benefits on sick leave, hours, health and safety protections; expanded rights to organize	Worker voice in all businesses; public support for worker cooperatives; growing public ownership; subsidies for childcare, health care, and transportation
Environment/ climate	Enforcement of existing environmental and climate regulations and standards; stronger emergency preparedness programs and funding; making New York City carbon neutral by 2050	Eliminate inequitable exposure to toxics, pollutants, and harmful impact of global warming; base environmental standards for safe air, water, and soil on precautionary principle*
Food	Protection and expansion of SNAP, Women, Infants, and Children (WIC), school meals, and other public food benefits; stronger and better-enforced rules to prevent misleading marketing of food, false health claims, or predatory pricing; more public support for urban and regional agriculture	Expand in new and significant ways public and nonprofit ownership of food retail and distribution; set policies, prices, and distribution of food retail to make it easier and less expensive to buy healthy than unhealthy food

TABLE 10.1 (*continued*)

SECTOR/ DOMAIN	SHORT-TERM CHANGES	LONG-TERM CHANGES
Transportation	Selected free bus or train routes; congestion pricing; added biking lanes and walking paths	All public transportation free; comfort, safety, and convenience of public transit significantly improved; added disincentives for car use; added train and ship lines to bring goods and services into the city
Criminal justice	Further reform of bail; close Rikers Island Detention Center; stricter rules around and enforcement of police accountability to end police abuse	New community safety and mental health services outside police department; policies to make incarceration rare and unnecessary through other social and safety policies; guaranteed rights to shelter, food, health care, and employment

* The precautionary principle posits that only policies and institutional practices whose safety has been proven should be implemented.

- By advocating for laws to ban discrimination against pregnant workers, A Better Balance advanced the value that both women and men were essential contributors to the New York City workforce and economy, and both deserved the same levels of protection against threats to health and safety, even when they faced different hazards based on their reproductive capacities.
- Through the mutual aid approach described in chapter 6, activist groups have combined direct services to people in need with embodying a vision of a more collective society where people caring for others is the norm (see figure 10.2).

By promoting ideas that challenge the status quo, activists can change public opinion, which in turn precipitates changes in policy. Activists have used mass media, social media, community forums, deep canvassing,

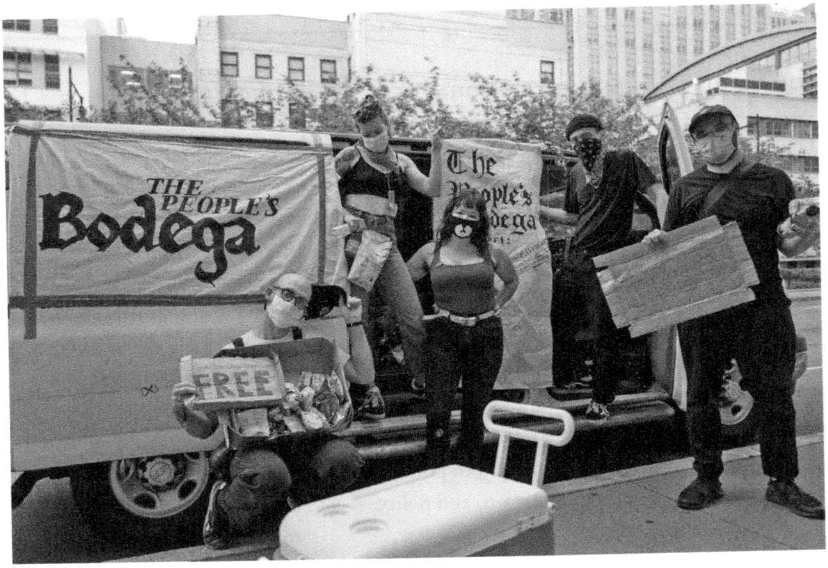

FIGURE 10.1 The "People's Bodega," a volunteer-led, mobile mutual aid initiative that provides essential supplies and resources to New York City protesters and those in need. It operates as a mobile store, delivering goods from a truck or van.

Source: Photo courtesy of Ian Reid. https://www.vogue.com/article/the-peoples-bodega-mutual-aid-nyc

ballot initiatives, public opinion polls, die-ins, posters, street demonstrations, and other methods to challenge conventional wisdom and to provoke informal conversations that lead to opinion change. Using these communications strategies, activists can shift public opinion to build deeper public understanding and support for proposed policy changes. In some cases, changes in policy and changes in public opinion can constitute a virtuous circle, each reinforcing the other.[44] New laws that enabled LGBTQI people to get married, for example, reflected and accelerated changes in public support for gay people.

In the next decade, a New York City health justice alliance and its member organizations can promote several cross-cutting actions to support the growth of this movement. These include the following activities:

- Defend science, fact-based evidence, and a commitment to truth to build support for healthier public policies.
- Affirm that all sectors of the population have a right to participate in making the decisions that shape their lives, an idea embodied in the slogan "nothing about us without us."
- Build the power and capacity of the labor movement, long a powerful actor in city politics and health care, to organize workers and influence public policies that support the well-being of workers and oppose those that undermine democracy and human rights.[45]
- Expand the public sector to create healthier and more affordable alternatives to the market-dominated sectors, such as food, housing, and medical care, that value profit over human well-being.
- Promote action to support the belief that the common good is as American as cherry pie, as valid a part of American culture as the veneration of individual responsibility.
- Combat the hopelessness promoted as the inevitable response to political or natural crises or hard times by powerful actors who benefit from the status quo.

A key role for social movements is to change public opinions that deter reforms.[46] By identifying the specific beliefs that support or challenge their goals, activists can make public opinion more favorable to their campaigns. The close Rikers campaigns, for example, portrayed mass incarceration as a threat rather than a boost to public safety, an idea that has won growing support from New Yorkers.

More broadly, urban health justice movements could bring together activist groups working across issues to identify the common beliefs that encourage or deter activism for health and to design coordinated, multifaceted strategies to build support for more favorable attitudes. Right-wing movements and their patrons in the United States have used this strategy successfully in recent decades.

In her book *Democracy in Chains*, the historian Nancy McLean describes how the Koch family foundations and the Atlas Network brought together think tanks, right-wing activists, wealthy individuals, foundations, and elected officials to define a common agenda and promote key ideas.[47] The Atlas Network seeks to "drive change in ideas, culture, and policy; remove barriers to opportunities; and empower individuals to live a life of choice." It partners with more than five hundred organizations around the world that share its commitment to market dominance, individual responsibility, low taxes, and limited regulation.[48] Since 1981, the network has played an important role in supporting the ideas and infrastructure of the radical right.

What might a hypothetical New York City–based Hygiea Network (named after the Greek goddess of health) designed to support the city's health justice alliance look like? It might include elements of some of the groups that have supported New York City activists since the 1960s—a few of which are described in chapter 8.

Like the Health Policy Advisory Center, the network could convene activists and academics from various health struggles to publish shared analyses. Like Popular Democracy, an outgrowth of Make the Road New York, such a network could provide economic analyses, policy reports, and guidance on communications to community organizations around the city and beyond, enabling cross-cutting learning across issues and places. Like Equity Advocates, a group that brings together those working on food justice in New York to exchange experiences and plan strategies, this network could convene groups across the many streams of health activism, thus helping to align equity-focused work across food, health care, housing, and sexual and reproductive justice.

Such a citywide network would of course require funding, leadership, and a vision. It is, however, a practical, feasible step toward a health movement for all of New York. By beginning to build this network, activists and their allies could create a common infrastructure and support system for the frequently siloed separate health campaigns. In the United States, previous movements like the civil rights movement, the women's movement, and the peace movement have benefited from such resources.[49] The World Social Forums have played a similar role on the global stage.[50]

ENGAGE MORE FULLY WITH GOVERNMENT AND POLITICAL SYSTEMS

Most of the activist campaigns for health in New York City have interacted with government in multiple ways, sometimes collaboratively, sometimes as adversaries. As Bradlow noted in his comparison of São Paulo and Johannesburg, the ongoing ties, the cross-cutting social networks, and the movement of activists into government positions and back to activism gave movements in São Paulo a greater ability to influence government policy than in Johannesburg, where activists were less engaged with government.

In New York, activists from health, housing, and other sectors have taken government-appointed positions as well as elected offices. Dr. Mary Bassett, a longtime health activist, worked as the New York City and State health commissioner before returning to human rights activism and scholarship. Dr. Helen Rodríguez followed her work with the Young Lords, CESA, and CARASA with a stint as the medical director of the New York AIDS Institute, the state agency that coordinated AIDS work.

On the electoral side, former Assembly Member Richard Gottfried served as an ongoing supporter and leader of the New York State universal health care campaign for decades (see figure 10.1). Julia Salazar, a housing organizer and a member of the Democratic Socialists of America, won election to the New York State Senate in 2018 and played an important role in steering new housing legislation through the state legislature in the following years. Ana Maria Archila, a founder of Make the Road New York, serves as codirector of the New York Working Families Party and (unsuccessfully) ran for lieutenant governor of New York in 2022.

Over the years, these and dozens of other activists have helped advocates to frame their asks in ways that legislators, mayors, and governors could hear. Working with other groups with relevant expertise and capacity, a New York City health justice alliance could build on this by pursuing the following goals:

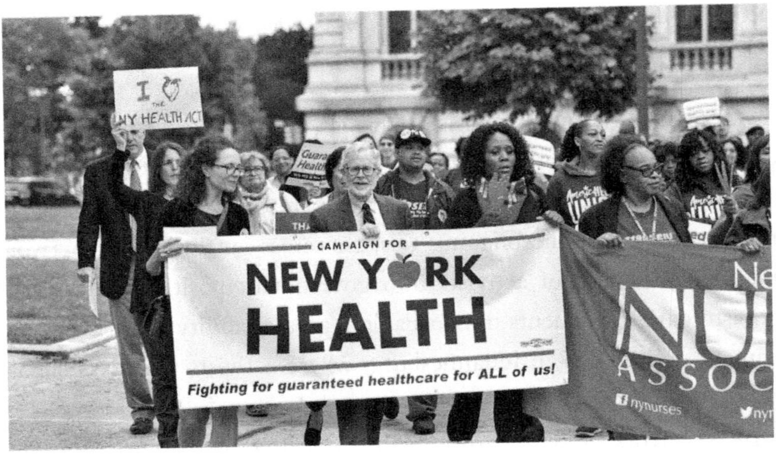
I THE NY HEALTH ACT
CAMPAIGN FOR
NEW YORK
HEALTH
Fighting for guaranteed healthcare for ALL of us!
ASSOC
nynurses

FIGURE 10.2 A 2019 demonstration in Albany in support of the New York State universal health care plan. New Yorkers have been organizing for a state universal health plan for more than thirty years. In the legislature, these efforts were led by now retired New York State Assembly Member and Health Committee Chair Richard Gottfried (at center of banner), the longest-serving member of the assembly at the time of his retirement. The New York State Nurses Association played a leading role in mobilizing support for the yet-to-be-passed legislation.

Source: https://www.metrohealthcare.net/end-of-session-health-care-bills-in-albany-part-3-expanding-health-insurance-coverage-may-19-2022/

- Training and supporting activists to run for elected office.
- Offering workshops and technical assistance to elected officials on health, health equity, and the various health issues facing government
- Partnering with the communications departments of Mayor Mamdani's office, the Health Department, and NYC Health + Hospitals to sponsor coordinated two-way informational campaigns during health emergencies.
- Developing a health platform and policy agenda for each election cycle, sponsoring candidate debates on the platform, and (within legal limits) endorsing candidates who sign on to this agenda.
- Inviting political parties to contribute to the platform and agenda and consider endorsing it.
- Conducting community forums and town hall meetings to discuss key health issues.

The goal of these activities is to build ongoing connections between activist organizations and the political system to facilitate collaborative action aimed at improving health and reducing health inequities.

ALIGN HEALTH, SOCIAL JUSTICE, AND DEMOCRACY FRAMES

From the 1960s to the 2020s, the city's activists pursued a complex blend of health, social justice, and democracy objectives. The Young Lords worked to prevent lead poisoning and tuberculosis; demand an end to discrimination against Puerto Ricans; and to claim a voice for neighborhood residents in running health centers, schools, and precincts. Sixty years later, Make the Road New York fought for a similar range of goals, adapted to the city's changing social, economic, and political conditions and the group's varied constituencies.

At best, these three intersecting goals widen a movement's base of support, open more doors to building power, and paint a more holistic vision of a better city and world. At worst, the multiplicity of aims confuses supporters, dissipates energy and momentum on any single issue, and makes it more difficult to achieve the consensus needed to move forward. How can activist campaigns find their sweet spot? How could urban health justice movements provide a framework for making wise strategic and tactical choices on aligning health, social justice, and democracy?

I suggest three ways to help activists answer these questions. First, activists should root their campaigns and messages in people's daily lives. Lead poisoning, for example, is experienced as a health problem for children, but it is also experienced as a social justice or educational problem. The parents of lead-poisoned children may have difficulty getting landlords to follow the law that requires them to clean up apartments or test for lead to prevent poisoning in the first place. Other tenants may resent landlords' failure to clean up buildings where children have previously been poisoned or the city's failure to enforce housing laws. Between 2017 and 2022, New York failed to collect $1.07 billion in fines from landlords for housing-law violations and unpaid property taxes,[51] a sum that could have repaired thousands of apartments to prevent poisoning.

Lead poisoning is a democracy problem too, as shown by the decades it took the New York City Council and various mayors to agree on strengthening laws to prevent lead poisoning, delays that were due primarily to lobbying by the real estate industry and landlords.[52] Even by 2025, lead poisoning laws did not adequately reflect scientific understanding of the best preventive practices.

Organizers can move away from the "one-size-fits-all" approach to a more layered one that incorporates the varied experiences and emotions of a range of supporters by offering multiple paths to action to reduce that problem. In childhood lead poisoning campaigns in New York City, some joined because their children were sick, others looked for a tool to pressure their landlord to make their home safer or for schools to better support their children with lead-induced learning problems, and still others sought to build the power of their tenants' union or neighborhood association.

To promote this approach, activists can train organizers to listen to their constituents and build coalitions with others who use health, social justice, and democracy frameworks. By doing so, health campaigns can create unified, coherent, and effective alliances and communications strategies to make compelling cases for policymakers, while simultaneously building the power that can force action.

A second reason to link these three frameworks is that the opponents of health activists' campaigns also link the three. The aggressive efforts of the Trump administration and its MAGA and Republican followers to cut health and social programs, repeal health and environmental regulations, demonize immigrants, shift the tax burden from the wealthy to the poor and working classes, and limit democratic rights such as voting and free speech provide current examples of coordinated attacks on health, social justice, and democracy, many informed by Project 2025, the Heritage Foundation's prescription for its right-wing vision for the nation.

In a similar effort from an earlier period, national and city business and political elites used the 1975 fiscal crisis to advance their efforts to cut back public health care, impose tuition at City University, implement the "planned withdrawal" of city services from low-income Black and Latiné neighborhoods, and delegate power from the mayor and the city council to an unelected Emergency Control Board of bankers and state officials.[53]

By showing the connections between policies that influence health, social justice, and democracy, activists can present a coherent explanation of why these threats emerge, provide a compelling alterative vision to the dark ones presented by political and business leaders, and invite a wide array of activists, civil society groups, and elected officials to join their movement.

A New York City health justice alliance could play a third role in aligning activism on health, social justice, and democracy by coordinating the practical division of labor across its members, reducing the time and energy needed from each individual organization. A cross-cutting communications team could develop shared messages to use across campaigns and issues. A movement coordinating committee could align communications from multiple streams of activism (e.g., housing, sexual and reproductive health, food) to emphasize its social justice aims, enabling a synergy of efforts that could amplify the cumulative impact of each group. By developing a common policy agenda, the alliance can create a system for endorsing candidates for city, state, and federal office who support its goals. Many individual groups already do this, but imagine the power of a health agenda supported by hundreds of activist organizations across the city.

EMBRACE A LONG-TERM PERSPECTIVE

Many activists in New York and around the country and world have been infected with the virus of hopelessness and despair since the 2016 and 2024 presidential victories of Donald Trump, the COVID pandemic, and the effort to roll back many of the accomplishments of the 1960s movements. They ask, If this man could be elected president not once but twice, and if we are moving backward confronting the global climate emergency, protecting democracy, and avoiding pandemics, what hope is there for our country?

While I understand this reaction and suffer myself from occasional bouts of gloom about the future of our world, in the lifetimes of those of us who are baby boomers, we have witnessed the elections of Richard Nixon, Ronald Reagan, and the two Bushes; unjust wars in Vietnam, Iraq, Palestine, and elsewhere; a pandemic or three; and the accelerating destruction of our environment. Our parents and older colleagues brought us up to recognize the violence of the anticolonial wars and the horrors triggered by the rise of Stalin, Nazism and fascism in Europe, the Cold War, the nuclear race, and the McCarthyism of the 1950s. So despair, hard times, and threats to survival are not new.

It is also true that in my lifetime, I have observed social movement victories that seemed unimaginable even a few years before they unfolded:

- The civil rights movement ended legal segregation in many of its most damaging forms.
- The environmental movement convinced many Americans and those in other countries to take action to protect human and planetary health from human-made threats.
- After a long period of decline, the labor movement has found new ways to organize precarious workers, immigrants, and women, and to build ties between community and labor organizing.
- The LGBTQI movement won the right of gay people to marry and popularized the value that these people should have the same rights as all Americans.
- The women's movement brought women into the workplace, moved women into leadership positions at every level of society, and normalized the belief that all people deserved the right to make their own decisions about sexuality and reproduction.

Of course, each of these movements had defeats as well as victories, and of course, every success was and continues to be challenged by a backlash from those who oppose these advances. But compared to the 1920s, the 1950s, or the 1970s, the successes of these and other social movements has made life better and improved health for millions of Americans.

From my perspective, two striking lessons from the history of activism in New York City are, first, how long it takes for simple ideas to be translated into practice, and second, how quickly, when conditions are right, ideas can move to policy and practice.

It took fifty years from the time the Black Panthers and the Young Lords raised the idea that children should not go to school hungry but ready to learn to 2017, when all New York City children were entitled to free lunches and breakfasts in their public schools.

Same-sex marriage had been an issue in New York State long before the Stonewall Uprising of 1969, and regained attention during the early days of AIDS. Despite several decades of organizing, court, and legislative decisions in 2006, 2007, and 2009 defeated efforts to legalize gay marriage in New York State. In 2011, however, the legislature approved and Governor Andrew Cuomo signed same-sex marriage legislation. Until that law passed, many observers believed that gay marriage could never be legal, but years of activism, changing windows of opportunity, and activist persistence led to a seemingly sudden victory.[54] In 2024, the New York State Constitution was amended to explicitly ban discrimination based on sexual orientation, further strengthening the state's legal recognition of same-sex marriage and the rights of LGTBQI people.

ACT UP members like Gregg Gonsalves, Sarah Schulman, Larry Kramer, and Maxine Wolfe, Helen Rodríguez of CESA and CARASA, WE ACT's Vernice Miller and Peggy Shepard, and dozens of other New York City activists provide a compelling argument for sticking with activist struggles. Over years, sometime decades, simply through their perseverance in making day-to-day decisions about how to cope with a specific defeat or leverage a specific victory, these leaders have served as role models for persistence and patience. They show that by playing the long game and being willing to modify tactics and strategy in the face of defeat, leaders of activist campaigns can inspire their members to find the endurance, determination, and courage to achieve success.

Like Alice in Wonderland, whom the White Queen urged to imagine several impossible tasks before breakfast, activists need to be able to master the seemingly impossible skill of operating simultaneously in two time frames—the hours, days, and weeks of the present, and the decades it often takes movements to achieve victories. By finding this two-track path, they maintain the impatience needed to pursue day-to-day opportunities for advancing their cause and develop the patience to wait for longer-term wins.

Every health campaign and every social movement in New York has left a record of its victories and defeats that can serve as a guide to action to overcome the health threats now on the city's horizon. In the coming years, a New York City health justice alliance can use this history to make the city a model for building an enduring movement that can advance well-being and promote social justice for all. Together, the activists, people, and institutions of New York can create another future for their city and other cities.

ACKNOWLEDGMENTS

It takes a movement or two to write a book like this. I am indebted to so many activists, scholars, health professionals, journalists, and organizations for the information and insights that informed *Fighting for New York*.

Over the years, I have had the privilege of observing, learning from, and in some cases interacting with many of the activists mentioned in this book. I especially thank Liz Accles, Mary Bassett, Joel Berg, Cecil Corbin, Kathy Goldman, Mark Hannay, Katrina Haslip, Iris Morales, Stanley Richards, Dr. Helen Rodrqiquez, Gabriel Sayegh, Peggy Shepard, and Cea Weaver for their inspiring work and words.

I have also had the good fortune to have academic colleagues, some at CUNY and others elsewhere, who have helped me shape the ideas in this book and whose work has informed my thinking over the years. These include Michelle Fine, Jerry Markowitz, and Jan Poppedieck, comrades of many decades, as well as Michael Carrera, Nevin Cohen, Josh Freeman, Sandro Galea, Alysha Galvez, Barbara Israel, Stephanie Luce, Terry McGovern, Meredith Minkler, Mark Naison, Marion Nestle, Ros Petchesky, Rayna Rapp, Diana Romero, David Vlahov, and Craig Willingham.

My students at CUNY have also been a vital source of information, through both their own activist and community experiences and the questions they raised in my classes. I am especially grateful to the PhD and master's students in my Health Activism in New York City courses in 2023 and 2024. Their case studies of activist campaigns in New York City deepened my understanding of a wide range of activism. I found the work of Juviza Rodriquez on campaigns to reduce maternal mortality, Sascha Garrey on PAIN's campaign against Purdue Pharmaceuticals, and Rachel Dannefer's work on the evaluation of activist campaigns especially helpful.

I have also relied on the many writers, activists, academics, and journalists who have written about health activism in New York City. Authors whose books, and subsequent conversation, have served as major influences on this work include Tamar Carroll, Susan Chambre, Johanna Fernández, Michelle Fine, Felicia Kornbluh, Stephanie Luce, Jerry Markowitz, Sandra Opdycke, Frances Fox Piven, Dana Lee Povitz, David Rosner, Sarah Schulman, Julie Sze, and Clarence Taylor.

Finally, friends and family have read and commented on earlier drafts, challenging me to refine and develop my ideas and words. Thanks to Nevin Cohen, Jerry Markowitz, Joanna Mishtal, Barbara Reisman, and Eric Scherzer, and Laurie Welch. My family—Wendy Chavkin, my partner, and Sasha, my son—are both skilled writers and editors, sometimes making our home seem like a writing workshop. For that feedback and everything else, I depend on these two unconditionally.

At Columbia University Press, Stephen Wesley and Alex Gupta provided unstinting support and guidance and Ryan Perks and Leslie Kriesel assisted in preparing the book for publication. Jonathan Cobb provided welcome additional editorial guidance. My deep thanks to them.

While this book depends on these and many others who gave generously of their ideas, experiences, and insights, the omissions and mistakes are mine. I look forward to seeing the revisions, corrections, and next chapters of this story that activists will create in the coming years.

NOTES

1. FRAMEWORKS FOR INVESTIGATING ACTIVISM FOR HEALTH AND SOCIAL JUSTICE IN NEW YORK CITY

1. See, for example, John Duffy, *A History of Public Health in New York City*, vol. 1, *1625–1866* (Russell Sage Foundation, 1968); John Duffy, *A History of Public Health in New York City*, vol. 2, *1866–1966* (Russell Sage Foundation, 1974); Lemuel Shattuck, Report of the Sanitary Commission of Massachusetts (1850; repr., Harvard University Press, 1948); George Rosen, *A History of Public Health* (MD Publications, 1958); David Rosner, ed., *Hives of Sickness: Public Health and Epidemics in New York City* (Rutgers University Press, 1995).
2. Theodore M. Brown and Elizabeth Fee, "Social Movements in Health," *Annual Review of Public Health* 35, no. 1 (2014): 385–398; Isa Susser, "Re-Envisioning Social Movements in the Global City: From Fordism to the Neoliberal Era," in *Worldwide Mobilizations: Class Struggles and Urban Commoning*, ed. Don Kalb and Massimiliano Mollona (Berghahn Books, 2018); Philipp Reick, "Toward a History of Urban Social Movements," *Moving the Social* 63 (2020): 147–162.
3. "Social Determinants of Health," World Health Organization, accessed November 27, 2025, https://www.who.int/health-topics/social-determinants-of-health#tab=tab_1.
4. Paula Braveman, Elaine Arkin, Tracy Orleans, Dwayne Proctor, Julia Acker, and Alonzo Plough, "What Is Health Equity?," *Behavioral Science & Policy* 4, no. 1 (2018): 1–14.
5. Nicholas Freudenberg, Sarah Picard Bradley, and Monica Serrano, "Public Health Campaigns to Change Industry Practices That Damage Health: An Analysis of 12 Case Studies," *Health Education & Behavior* 36, no. 2 (2009): 230–249.

6. Joshua D. Atkinson, "Activist Organizations," in *Journey into Social Activism: Qualitative Approaches* (Fordham University Press, 2017).
7. Matthew E. Archibald and Charity Crabtree, "Health Social Movements in the United States: An Overview," *Sociology Compass* 4, no. 5 (2010): 334–343.
8. Kimberlé Crenshaw, "Demarginalizing the Intersection of Race and Sex: A Black Feminist Critique of Antidiscrimination Doctrine, Feminist Theory and Antiracist Politics," *University of Chicago Legal Forum* 1989, no. 1 (1989): 149.
9. Barbara Klugman, "Effective Social Justice Advocacy: A Theory-of-Change Framework for Assessing Progress," *Reproductive Health Matters* 19, no. 38 (2011): 146–162.
10. Nancy Fraser, "Social Justice in the Age of Identity Politics: Redistribution, Recognition, and Participation," in *Geographic Thought: A Praxis Perspective*, ed. George Henderson and Marvin Waterstone (Routledge, 2009).
11. Horst Brand, *The New York Puerto Rican: Patterns of Work Experience* (Bureau of Labor Statistics, 1971), https://files.eric.ed.gov/fulltext/ED053226.pdf.
12. Judson Jeffries, "From Gang-Bangers to Urban Revolutionaries: The Young Lords of Chicago," *Journal of the Illinois State Historical Society* 96, no. 3 (2003): 288–304.
13. Jama Lazerow and Yohuru Williams, eds., *In Search of the Black Panther Party: New Perspectives on a Revolutionary Movement* (Duke University Press, 2006); Joshua Bloom and Waldo E. Martin Jr., *Black Against Empire: The History and Politics of the Black Panther Party* (University of California Press, 2013); Kathleen Cleaver and George Katsiaficas, eds., *Liberation, Imagination, and the Black Panther Party: A New Look at the Panthers and Their Legacy* (Routledge, 2001); Alondra Nelson, *Body and Soul: The Black Panther Party and the Fight Against Medical Discrimination* (University of Minnesota Press, 2011).
14. Peter B. Levy, *The Great Uprising: Race Riots in Urban America During the 1960s* (Cambridge University Press, 2018).
15. Johanna Fernández, *The Young Lords: A Radical History* (University of North Carolina Press, 2019), 52.
16. Daniel Burnstein, *Next to Godliness: Confronting Dirt and Despair in Progressive Era New York City* (University of Illinois Press, 2006).
17. Johanna Fernández, "When the Young Lords Put Garbage on Display to Demand Change," History Channel, September 15, 2021, https://www.history.com/news/young-lords-garbage-offensive.
18. Fernández.
19. Daniel José Older, "Garbage Fires for Freedom: When Puerto Rican Activists Took Over New York's Streets," *New York Times*, October 26, 2019, A19.
20. Fernández, "When the Young Lords Put Garbage on Display."
21. Darrel Enck-Wanzer, "Trashing the System: Social Movement, Intersectional Rhetoric, and Collective Agency in the Young Lords Organization's Garbage Offensive," *Quarterly Journal of Speech* 92, no. 2 (2006): 174–201.
22. Fernández, *The Young Lords*, 91.
23. Fernández, 99.

24. Gerald Markowitz and David Rosner, *Lead Wars: The Politics of Science and the Fate of America's Children* (University of California Press, 2014).
25. Fernández, *The Young Lords*, 146–149.
26. Gary Eidsvold, Anthony Mustalish, and Lloyd F. Novick, "The New York City Department of Health: Lessons in a Lead Poisoning Control Program," *American Journal of Public Health* 64, no. 10 (1974): 956–962.
27. Young Lords Party and Michael Abramson, *Palante: Voices and Photographs of the Young Lords, 1969–1971* (Haymarket Books, 2011), 135.
28. Nicholas Freudenberg and Maxine Golub, "Health Education, Public Policy and Disease Prevention: A Case History of the New York City Coalition to End Lead Poisoning," *Health Education Quarterly* 14, no. 4 (1987): 387–401.
29. Susan Klitzman and Jessica Leighton, "Decreasing Childhood Lead Poisoning in New York City: 1970–1998," *Journal of Urban Health: Bulletin of the New York Academy of Medicine* 76, no. 4 (1999): 542–545.
30. Fernández, *The Young Lords*, 296–297.
31. Fernández, 296.
32. Fernández, 289–290.
33. Sessi Kuwabara Blanchard, "How the Young Lords Took Lincoln Hospital, Left a Health Activism Legacy," *Filter*, October 30, 2018, https://filtermag.org/how-the-young-lords-took-lincoln-hospital-and-left-a-health-activism-legacy/.
34. Olga Khazan, "How Racism Gave Rise to Acupuncture for Addiction Treatment," *Atlantic*, August 3, 2018, https://www.theatlantic.com/health/archive/2018/08/acupuncture-heroin-addiction/566393/.
35. Carlito Rovira, "Crime Against Our Youth," *Palante*, May 8, 1970, 9.
36. Iris Morales, *Through the Eyes of Rebel Women: The Young Lords 1969–1976* (Red Sugarcane Press, 2016), 18.
37. Young Lords Organization, "Ten Point Health Program" (1970), from *Caring Labor: An Archive* (blog), December 4, 2010, https://caringlabor.wordpress.com/2010/12/04/the-young-lords-reader-health-and-hospitals/.
38. Young Lords Organization.
39. Fernández, *The Young Lords*, 136.
40. Bernie Sanders, "Why We Need Medicare for All," *New York Times*, September 13, 2017, A27.
41. WHO Commission on Social Determinants of Health, World Health Organization, *Closing the Gap in a Generation: Health Equity Through Action on the Social Determinants of Health: Commission on Social Determinants of Health Final Report* (World Health Organization, 2008).
42. World Health Organization, *Constitution* (World Health Organization, 1948).
43. Young Lords Organization, "Ten Point Health Program."
44. "Poster for Housing Crimes Trial (1970)," Metropolitan Council on Housing, accessed November 30, 2025, https://www.metcouncilonhousing.org/about-us/history/grassroots-political-action-of-the-70s-and-80s/.

45. Johanna Fernández, "Learning from the Young Lords," interview by Nathan J. Robinson, *Current Affairs* 8, no. 3 (2023): 59–64.
46. Simon Szreter, "The Importance of Social Intervention in Britain's Mortality Decline c. 1850–1914: A Reinterpretation of the Role of Public Health," *Social History of Medicine* 1, no. 1 (1988): 1–38.
47. David Rosner and Gerald Markowitz, "A Short History of Occupational Safety and Health in the United States," *American Journal of Public Health* 110, no. 5 (2020): 622–628.
48. Michel Sidibé, Shigekazu Tanaka, and Kent Buse, "People, Passion & Politics: Looking Back and Moving Forward in the Governance of the AIDS Response," *Global Health Governance* 4, no. 1 (2010): 1–17.
49. Meredith Turshen and Michele Berger, "Feminist Health Movements," in *Companion to Feminist Studies*, ed. Nancy A. Naples (Wiley, 2020).
50. David Schlosberg and Lisabeth B. Collins, "From Environmental to Climate Justice: Climate Change and the Discourse of Environmental Justice," *Wiley Interdisciplinary Reviews: Climate Change* 5, no. 3 (2014): 359–374.
51. See, for example, John Walter Kerr, *The History, Development, and Statistics of Milk Charities in the United States* (US Government Printing Office, 1910); Diane Allensworth, Elaine Lawson, Lois Nicholson, and James Wyche, "Evolution of School Health Programs," in *Schools & Health: Our Nation's Investment* ed. Diane Allensworth, Elaine Lawson, Lois Nicholson, and James Wyche (National Academies Press, 1997); John L. Holloman Jr., "Plans and Policies for the Operation of the Health and Hospitals Corporation," *Bulletin of the New York Academy of Medicine* 51, no. 8 (1975): 967; James Colgrove, *Epidemic City: The Politics of Public Health in New York* (Russell Sage Foundation, 2011), 237–246.
52. For descriptions of the rise of neoliberalism in New York City, see David Harvey, "Neoliberalism and the City," *Studies in Social Justice* 1, no. 1 (2007): 2–13; Kim Phillips-Fein, *Fear City: New York's Fiscal Crisis and the Rise of Austerity Politics* (Metropolitan Books, 2017); Benjamin Holtzman, *The Long Crisis: New York City and the Path to Neoliberalism* (Oxford University Press, 2021).
53. Daniel E. Dawes, *The Political Determinants of Health* (Johns Hopkins University Press, 2020).
54. Anna B. Gilmore, Amanda Fabbri, Fran Baum, Alexa Bertscher, Krista Bondy, Hyun J. Chang, et al. "Defining and Conceptualising the Commercial Determinants of Health." *Lancet* 401, no. 10383 (2023): 1194–1213.
55. Nicholas Freudenberg, "Integrating Social, Political and Commercial Determinants of Health Frameworks to Advance Public Health in the Twenty-First Century," *International Journal of Social Determinants of Health and Health Services* 53, no. 1 (2023): 4–10.
56. Charles Perrow and Mauro F. Guillen, *The AIDS Disaster: The Failure of Organizations in New York and the Nation* (Yale University Press, 1990); Deborah Wallace and Rodrick Wallace, *A Plague on Your Houses: How New York Was Burned Down and National Public Health Crumbled* (Verso, 1998); Nicholas Freudenberg, Marianne Fahs, Sandro Galea,

and Andrew Greenberg, "The Impact of New York City's 1975 Fiscal Crisis on the Tuberculosis, HIV, and Homicide Syndemic," *American Journal of Public Health* 96, no. 3 (2006): 424–434; Karen DeSalvo, Bob Hughes, Mary Bassett, Georges Benjamin, Michael Fraser, Sandro Galea, et al., "Public Health COVID-19-19 Impact Assessment: Lessons Learned and Compelling Needs," *NAM Perspectives*, April 7, 2021, https://nam.edu/perspectives/public-health-covid-19-impact-assessment-lessons-learned-and-compelling-needs/.

57. Simon Szreter, "The Importance of Social Intervention in Britain's Mortality Decline c. 1850–1914: A Re-Interpretation of the Role of Public Health," *Social History of Medicine* 1, no. 1 (1988): 1–38; Amy L. Fairchild, David Rosner, James Colgrove, Ronald Bayer, and Linda P. Fried, "The EXODUS of Public Health What History Can Tell Us About the Future," *American Journal of Public Health* 100, no. 1 (2010): 54–63; Theodore M. Brown and Elizabeth Fee, "Social Movements in Health," *Annual Review of Public Health* 35, no. 1 (2014): 385–398.
58. Abigail Watts, Anna L. Araiza, Cristina R. Fernández, Leslie Rosenthal, Ileana Vargas-Rodriguez, Nathalie Duroseau, et al., "The Campaign for Universal Free Lunch in New York City: Lessons Learned," *Pediatrics* 148, no. 4 (2021): e2020049734, https://doi.org/10.1542/peds.2020-049734.
59. Marian McDonald, "AntiSterilization Abuse Organizing: A Retrospective Examination," *International Quarterly of Community Health Education* 9, no. 2 (1988): 111–124.
60. Nicholas Freudenberg, Sarah Picard Bradley, and Monica Serrano, "Public Health Campaigns to Change Industry Practices That Damage Health: An Analysis of 12 Case Studies," *Health Education & Behavior* 36, no. 2 (2009): 230–249.
61. Saul Alinsky, *Rules for Radicals: A Pragmatic Primer for Realistic Radicals* (Vintage, 1989), and Saul Alinsky, *Reveille for Radicals* (Vintage, 1989).
62. Prerna Sharma, "Saul Alinsky Model of Community Organization Practice," in *Community Organization & Development in the Context of Literacy* (INFLIBNET Centre, n.d.), https://ebooks.inflibnet.ac.in/aep05/chapter/saul-alinsky-model-of-community-organisation-practice/.
63. Henry Scott-Stokes, "The Alinsky Theory of Protest, Its Application in Queens," *New York Times*, March 7, 1978, 74.
64. Kelly Hayes, "On Activism and Organizing: There Is a Distinction," Transformative Spaces, October 18, 2016, https://transformativespaces.org/2016/10/18/on-activism-and-organizing-there-is-a-distinction/.
65. For a background in these discussions, see Phil Brown and Stephen Zavestoski, eds., *Social Movements in Health* (Wiley, 2005); Theodore M. Brown and Elizabeth Fee, "Social Movements in Health," *Annual Review of Public Health* 35 (2014): 385–398; Catherine Campbell, "Social Capital, Social Movements, and Global Public Health: Fighting for Health-Enabling Contexts in Marginalised Settings," *Social Science & Medicine* 257 (2020): 112153; Nisha Goel, Alina Baciu, and Alison Mack, eds., *Supporting a Movement for Health and Health Equity: Lessons from Social Movements: Workshop Summary* (National Academies Press, 2014); Robert H. Keefe, Sandra D. Lane, and Heidi J.

Swarts, "From the Bottom Up: Tracing the Impact of Four Health-Based Social Movements on Health and Social Policies," *Journal of Health & Social Policy* 21, no. 3 (2006): 55–69; Connie Musolino, Fran Baum, Toby Freeman, Ronald Labonté, Chiara Bodini, and David Sanders, "Global Health Activists' Lessons on Building Social Movements for Health for All," *International Journal for Equity in Health* 19 (2020): 1–4; James Orbinski, "Global Health, Social Movements, and Governance," in *Governing Global Health*, ed. John Kirton (Routledge, 2007).

66. Phil Brown and Stephen Zavestoski, "Social Movements in Health: An Introduction," *Sociology of Health & Illness* 26, no. 6 (2004): 679–694.
67. Joshua B. Freeman, *Working-Class New York: Life and Labor Since World War II* (New Press, 2021); Lowell Turner and Richard W. Hurd, "Building Social Movement Unionism," in *Rekindling the Movement: Labor's Quest for Relevance in the Twenty-First Century*, ed. Lowell Turner, Harry C. Katz, and Richard W. Hurd (Cornell University Press, 2018); Ruth Milkman and Ed Ott, eds., *New Labor in New York: Precarious Workers and the Future of the Labor Movement* (Cornell University Press, 2014).
68. Garrett Chase, "The Early History of the Black Lives Matter Movement, and the Implications Thereof," *Nevada Law Journal* 18 (2017): 1091.
69. Clarence Taylor, *Fight the Power: African Americans and the Long History of Police Brutality in New York City* (NYU Press, 2018).
70. Jennifer Nelson, *More Than Medicine: A History of the Feminist Women's Health Movement* (NYU Press, 2015).
71. John D'Emilio, "Cycles of Change, Questions of Strategy: The Gay and Lesbian Movement After Fifty Years," in *The Politics of Gay Rights* (University of Chicago Press, 2000).
72. Robert D. Bullard, "Anatomy of Environmental Racism and the Environmental Justice Movement," in *Confronting Environmental Racism: Voices from the Grassroots*, ed. Robert D. Bullard (South End Press, 1993).
73. Mayra D. Mora, Rodrigo Rodriguez, Alma Zermeño, and Paul Almeida, "Immigrant Rights and Social Movements," *Sociology Compass* 12, no. 8 (2018): e12599.
74. Lindsey Patterson, "The Disability Rights Movement in the United States," in *Oxford Handbook of Disability History*, ed. Michael Rembis, Catherine Kudlick, and Kim E. Nielsen (Oxford Academic, 2018), 439–458.
75. Brian Tokar, "Movements for Climate Justice in the US and Worldwide," in *Routledge Handbook of the Climate Change Movement*, ed. Matthias Dietz and Heiko Garrelts (Routledge, 2014).
76. Alex Karner, Tierra Bills, and Aaron Golub, "Emerging Perspectives on Transportation Justice," *Transportation Research Part D: Transport and Environment* 116 (2023): 103618.
77. Cassie Schwerner, "Building the Movement for Education Equity," in *Rhyming Hope and History: Activists, Academics, and Social Movement Scholarship*, ed. David Croteau, William Hoynes, and Charlotte Ryan (University of Minnesota Press, 2005).
78. Julia C. Sudbury, "Toward a Holistic Antiviolence Agenda: Women of Color as Radical Bridge-Builders," *Social Justice* 30, no. 3 (93 (2003): 134–140.

79. "The Fight for Sydenham Hospital," *Shoe Leather*, podcast, Columbia University Libraries, May 17, 2021, https://shoeleather.podcasts.library.columbia.edu/podcast/the-fight-for-sydenham-hospital/.

80. Gary Chartier, "Civil Rights and Economic Democracy," *Washburn Law Journal* 40 (2000): 267; Janette A. Clements, "Participatory Democracy: The Bridge from Civil Rights to Women's Liberation," *Annual Meeting of the American Political Science Association* (2003): 5–24; Students for a Democratic Society, *The Port Huron Statement* (1964), from *Progressive Fox* (blog), accessed November 30, 2025, http://www.progressivefox.com/misc_documents/PortHuronStatement.pdf; Lillian B. Rubin, "Maximum Feasible Participation: The Origins, Implications, and Present Status," *Annals of the American Academy of Political and Social Science* 385, no. 1 (1969): 14–29.

81. City of New York, *Summary of Vital Statistics 1970* (Department of Health and Mental Hygiene, 1970), https://www.nyc.gov/assets/doh/downloads/pdf/vs/1970sum.pdf; City of New York, *Summary of Vital Statistics 2019* (Department of Health and Mental Hygiene, 2019), https://www.nyc.gov/assets/doh/downloads/pdf/vs/2019sum.pdf.

82. Jason M. Barr, "Disease and Unease in New York City (Part I): Mortality Rates Since 1800," *Skynomics Blog*, June 16, 2020, https://buildingtheskyline.org/mortality-nyc-1/.

2. HOW NEW YORK CITY'S POLITICS AND ECONOMY SHAPE ACTIVISM

1. Mark Levitan and Susan S. Wieler, "Poverty in New York City, 1969–99: The Influence of Demographic Change, Income Growth, and Income Inequality," *FRBNY Economic Policy Review*, July 2008, 13–30, https://www.newyorkfed.org/medialibrary/media/research/epr/08v14n1/0807levi.pdf.

2. Poverty Tracker Research Group at Columbia University, *The State of Poverty and Disadvantage in New York City*, vol. 7 (Robin Hood, 2025), https://robinhood.org/wp-content/uploads/2025/02/PT_Annual24_final_digital.pdf.

3. "Population Density Dataset," Kontur, accessed November 30, 2025, https://www.kontur.io/portfolio/population-dataset/.

4. John Cassel, "Health Consequences of Population Density and Crowding," in *People and buildings*, ed. Robert Gutman (Routledge, 2017).

5. James N. Gregory, *The Southern Diaspora: How the Great Migrations of Black and White Southerners Transformed America* (University of North Carolina Press, 2006).

6. "New York—Race and Hispanic Origin for Selected Large Cities and Other Places: Earliest Census to 1990," US Census Bureau, accessed November 30, 2025, https://www2.census.gov/library/working-papers/2005/demo/pop-twps0076/nytab.pdf.

7. Isabel Wilkerson, *The Warmth of Other Suns: The Epic Story of America's Great Migration* (Random House, 2010).

8. "Immigration to New York, 1900–2000," *American Experience*, PBS.org, accessed November 30, 2025, https://www.pbs.org/wgbh/americanexperience/features/newyork-immigration/.
9. Kasey Zapatka and Van C. Tran, "New Frontiers of Integration: Convergent Pathways of Neighborhood Diversification in Metropolitan New York," *RSF: The Russell Sage Foundation Journal of the Social Sciences* 9, no. 1 (2023): 52–83.
10. Arya Sundaram, "African and Asian Newcomers Are the New Face of Migrants in NYC," *Gothamist*, March 26, 2024, https://gothamist.com/news/african-and-asian-newcomers-are-the-new-face-of-migrants-in-nyc?.
11. J. David Goodman, Keith Collins, Edgar Sandoval, and Jeremy White, "Bus by Bus, Texas' Governor Changed Migration Across the U.S.," *New York Times*, July 20, 2024, https://www.nytimes.com/2024/07/20/us/abbott-texas-migrant-buses.html.
12. Dave Davies, "How NYC Is Coping with 175,000 Migrants from the Southern Border," *Fresh Air*, NPR, February 15, 2024, https://www.npr.org/2024/02/15/1231712535/how-nyc-is-coping-with-175-000-migrants-from-the-southern-border.
13. Joseph Berger, "Study Reports Exodus of Affluent and Educated New Yorkers in the Late 70s," *New York Times*, September 19, 1984, B1.
14. Samuel Ehrenhalt, "Economic and Demographic Change: The Case of New York City," *Monthly Labor Review* 47 (1993): 40–50.
15. Justin Gest, *Majority Minority* (Oxford University Press, 2022).
16. Jason Hackworth, "Postrecession Gentrification in New York City," *Urban Affairs Review* 37, no. 6 (2002): 815–843.
17. Alina S. Schnake-Mahl, Jaquelyn L. Jahn, S. V. Subramanian, Mary C. Waters, and Mariana Arcaya. "Gentrification, Neighborhood Change, and Population Health: A Systematic Review," *Journal of Urban Health* 97 (2020): 1–25.
18. Lance Freeman and Frank Braconi, "Gentrification and Displacement New York City in the 1990s," *Journal of the American Planning Association* 70, no. 1 (2004): 39–52.
19. Marianne Maeckelbergh, "Mobilizing to Stay Put: Housing Struggles in New York City," *International Journal of Urban and Regional Research* 36, no. 4 (2012): 655–673.
20. Daniel Bates, "The Lessons NYC Activists Have for Those Fighting Displacement the World Over," *City Limits*, May 4, 2018, https://citylimits.org/2018/05/04/2365413/.
21. James Parrott, "As Incomes Gap Widens, New York Grows Apart," *Gotham Gazette*, 2019, https://www.gothamgazette.com/49-topics/economy/683-as-incomes-gap-widens-new-york-grows-apart.
22. New York City Economic Development Corporation, *State of the New York City Economy 2024* (New York City Economic Development Corporation, 2025), https://edc.nyc/sites/default/files/2025-01/NYCEDC-State-of-the-NYC-Economy-2024-v3.pdf.
23. Mohamed Obaidy, James Parrott, and Apurva Mehrotra, "Wage Compression or Wage Divergence? Real Wage Growth Comparison Between New York City and the U.S., 2019–2023," Center for New York City Affairs, October 9, 2024, https://www.centernyc.org/reports-briefs/wage-compression-or-wage-divergence-real-wage-growth-comparison-between-new-york-city-and-the-us-2019-2023.

24. Anastasia Koutavas, Sophie Collyer, Yajun Jia, and Christopher Wimer, "Spotlight On: The Racial Wealth Gap in New York City," Poverty Tracker, February 2025, https://robinhood.org/reports/poverty-tracker-spotlight-racial-wealth-gap-january-2025/.
25. Stephen Bezruchka, *Inequality Kills Us All: COVID-19's Health Lessons for the World* (Taylor and Francis, 2023), 47–71.
26. Xiaobo Zhong, Ziqi Zhou, Guohua Li, Muhire H. Kwizera, Peter Muennig, and Qixuan Chen, "Neighborhood Disparities in COVID-19 Outcomes in New York City Over the First Two Waves of the Outbreak," *Annals of Epidemiology* 70 (2022): 45–52, https://doi.org/10.1016/j.annepidem.2022.04.008.
27. Ellen Durkin, "NYC's Poorest Neighborhoods Have Highest Death Rates from Coronavirus," *Politico*, May 18, 2020, https://www.politico.com/states/new-york/city-hall/story/2020/05/18/nycs-poorest-neighborhoods-have-highest-death-rates-from-coronavirus-1284519.
28. Center for Research on Housing Opportunity, Mobility and Equity, *Essential Every Day: The Lives of NYC's Essential Workforce During COVID-19* (New York City Department of Housing Preservation and Development, 2021), https://www.nyc.gov/assets/hpd/downloads/pdfs/about/nyc-home-essential-workers.pdf.
29. For examples of the few descriptions of COVID-19 activism in New York City, see Rita Charon, *A Pandemic Chronicle: Harnessing Narrative Fusion, in Pandemic Storytelling* (Brill, 2024), 15–26; "Guide to the New York City COVID-19 Web Activism Collection TAM.798," NYU Libraries, accessed November 30, 2025, https://findingaids.library.nyu.edu/tamwag/tam_798/all/?form=MG0AV3; "NYC COVID-19 Oral History, Narrative, and Memory Project," Columbia University Center for Oral History Research, accessed November 30, 2025, https://incite.columbia.edu/projects/nyc-COVID-19-oral-history-narrative-and-memory-project?form=MG0AV3.
30. Lindsay Schachnow, " 'Mixed Signals': New York City's Precarious Economic Recovery," Gotham Gazette, August 17, 2022, https://www.gothamgazette.com/city/11523-nyc-economic-recovery-august-2022-jobs.
31. Susan Klitzman and Nicholas Freudenberg, "Implications of the World Trade Center Attack for the Public Health and Health Care Infrastructures," *American Journal of Public Health* 93, no. 3 (2003): 400–406.
32. Roger Waldinger and Thomas Bailey, "The Youth Employment Problem in the World City," *Social Policy* 16, no. 1 (1985): 55–59.
33. "New York City's Millennials in Recession and Recovery," New York City Comptroller's Office, April 26, 2016, https://comptroller.nyc.gov/reports/new-york-citys-millennials-in-recession-and-recovery/.
34. Bruce Johnson, Andrew Golub, and Eloise Dunlap, "The Rise and Decline of Hard Drugs, Drug Markets, and Violence in Inner-City New York," in *The Crime Drop in America*, ed. Bruce Johnson, Andrew Golub, and Eloise Dunlap (Cambridge University Press, 2000).

35. John Bacheller, "The Decline of Manufacturing in New York and the Rust Belt," *Policy by Numbers New York* (blog), October 4, 2016, https://policybynumbers.com/the-decline-of-manufacturing-in-new-york-and-the-rust-belt.
36. "Recent NYC Job Growth Concentrated in Low- and Moderate-Wage Industries," Center for New York City Affairs, February 23, 2023, https://www.centernyc.org/reports-briefs/recent-nyc-job-growth-concentrated-in-low-and-moderate-wage-industries-long-term-employment-growth-prediction-suggests-job-quality-should-be-a-top-policy-priority.
37. "Pandemic Wage Gains in New York City's High-Wage Industries Outpace Gains for Low- and Middle-Wage Industry Workers," Center for New York City Affairs, August 23, 2023, https://www.centernyc.org/reports-briefs/pandemic-wage-gains-in-new-york-citys-high-wage-industries-outpace-gains-for-low-and-middle-wage-industry-workers.
38. Felicia Kornbluh, "Poverty Rights Activism," in *Speaking Out: Activism and Protest in the 1960s and 1970s*, ed. Heather Ann Thompson (Prentice Hall, 2020), 173–177.
39. Richard Rothstein, *The Color of Law: A Forgotten History of How Our Government Segregated America* (Liveright Publishing, 2017).
40. Joseph P. Fried, "Housing Abandonment Spreads in Bronx and Parts of Brooklyn," *New York Times*, April 12, 1976, 1.
41. Vivian Vázques Irizarry, dir., *Decade of Fire* (n.p., 2019), https://decadeoffire.com/.
42. Deborah Wallace and Rodrick Wallace, *A Plague on Your Houses: How New York Was Burned Down and National Public Health Crumbled* (Verso, 1998).
43. Mark Naison, "Why Environmental Racism in the Bronx May Be a More Pressing Issue than Gentrification," *Bronx American History Project*, Fordham Research Commons, August 2, 2022, https://research.library.fordham.edu/cgi/viewcontent.cgi?article=1018&context=baahp_essays.
44. Tom Angotti, *New York for Sale: Community Planning Confronts Global Real Estate* (MIT Press, 2011).
45. Stacey Sutton, "Gentrification and the Increasing Significance of Racial Transition in New York City 1970–2010," *Urban Affairs Review* 56, no. 1 (2020): 65–95.
46. Ingrid Gould Ellen, Michael H. Schill, Amy Ellen Schwartz, and Ioan Voicu, "Housing Production Subsidies and Neighborhood Revitalization: New York City's Ten-Year Capital Plan for Housing," *FRBNY Economic Policy Review* 9, no. 2 (2003): 71–85.
47. Desiree Fields and Sabina Uffer, "The Financialisation of Rental Housing: A Comparative Analysis of New York City and Berlin," *Urban Studies* 53, no. 7 (2016): 1486–1502.
48. "Mapping Displacement and Gentrification in the New York Metropolitan Area," Urban Displacement Project, accessed November 30, 2025, https://www.urbandisplacement.org/maps/new-york-gentrification-and-displacement/.
49. Andy Newman, "How a Once-Loathed Arena in Brooklyn Became a Center for Protests," *New York Times*, June 17, 2020, A17.
50. "Real Estate," New York City Economic Development Corporation, accessed November 30, 2025,https://edc.nyc/industry/real-estate#:~:text=Real%20estate%20is%20in%20New,and%20work%20in%20our%20city.

2. HOW POLITICS AND ECONOMY SHAPE ACTIVISM

51. Ronald Lawson, ed., *The Tenant Movement in New York City, 1904–1980* (Rutgers University Press, 1986); Nicholas Dagen Bloom, *Public Housing That Worked: New York in the Twentieth Century* (University of Pennsylvania Press, 2008).
52. Michael K. Gusmano, Victor G. Rodwin, and Daniel Weisz, "Persistent Inequalities in Health and Access to Health Services: Evidence from New York City," *World Medical & Health Policy* 9, no. 2 (2017): 186–205; Kate E. Pickett and Richard G. Wilkinson, "Income Inequality and Health: A Causal Review," *Social Science & Medicine* 128 (2015): 316–326.
53. Julia Lynch, "The Political Economy of Health: Bringing Political Science In," *Annual Review of Political Science* 26, no. 1 (2023): 389–410.
54. George E. Peterson, "Finance," in *The Urban Predicament*, ed. William Gorham and Nathan Glazer (Urban Institute, 1976), 60.
55. J. Ward Wright, *New York City and the Urban Fiscal Predicament* (Municipal Officers Finance Association, 1976), https://www.baruch.cuny.edu/mac/Economic_Reports/04-01-76.pdf.
56. "The Fight for Sydenham Hospital," *Shoe Leather*, podcast, Columbia University Libraries, May 17, 2021, https://shoeleather.podcasts.library.columbia.edu/podcast/the-fight-for-sydenham-hospital/.
57. Aisla Chang, "Council Members Push NYPD Reform to Curb Stop-and-Frisk Practice," *WNYC News Blog*, February 29, 2012, https://www.changethenypd.org/media/council-members-push-nypd-reform-curb-stop-and-frisk-practice.
58. Bill Bradley, "Bill de Blasio Vows to Reform Stop-and-Frisk Tactics in New York," *Next City*, January 31, 2014, https://nextcity.org/urbanist-news/bill-de-blasio-vows-to-reform-stop-and-frisk-tactics-in-new-york?.
59. Michelle Shames and Simon McCormack, "Stop and Frisks Plummeted Under New York Mayor Bill de Blasio, but Racial Disparities Haven't Budged," ACLU, March 14, 2019, https://www.aclu.org/news/criminal-law-reform/stop-and-frisks-plummeted-under-new-york-mayor.
60. John Kingdon, *Agendas, Alternatives, and Public Policies*, 2nd ed. (Pearson, 2003).
61. William Clinton, "Executive Order 12898 of February 11, 1994: Federal Actions to Address Environmental Justice in Minority Populations and Low-Income Populations," *Federal Register* 59, no. 32 (February 16, 1994), https://www.archives.gov/files/federal-register/executive-orders/pdf/12898.pdf
62. Joy Ang, Rob Galbraith, and Alison Wilkey, *Pay to Play: How Big Real Estate Money Is Leaving New York' Tenants in the Dust* (Housing Justice for All, Public Accountability Initiative, and Community Voices Heard, 2022), https://housingjusticeforall.org/wp-content/uploads/2022/04/Pay-to-Play-Report.pdf.
63. Antonio Machado, *Lands of Castile*, trans. Paul Burns and Salvador Ortiz-Carboneres (Oxford University Press, 2002), 143.
64. "Make the Road New York," Nonprofit Explorer, *ProPublica*, accessed November 30, 2025, https://projects.propublica.org/nonprofits/organizations/113344389.

65. Make the Road New York, *Respect and Dignity for All: Make the Road New York's 2023–24 State Policy Platform* (Make the Road New York, March 2023), https://maketheroadny.org/wp-content/uploads/2023/03/Make-the-Road-NY-2023-24-State-Platform.pdf.
66. See Jane McAlevey, "Make the Road New York: Success Through 'Love and Agitation,' " *Nation*, May 13, 2013, https://www.thenation.com/article/archive/make-road-new-york-success-through-love-and-agitation/; Jane McAlevey, "Make the Road New York's Participatory Approach to Immigrant Organizing," in *New Labor in New York: Precarious Workers and the Future of the Labor Movement*, ed. Ruth Milkman and Edward Ott (ILR Press, 2014): 173–186; Jane McAlevey, *No Shortcuts: Organizing for Power in the New Gilded Age* (Oxford University Press, 2016), 179–198. See also Deborah Axt, Amy Carroll, and Andrew Friedman, "The Campaign to Pass New York's Wage Theft Prevention Act: Advocacy Stories," *Clearinghouse Review Journal of Poverty Law and Policy* 154 (2011–2012): 942–949; Marika Dias, "Stepping Aside, Standing Back, and Raising Up: Lawyering Within Grassroots Community Movements," *Georgetown Journal on Poverty Law and Policy* 22 (2014): 405; David Dyssegaard Kallick, "New York's Pandemic Aid for Undocumented Immigrants: A Model for Other States," Economic Policy Institute, accessed November 30, 2025, https://coilink.org/20.500.12592/x3z18j.
67. McAlevey, *No Shortcuts*, 188.
68. McAlevey, 187.
69. Kirk Semple, "Cuomo Ends State's Role in Checking Immigrants," *New York Times*, June 2, 2011, A21.
70. "Diverse Chorus Applauds as Mayor Bloomberg Signs Two Bills Limiting NYC's Participation in Widely Discredited Immigration Enforcement Programs," Center for Popular Democracy, November 22, 2011, https://www.populardemocracy.org/news/diverse-chorus-applauds-mayor-bloomberg-signs-two-bills-limiting-nyc-s-participation-widely.
71. Asawin Suebsaeng, "These Are the Groups Behind Those 'Spontaneous' Anti-Trump-Ban Protests," *Daily Beast*, February 2, 2017, https://www.thedailybeast.com/these-are-the-groups-behind-those-spontaneous-anti-trump-ban-protests/.
72. Axt et al., "The Campaign to Pass New York's Wage Theft Prevention Act."
73. Interview cited in McAlevey, *No Shortcuts*, 184.
74. Kallick, "New York's Pandemic Aid for Undocumented Immigrants."
75. "Health Access Programs," Make the Road New York, accessed December 1, 2025, https://maketheroadny.org/program/health-access/.
76. McAlevey, *No Shortcuts*, 179–198.
77. Mason B. Williams, *City of Ambition: FDR, LaGuardia, and the Making of Modern New York* (W. W. Norton & Company, 2013).
78. "Welcome NYWFP Co-Directors Ana María Archila and Jasmine Gripper!," Working Families Party, October 16, 2023, https://workingfamilies.org/2023/10/welcome-nywfp-co-directors-ana-maria-archila-and-jasmine-gripper/.

79. Joan Walsh, "New York's Working Families Party Came Back From the Brink. Its Departing Leader Recalls the Battle," *Nation*, May 1, 2023, https://www.thenation.com/article/politics/working-families-party-new-york/.
80. Peter Dreier, "Philanthropy's Misguided Ideas for Fixing Ghetto Poverty: The Limits of Free Markets and Place-Based Initiatives," *NP Quarterly*, March 19, 2015, https://nonprofitquarterly.org/philanthropy-ideas-for-fixing-ghetto-poverty-the-limits-of-free-markets-and-place-based-initiatives/.
81. "About Us," Center for Popular Democracy, accessed December 1, 2025, https://www.populardemocracy.org/about-us.

3. HOW ACTIVISTS DEFINE THE PROBLEM

1. Useful sources on the history of housing organizing in New York City include Nicholas D. Bloom, *Public Housing That Worked: New York in the Twentieth Century* (University of Pennsylvania Press, 2008); Jared N. Day, *Urban Castles: Tenement Housing and Landlord Activism in New York City, 1890–1943* (Columbia University Press, 1999); Roberta Gold, *When Tenants Claimed the City: The Struggle for Citizenship in New York City Housing* (University of Illinois Press, 2014); Ronald Lawson, ed., *The Tenant Movement in New York City, 1904–1980* (Rutgers University Press, 1986); Thomas J. Main, *Homelessness in New York City: Policymaking from Koch to DeBlasio* (New York University Press, 2016); Richard Plunz, *A History of Housing in New York City* (Columbia University Press, 2016).
2. Recent reviews that summarize this evidence include Kiana D. Bess, Alison L. Miller, and Roshanak Mehdipanah, "The Effects of Housing Insecurity on Children's Health: A Scoping Review," *Health Promotion International* 38, no. 3 (2023): daac006; Philippa Howden-Chapman, Julie Bennett, Richard Edwards, David Jacobs, Kim Nathan, and David Ormandy, "Review of the Impact of Housing Quality on Inequalities in Health and Well-Being," *Annual Review of Public Health* 44, no. 1 (2023): 233–254; Danya E. Keene and Kim M. Blankenship, "The Affordable Rental Housing Crisis and Population Health Equity: A Multidimensional and Multilevel Framework," *Journal of Urban Health* 100, no. 6 (2023): 1212–1223; Carolyn B. Swope and Diana Hernández, "Housing as a Determinant of Health Equity: A Conceptual Model," *Social Science & Medicine* 243 (2019): 112571.
3. "Who We Are," Housing Justice for All, accessed December 2, 2025, https://housingjusticeforall.org/who-we-are/.
4. See "Housing Justice for All in New York State: Citizen Action of New York & the Upstate Downstate Housing Alliance," in "Case Studies," Public Reconstruction, accessed December 2, 2025, https://www.publicreconstruction.org/case-studies/.
5. "Our Members," Housing Justice for All, accessed December 2, 2025, https://housingjusticeforall.org/members/.

6. "Senate Deputy Leader Gianaris Rallies With More than 1,000 Tenants for Stronger Rent Laws," press release, New York State Senate, May 14, 2019, https://www.nysenate.gov/newsroom/press-releases/2019/michael-gianaris/senate-deputy-leader-gianaris-rallies-more-1000.
7. Molly Crabapple, "The Revolution Against Shady Landlords Has Begun," Economic Hardship Reporting Project, April 3, 2023, https://economichardship.org/2023/04/the-revolution-against-shady-landlords-has-begun/.
8. Austin C. Jefferson, "Q&A: Julia Salazar on 'Good Cause' Negotiations and Why Solidarity PAC Is Nothing New," City & State, March 30, 2024, https://www.cityandstateny.com/personality/2024/03/julia-salazar-good-cause-negotiations-and-why-solidarity-pac-nothing-new/395364/.
9. Joy Ang, Rob Galbraith, and Alison Wilkey, *Pay to Play: How Big Real Estate Money Is Leaving New York' Tenants in the Dust* (Housing Justice for All, Public Accountability Initiative, and Community Voices Heard, 2022), https://housingjusticeforall.org/wp-content/uploads/2022/04/Pay-to-Play-Report.pdf.
10. "Statement: Housing Justice for All Responds to Collapse of Housing Deal," Housing Justice for All, June 9, 2023, https://housingjusticeforall.org/statement-housing-justice-for-all-responds-to-collapse-of-housing-deal/.
11. "Housing Justice Hub," Urban Institute, accessed December 2, 2025, https://www.urban.org/projects/housing-justice-hub#.
12. Oksana Mironova, "Defensive and Expansionist Struggles for Housing Justice: 120 Years of Community Rights in New York City," *Radical Housing Journal* 9, no. 2 (2019): 137–152.
13. Cassim Shepard, "Justice Supply," *Places Journal*, August 2024, https://placesjournal.org/article/justice-supply-pro-housing-movement/?
14. "All About the Right to Counsel for Evictions in NYC," National Coalition for a Civil Right to Counsel, March 7, 2024, https://civilrighttocounsel.org/major_developments/all-about-the-right-to-counsel-for-evictions-in-nyc/.
15. Vivian Wang, "In a Victory for Tenants, Sweeping Rent Laws Pass," *New York Times*, June 14, 2019, A19.
16. Dana Rubinstein, "New York Bans Most Evictions in Sweeping Law," *New York Times*, December 28, 2020, A1.
17. National Coalition for a Civil Right to Counsel, "All About the Right to Counsel for Evictions in NYC."
18. "New York Tenants Have New Protections from Unfair Evictions & Rent Hikes," Housing Justice for All, accessed December 3, 2025, https://housingjusticeforall.org/kyr-good-cause/.
19. Juan Pablo Garnham, "In the Most Expensive City in the Country, Evictions Remain Lower than Before COVID-19," Eviction Lab, January 14, 2025, https://evictionlab.org/in-the-most-expensive-city-in-the-country-evictions-remain-lower-than-before-covid-19/.

3. HOW ACTIVISTS DEFINE THE PROBLEM

20. Young Lords Party and Michael Abramson, *Palante: Voices and Photographs of the Young Lords, 1969–1971* (Haymarket Books, 2011), 97.
21. Make the Road New York, *Excluded in the Epicenter: Impacts of the COVID Crisis on Working-Class, Immigrant, Black and Brown New Yorkers* (Make the Road New York, May 2020), https://maketheroadny.org/wp-content/uploads/2020/05/MRNY_SurveyReport_small.pdf.
22. "52 State Lawmakers Reject Housing Deal That Would Gut Rent Stabilization and Good Cause Eviction," Housing Justice for All, April 12, 2024, https://housingjusticeforall.org/new-50-state-lawmakers-reject-housing-deal-that-would-gut-rent-stabilization-and-good-cause-eviction/.
23. Horst W. J. Rittel and Melvin M. Webber, "Dilemmas in a General Theory of Planning," Policy Sciences 4, no. 2 (1973): 155–169.
24. Mark Purcell, "Urban Democracy and the Local Trap," *Urban Studies* 43, no. 11 (2006): 1921–1941.
25. Allyn L. Taylor and Douglas W. Bettcher, "WHO Framework Convention on Tobacco Control: A Global 'Good' for Public Health," *Bulletin of the World Health Organization* 78 (2000): 920–929.
26. Julie Ayling and Neil Gunningham, "Non-State Governance and Climate Policy: The Fossil Fuel Divestment Movement," *Climate Policy* 17, no. 2 (2017): 131–149.
27. Mark Heywood, "South Africa's Treatment Action Campaign: Combining Law and Social Mobilization to Realize the Right to Health," *Journal of Human Rights Practice* 1, no. 1 (2009): 14–36.
28. Jared Malsin, "Best of Enemies: Why Occupy Activists Are Working with New York City's Government," *Time*, November 13, 2012, https://nation.time.com/2012/11/13/best-of-enemies-why-occupy-activists-are-working-with-new-york-citys-government/.
29. Laura Landau, "Mutual Aid as Disaster Response in NYC: Hurricane Sandy to COVID-19," *Journal of Extreme Events* 9, no. 02n03 (2022): 2241001.
30. Bill de Blasio, *Built to Last: Transforming New York City's Buildings for a Low-Carbon Future* (Office of the Mayor, September 2014), https://www.nyc.gov/assets/builttolast/downloads/OneCity.pdf.
31. "Dirty Buildings Campaign," Climate Works for All, accessed December 3, 2025, https://www.nyclimateworks.org/dirty-buildings-campaign.
32. "Climate Works for All's Local Law 97 Implementation Priorities," Climate Works for All, January 2023, https://docs.google.com/document/d/1tBRqekqef5Qx3_PnxYh2NJDDxUnpmNzEfbxvTDSTDhA/edit?tab=t.0.
33. Diana R. Gordon, *City Limits: Barriers to Change in Urban Government* (Charterhouse, 1973), 44.
34. Nicholas Freudenberg and Maxine Golub, "Health Education, Public Policy and Disease Prevention: A Case History of the New York City Coalition to End Lead Poisoning," *Health Education Quarterly* 14, no. 4 (1987): 387–401.

35. Thomas P. DiNapoli, *Childhood Lead Poisoning* (Office of the New York State Comptroller, June 2007), https://www.osc.state.ny.us/files/reports/special-topics/pdf/childhood-lead-poisoning-2007-06.pdf.
36. Freudenberg and Golub, "Health Education, Public Policy and Disease Prevention."
37. Freudenberg and Golub.
38. DiNapoli, *Childhood Lead Poisoning*.
39. "The Comprehensive Guide to New York City's Lead Laws and Their Evolution," Frankel Law Firm, accessed December 3, 2025, https://frankellawfirm.com/the-comprehensive-guide-to-new-york-citys-lead-laws-and-their-evolution/.
40. "Lead Poisoning in NYC Kids at Record Low," NBC 4 New York, October 4, 2013. https://www.nbcnewyork.com/news/local/lead-poisoning-children-statistics-new-york-city-health-department/1986469/.
41. Jeffery C. Mays, "Tenants Sue New York City Housing Authority: 'We Have Let Other People Speak for Us for Too Long,' " *New York Times*, February 27, 2018, https://www.nytimes.com/2018/02/27/nyregion/nycha-lawsuit-nyc-housing.html.
42. Greg B. Smith, "NYCHA'S Lead Paint Crisis Explodes as Known Number of Apartments Where Kids Risk Exposure Triples," *The City*, October 22, 2020, https://www.thecity.nyc/2020/10/22/nycha-lead-paint-more-apartments-identified/.
43. "HPD Joins AG James as She Takes Action to Protect Tenants from Lead Poisoning," NYC Housing Preservation and Development, February 27, 2020, https://www.nyc.gov/site/hpd/news/013-20/hpd-joins-ag-james-she-takes-action-protect-tenants-lead-poisoning#/0.
44. "Attorney General James and HPD Take Action to Protect Children and Families from Lead Poisoning in NYC," Office of New York State Attorney General, September 23, 2021, https://www.nyc.gov/site/hpd/news/047-21/attorney-general-james-hpd-take-action-protect-children-families-lead-poisoning-in.
45. Speaker Cory Johnson, hearing of the New York City Council Committees on Housing, Buildings, Public Housing, Education, and Health, November 13, 2019, video, https://legistar.council.nyc.gov/MeetingDetail.aspx?ID=724806&GUID=41EAC120-525D-4F22-A0EC-86385F60A8BA.

4. HOW ACTIVISTS DECIDE TO TAKE ON THE PROBLEM THEY IDENTIFY

1. Susan M. Chambré, *Fighting for Our Lives: New York's AIDS Community and the Politics of Disease* (Rutgers University Press, 2006).
2. See, for example, Chambré, *Fighting for Our Lives*; Tamar W. Carroll, *Mobilizing New York: AIDS, Antipoverty, and Feminist Activism* (University of North Carolina Press, 2015); David France, *How to Survive a Plague: The Inside Story of How Citizens and Science Tamed AIDS* (Knopf, 2016); Aisha Harris and OmiSoore H. Dryden, *Womanist AIDS Activism in*

the United States: "It's Who We Are" (Lexington Books, 2022); Charles Perrow and Mauro F. Guillén, *The AIDS Disaster: The Failure of Organizations in New York and the Nation* (Yale University Press, 1990); Darrel Royles, *To Make the Wounded Whole: The African American Struggle Against HIV/AIDS* (University of North Carolina Press, 2020).

3. Sarah Schulman, *Let the Record Show: A Political History of ACT UP New York, 1987–1993* (Farrar, Straus and Giroux, 2021).
4. Nora Neus, "The Start of the National Aids Movement': Act Up's Defining Moment in Queer Protest History," *Guardian*, October 11, 2023, https://www.theguardian.com/society/2023/oct/11/act-up-hiv-aids-1988-fda-protest#.
5. Schulman, *Let the Record Show*, 122.
6. Philip J. Hilts, "FDA, in Big Shift, Will Permit Use of Experimental AIDS Drug," *New York Times*, September 29, 1989, A1.
7. Schulman, *Let the Record Show*, 86.
8. Schulman, 86–89, 173–174, and 215–217.
9. Lorraine Boissoneault, "How the New York Stock Exchange Gave Abbie Hoffman His Start in Guerrilla Theater," Smithsonian Magazine, August 24, 2017, https://www.smithsonianmag.com/history/how-new-york-stock-exchange-gave-abbie-hoffman-his-start-guerrilla-theater-180964612/.
10. John Darnton, "Civil Service Rally Assails Bank's Role in City Crisis," *New York Times*, June 5, 1975, 31.
11. Celia Farber, "Sins of Omission," *Spin*, no. 8 (November 1989): 185–186.
12. Schulman, *Let the Record Show*, 209–212.
13. Philip J. Hilts, "AIDS Drug's Maker Cuts Price By 20%," *New York Times*, September 19, 1989, A1. Schulman, *Let the Record Show*, 206.
14. "A Rationale for the AIDS Cure Project" (1994), ACT UP, accessed December 5, 2025, https://actupny.org/ACP/ACPback.html.
15. "Pharma Industry at a 'Once in a Generation' Inflection Point," Harris Poll, July 2, 2020, https://theharrispoll.com/briefs/pharma-industry-at-a-once-in-a-generation-inflection-point/.
16. Justin McCarthty, "Big Pharma Sinks to the Bottom of U.S. Industry Rankings," Gallup News, September 3, 2019, https://news.gallup.com/poll/266060/big-pharma-sinks-bottom-industry-rankings.aspx.
17. Nicholas Freudenberg, "The Role of Social Movements in Reducing Harmful Corporate Practices; Comment on 'National Public Health Surveillance of Corporations in Key Unhealthy Commodity Industries–A Scoping Review and Framework Synthesis,'" *International Journal of Health Policy and Management* 13, no. 1 (2024): 8664; G. Mahood, *"Tobacco Industry Denormalization": Telling the Truth About the Tobacco Industry's Role in the Tobacco Epidemic* (Nonsmokers' Rights Association, 2004).
18. Carroll, *Mobilizing New York*, 155–161.
19. Jason Deparle, "111 Held in St. Patrick's Day Protest," *New York Times*, December 11, 1989, B3.

20. Stop the Church flyer in Schulman, *Let the Record Show*, 152.
21. Schulman, 146–147.
22. Schulman, 161.
23. Schulman, 140.
24. Schulman, 160.
25. Schulman, 27–30 and 182–184.
26. Schulman.
27. Schulman, 498.
28. Schulman, 159.
29. Schulman, 146.
30. Karen J. Alter and Michael Zürn, "Conceptualising Backlash Politics: Introduction to a Special Issue on Backlash Politics in Comparison," *British Journal of Politics and International Relations* 22, no. 4 (2020): 563–584.
31. Mark Harrington, "Organizers Learning from the HIV/AIDS Treatment Movement," Panel Discussion with Organizers for Health Justice, October 15, 2024, author's notes from unrecorded session.
32. Gregg Gonsalves, "Organizers Learning from the HIV/AIDS Treatment Movement," Panel Discussion with Organizers for Health Justice, October 15, 2024, author's notes from unrecorded session.
33. Schulman, *Let the Record Show*, 10.
34. Nicholas Freudenberg, "Why Do We Ignore Capitalism When We Examine the Health Crises of Our Time," *BMJ Opinion*, May 6, 2021, https://blogs.bmj.com/bmj/2021/05/06/why-do-we-ignore-capitalism-when-we-examine-the-health-crises-of-our-time/.
35. "Who We Are," VOCAL-NY, accessed December 5, 2025, https://www.vocal-ny.org/about-us/#mission-vision.
36. Doug Osborne, "The Small Agency with a Big Voice," *Gay City News*, September 1, 2016, https://gaycitynews.com/the-small-agency-with-a-big-voice/.
37. "Governor Cuomo Announces Second Round of Awards for Development of Supportive Housing Units Across New York State," New York State Governor's Office, October 11, 2017, https://hcr.ny.gov/governor-cuomo-announces-second-round-awards-development-supportive-housing-units-across-new-york-0.
38. Erik W. Wiewel, Yijia Zhong, Qi Xia, Claire M. Beattie, Paul A. Brown, Peter X. Farquhar, and Jose F. Rojas, "Homelessness and Housing Assistance Among Persons with HIV, and Associations with HIV Care and Viral Suppression, New York City 2018," *PLoS One* 18, no. 5 (May 12, 2023): e0285765, https://journals.plos.org/plosone/article?id=10.1371/journal.pone.0285765.
39. Paulette Soltani, "Budget Can Offer a Down Payment Towards a Caring and Compassionate New Deal for NYC," *City Limits*, May 3, 2021, https://citylimits.org/2021/05/03/opinion-budget-can-offer-a-down-payment-towards-a-caring-and-compassionate-new-deal-for-nyc/.

40. Karen Yi, "Many NYC Homeless Shelter Residents Can't Access Wi-Fi. 2 New Bills Hope to Change That," *Gothamist*, June 8, 2025, https://gothamist.com/news/many-nyc-homeless-shelter-residents-cant-access-wi-fi-2-new-bills-hope-to-change-that.
41. VOCAL-NY (@vocalnewyork), "VOCAL-NY Applauds Mayor-Elect Mamdani for Vowing to End Encampment Sweeps," Instagram, December 8, 2025, https://www.instagram.com/p/DSAnOR6FeIA/.
42. VOCAL-NY, *Annual Report 2022* (VOCAL-NY, 2023), https://www.vocal-ny.org/resource/vocal-ny-2022-annual-report/.
43. "Power Mapping to Design a Winning Campaign Strategy," Beautiful Trouble, accessed December 5, 2025, https://beautifultrouble.org/toolbox/tool/power-mapping.
44. "Process Guide: Power Mapping," Change Agency, accessed December 5, 2025, https://thechangeagency.org/power-mapping/.
45. Peggy Shepard, presentation at the CUNY School of Public Health, March 13, 2023.
46. Manissa M. Maharawal and Erin McElroy, "Reflections on Doing the Work: City Life / Vida Urbana and the AntiEviction Mapping Project," *Radical Housing Journal* 3, no. 1 (2021): 267–276.
47. "Eviction Lawsuits from March 2020 to September 2021," AntiEviction Mapping Project, accessed December 5, 2025, https://www.worstevictorsnyc.org/map.
48. Steven Lukes, *Power: A Radical View*, 2nd ed. (Palgrave McMillan, 2004).
49. John Gaventa, "Linking the Prepositions: Using Power Analysis to Inform Strategies for Social Action," *Journal of Political Power* 14, no. 1 (2021):109–130, https://doi.org/10.1080/2158379X.2021.1878409.
50. Deepak Bhargava and Stephanie Luce, *Practical Radicals: Seven Strategies to Change the World* (New Press, 2023), 51–54.
51. Frances Fox Piven and Richard Cloward, *Poor People's Movements: Why They Succeed, How They Fail* (Vintage, 1977).
52. Lisa VeneKlasen and Valerie Miller, *A New Weave of Power People and Politics: The Action Guide for Advocacy and Citizen Participation* (World Neighbors, 2002).
53. Jack Newfield and Paul Du Brul, *The Permanent Government: Who Really Rules New York?* (Pilgrim Press, 1981).
54. Newfield and DuBrul, 32.
55. Mayer N. Zald and Roberta Ash, "Social Movement Organizations: Growth, Decay and Change," *Social Forces* 44, no. 3 (1966): 327–341.
56. Kirk Semple, "Cuomo Ends State's Role in Checking Immigrants," *New York Times*, June 2, 2011, A21; "Diverse Chorus Applauds as Mayor Bloomberg Signs Two Bills Limiting NYC's Participation in Widely Discredited Immigration Enforcement Programs," Center for Popular Democracy, November 22, 2011, https://www.populardemocracy.org/news/diverse-chorus-applauds-mayor-bloomberg-signs-two-bills-limiting-nyc-s-participation-widely.
57. Make the Road New York, *Protect Our Futures: Make the Road New York's 2025–26 State Policy Platform* (Make the Road New York, 2025), https://maketheroadny.org/2025-26-state-policy-platform/.

5. HOW ACTIVISTS ENGAGE PEOPLE IN THEIR CAMPAIGNS

1. Marshall Ganz, *People, Power, Change: Organizing for Democratic Renewal* (Oxford University Press, 2024), 19.
2. Lana D. Povitz, *Stirrings: How Activist New Yorkers Ignited a Movement for Food Justice* (University of North Carolina Press, 2019), 31–33.
3. "Uprose: Elizabeth Yeampierre," Women's Leadership in Community Development, August 5, 2020, https://www.womenbuildcommunity.org/case/uprose/.
4. "The History of Plumbing in New York City," Omnia Mechanical Group, October 1, 2020, https://sanitary.nyc/the-history-of-plumbing-in-new-york-city/#.
5. Vernice D. Miller, "Planning, Power and Politics: A Case Study of the Land Use and Siting History of the North River Water Pollution Control Plant," *Fordham Urban Law Journal* 21 (1993): 707–722.
6. Miller.
7. Miller.
8. Miller.
9. Marco Martuzzi and Joel A. Tickner, eds., *The Precautionary Principle: Protecting Public Health, the Environment and the Future of Our Children* (World Health Organization, Regional Office for Europe, 2004).
10. Miller, "Planning, Power and Politics."
11. Vernice Miller, Moya Hallstein, and Susan Qyass, "Feminist Politics and Environmental Justice: Women's Community Activism in West Harlem, New York," in *Feminist Political Ecology*, ed. Dianne Rocheleau, Barbara Thomas-Slayter, and Esther Wangari (Routledge, 1996).
12. Miller et al., "Feminist Politics and Environmental Justice."
13. Seth S. King, "Sewage Plant Voted Over Harlem Protest," *New York Times*, April 26, 1968, 45.
14. Barry Commoner, "Report on the North River Sewage Treatment Plant," unpublished report, 1987.
15. Miller et al., "Feminist Politics and Environmental Justice."
16. Miller, "Planning, Power and Politics."
17. Alex Karner, Jonathan London, Dana Rowangould, and Kevin Manaugh, "From Transportation Equity to Transportation Justice: Within, Through, and Beyond the State," *Journal of Planning Literature* 35, no. 4 (2020): 440–459.
18. Charles R. Johnson Jr. and Glenn S. Johnson, "Environmental Justice and Title VI of the Civil Rights Act of 1964: A Case Study on the Siting of MTA's Bus Depot in Harlem, New York," *Race, Gender & Class* 19, nos. 3–4 (2012): 196–216.
19. Peggy Shepard, "Breathe at Your Own Risk: Transit Justice in West Harlem," *Race, Poverty & the Environment* 12, no. 1 (2005): 51–53; Luz Claudio, Leon Tulton, John Doucette, and Philip J. Landrigan, "Socioeconomic Factors and Asthma Hospitalization Rates in New York City," *Journal of Asthma* 36, no. 4 (1999): 343–350.

20. John B. Faust, "Perspectives on Cumulative Risks and Impacts," *International Journal of Toxicology* 29, no. 1 (2010): 58–64.
21. Shepard, "Breathe at Your Own Risk," 52.
22. Johnson Jr. and Johnson, "Environmental Justice and Title VI of the Civil Rights Act of 1964."
23. Peggy Shepard, presentation at the CUNY School of Public Health, March 13, 2023.
24. Patrick L. Kinney, Maneesha Aggarwal, Mary E. Northridge, Nicole A. Janssen, and Peggy Shepard, "Airborne Concentrations of PM (2.5) and Diesel Exhaust Particles on Harlem Sidewalks: A Community-Based Pilot Study," *Environmental Health Perspectives* 108, no. 3 (2000): 213–218.
25. "Governor Hochul Signs Landmark Environmental Justice Legislation Reducing the Cumulative Impacts of Pollution on Disadvantaged Communities," WE ACT, December 31, 2022, https://www.weact.org/2022/12/governor-hochul-signs-landmark-environmental-justice-legislation-reducing-the-cumulative-impacts-of-pollution-on-disadvantaged-communities/.
26. Robert D. Bullard, "The Threat of Environmental Racism," *Natural Resources & Environment* 7, no. 3 (1993): 23–56.
27. Ryan Holifield, "Defining Environmental Justice and Environmental Racism," *Urban Geography* 22, no. 1 (2001): 78–90.
28. Kinney et al., "Airborne Concentrations of PM (2.5) and Diesel Exhaust Particles on Harlem Sidewalks."
29. Kimberlé Crenshaw, "Demarginalizing the Intersection of Race and Sex: A Black Feminist Critique of Antidiscrimination Doctrine, Feminist Theory and Antiracist Politics," *University of Chicago Legal Forum* 1, no. 8 (1989): 139–168.
30. Miller et al. "Feminist Politics and Environmental Justice."
31. Kathy Boudin, "The Resilience of the Written Off: Women in Prison as Women of Change," *Women's Rights Law Reporter* 29, no. 1 (2007): 15–22.
32. Mireya Navarro, "Conversations: Katrina Haslip; An AIDS Activist Who Helped Women Get Help Earlier," *New York Times*, November 15, 1992, Section 4, 9.
33. AIDS Education and Counseling Program, *Breaking the Walls of Silence: AIDS and Women in a New York Maximum Security Prison* (Overlook Books, 1998), 9–10.
34. Bert P. G. Klandermans, "Identity Politics and Politicized Identities: Identity Processes and the Dynamics of Protest," *Political Psychology* 35, no. 1 (February 2014): 1–22.
35. Mary Bernstein, "Identity Politics," *Annual Review of Sociology* 31, no. 1 (2005): 47–74.
36. Walter Benn Michaels, *The Trouble with Diversity: How We Learned to Love Identity and Ignore Inequality* (Metropolitan Books, 2007).
37. Jane McAlevey, "The High-Touch Model: Make the Road New York's Participatory Approach to Immigrant Organizing," in *New Labor in New York: Precarious Workers and the Future of the Labor Movement*, ed. Ruth Milkman and Ed Ott (Cornell University Press, 2014).

38. William Brennan and Margo A. Jackson, "A Qualitative Examination of Dialogical Elements in Antiracist Deep Canvassing Conversations," *Counseling Psychologist* 50, no. 2 (2022): 177–211.
39. Jennifer Nelson, *Women of Color and the Reproductive Rights Movement* (NYU Press, 2003), 140–142.
40. Felicia Kornbluh, *A Women's Life is a Human Life* (Grove Press, 2023), 306.
41. Kornbluh, 243–249.
42. Taahira Thompson, "NYPD's Infamous Stop-and-Frisk Policy Found Unconstitutional," Leadership Conference Education Fund, August 21, 2013, https://civilrights.org/edfund/resource/nypds-infamous-stop-and-frisk-policy-found-unconstitutional/.
43. Joseph Goldstein, "Judge Rejects New York's Stop-and-Frisk Policy," *New York Times*, August 13, 2013, A1.
44. "Stop-and-Frisk Data," New York Civil Liberties Union, March 14, 2019, https://www.nyclu.org/data/stop-and-frisk-data#admin.
45. Joe Sexton, "In New York, Crime Falls Along with Police Stops," *ProPublica*, January 16, 2018, https://www.propublica.org/article/in-new-york-crime-falls-along-with-police-stops.
46. Kyle Smith, "We Were Wrong About Stop-and-Frisk," *National Review*, January 1, 2018, https://www.nationalreview.com/2018/01/new-york-city-stop-and-frisk-crime-decline-conservatives-wrong/.
47. Communities United for Police Reform et al., letter to Mayor de Blasio and Speaker Johnson, April 30, 2020, https://www.changethenypd.org/sites/default/files/letter-mayor_-speaker-nypd_budget4-30-2020.pdf.
48. Sophie Dorn, "Was the NYPD Budget Increased This Year? Yes—but It's Complicated," City and State New York, June 15, 2022, https://www.cityandstateny.com/policy/2022/06/was-nypd-budget-increased-year-yes-its-complicated/368239/.
49. Emma Umansky, "The NYPD Is Tossing Out Hundreds of Misconduct Cases—Including Stop-and-Frisks—Without Even Looking at Them," *ProPublica*, September 11, 2024, https://www.propublica.org/article/nypd-tossed-out-police-misconduct-discipline-cases-edward-caban.
50. Heather McGhee, *The Sum of Us: What Racism Costs Everyone and How We Can Prosper Together* (One World, 2022).
51. Johanna Fernández, *The Young Lords: A Radical History* (University of North Carolina Press, 2019), 273–277.
52. Julie Sze, *Noxious New York: The Racial Politics of Urban Health and Environmental Justice* (NYU Press, 2003), 115.
53. Eddie Bautista, Eva Hanhardt, Juan Camilo Osorio, and Natasha Dwyer, "New York City Environmental Justice Alliance Waterfront Justice Project," *Local Environment* 20, no. 6 (2015): 664–682.
54. "Federal Policy Office," WE ACT for Environmental Justice, accessed December 8, 2025, https://www.weact.org/federal-policy-office/.

55. "Peggy Shepard Criticizes Trump's Executive Orders in CNN Story," We Act for Environmental Justice, January 26, 2025, https://weact.org/updates/peggy-shepard-criticizes-trumps-executive-orders-in-cnn-story/.

6. HOW ACTIVISTS CHOOSE STRATEGIES AND TACTICS

1. Lana D. Povitz, "Hunger Doesn't Take a Vacation: The Food Activism of United Bronx Parents," in *Women's Activism and "Second Wave" Feminism: Transnational Histories*, ed. Barbara Molony and Jennifer Nelson (Bloomsbury Academic, 2017).
2. Bianca Fortis, "Hochul Unveils Universal Free School Meals Program Across New York," The 74, January 17, 2025, https://www.the74million.org/article/hochul-unveils-universal-free-school-meals-program-across-new-york/.
3. Deepak Bhargava and Stephanie Luce, *Practical Radicals: Seven Strategies to Change the World* (New Press, 2023), 35.
4. Hunger Free America, *New York State and New York City Hunger Survey Report, 2024: Aid Denied, Hunger Increased: Cutbacks Fuel New U.S. Hunger Crises* (Hunger Free America, 2024), https://hfa-website.cdn.prismic.io/hfa-website/ZoS6Gq8jQArT1SiR_2024NY_NYCReportFinal.pdf.
5. "Diabetes," NYC Health, accessed December 10, 2025, https://www.nyc.gov/site/doh/health/health-topics/diabetes.page.
6. "Overweight," Environmental & Health Data Portal, NYC Health, accessed December 10, 2025, https://a816-dohbesp.nyc.gov/IndicatorPublic/beta/data-explorer/overweight/?id=2062#display=summary.
7. Sarah Angell, "Generating Health in New York City," *Journal of Health Inequalities* 5, no. 1 (2019): 48.
8. See, for example, Michael Pollan, "Food Movement Rising," *New York Review of Books* 57, no. 10 (2010): 31–33; Nicholas Freudenberg, John McDonough, and Emma Tsui, "Can a Food Justice Movement Improve Nutrition and Health? A Case Study of the Emerging Food Movement in New York City," *Journal of Urban Health* 88 (August 2011): 623–636; Kristin Reynolds and Nevin Cohen, *Beyond the Kale: Urban Agriculture and Social Justice Activism in New York City* (University of Georgia Press, 2016); Nicholas Freudenberg, Nevin Cohen, Janet Poppendieck, and Craig Willingham, "Ten Years of Food Policy Governance in New York City: Lessons for the Next Decade," *Fordham Urban Law Journal* 45 (2017): 951–994; Lana D. Povitz, *Stirrings: How Activist New Yorkers Ignited a Movement for Food Justice* (University of North Carolina Press, 2019); "Speaker Corey Johnson Unveils Plan to Combat Food Inequity in New York City," City Council Speaker's Office, August 1, 2019. https://council.nyc.gov/press/2019/08/01/1786/; Nevin Cohen, "Food Crisis as a Tool for Social Change: Lessons from New York City's COVID-19 Response," *Urban Governance* 2, no. 1 (2022): 173–177.

9. Prem Thakker, "Republicans Declare Banning Universal Free School Meals a 2024 Priority," *New Republic*, June 15, 2023, https://newrepublic.com/post/173668/republicans-declare-banning-universal-free-school-meals-2024-priority.
10. Susan Levine, *School Lunch Politics: The Surprising History of America's Favorite Welfare Program* (Princeton University Press, 2008), 109.
11. Janet Poppendieck, *Sweet Charity? Emergency Food and the End of Entitlement* (Penguin, 1999).
12. Jennifer E. Gaddis, *The Labor of Lunch: Why We Need Real Food and Real Jobs in American Public Schools* (University of California Press, 2019).
13. Sarah R. Stapleton, "Nevertheless, They Persisted: How a Group of 'Noisy Moms' Overcame Dismissal and Helped to Improve School Food in a US Small City School District," *Gender, Place & Culture* 28, no. 1 (2021): 88–108.
14. Johanna Fernández, *The Young Lords: A Radical History* (University of North Carolina Press, 2019), 123.
15. Fernández, 100.
16. Fernández, 178.
17. Povitz, "Hunger Doesn't Take a Vacation."
18. Povitz.
19. Povitz, 31–33.
20. Povitz, 36.
21. Povitz, 36.
22. Povitz.
23. Povitz.
24. Povitz.
25. Aurora Flores-Hostos, " 'I'm a Mother, and I'm a Mother': A Eulogy for Evelina, the Hell Lady of the Bronx," Latinx Project, September 16, 2022, https://www.latinxproject.nyu.edu/intervenxions/1wyt8fmrwrsdsyf3z745mjpjzl549p.
26. Povitz, 24.
27. Povitz, 25.
28. Rachel Leah, "All kids at New York City Public Schools Will Now Get Free Lunch," *Salon*, September 7, 2017, https://www.salon.com/2017/09/07/all-kids-at-new-york-city-public-schools-will-now-get-free-lunch/.
29. Angela Watts, Ana L. Araiza, Carmen R. Fernández, Lori Rosenthal, Ingrid Vargas-Rodriguez, Nicole Duroseau et al., "The Campaign for Universal Free Lunch in New York City: Lessons Learned," *Pediatrics* 148, no. 4 (2021): e2020049734.
30. Liz Accles, presentation on Lunch for Learning Campaign to CUNY Public Health Students, March 6, 2023.
31. Watts et al., "The Campaign for Universal Free Lunch in New York City."
32. Accles, presentation on Lunch for Learning Campaign to CUNY Public Health Students Campaign.
33. Accles.

34. Aminata Abdouramane, "First Person: How the Shame of 'Free-Free' Inspired My Push for Universal Free Lunch," Chalkbeat, April 27, 2016, https://www.chalkbeat.org/newyork/2016/4/27/21098156/first-person-how-the-shame-of-free-free-inspired-my-push-for-universal-free-lunch/.
35. Kate Lisa, "Advocates Eye Federal Solution to Achieve Universal Free School Meals in N.Y.," Spectrum News, September 5, 2023, https://spectrumlocalnews.com/nys/central-ny/politics/2023/09/06/advocates-eye-federal-solution-for-universal-free-school-meals-in-ny.
36. Jennifer Lewke, "Coalition of 200+ Groups Urges Gov. Hochul to Fund Free School Meals for All New York Students," News10NBC, October 24, 2024, https://www.whec.com/local/coalition-of-200-groups-urges-gov-hochul-to-fund-free-school-meals-for-all-new-york-students/.
37. Benjamin Oreskes and Jay Root, "Hochul's Budget Plan Aims More at Pocketbook Issues Than at Trump," *New York Times*, January 21, 2025, A19.
38. See, for example, Janet Poppendieck, *Free for All: Fixing School Food in America* (University of California Press, 2010); Freudenberg et al., "Ten Years of Food Policy Governance in New York City"; Povitz, *Stirrings*; Watts et al., "The Campaign for Universal Free Lunch in New York City."
39. Povitz, *Stirrings*, 76.
40. World Health Organization, *Constitution of the World Health Organization* (World Health Organization, 1948).
41. WHO Commission on Social Determinants of Health, *Closing the Gap in a Generation: Health Equity Through Action on the Social Determinants of Health: Commission on Social Determinants of Health Final Report* (World Health Organization, 2008).
42. Fernández, *The Young Lords*, 178.
43. Povitz, *Stirrings*, 76.
44. "Universal School Meals: Governor Hochul Announces Free Breakfast and Lunch for More Than 2.7 Million Students in New York as Part of the 2025 State of the State," New York State, January 10, 2025, https://www.governor.ny.gov/news/universal-school-meals-governor-hochul-announces-free-breakfast-and-lunch-more-27-million.
45. Bhargava and Luce, *Practical Radicals*, 209–227.
46. John Krinsky and Hannah Caldwell, "New York City's Movement Networks: Resilience, Reworking, and Resistance in a Time of Distancing and Brutality," Open Democracy, April 28, 2020, https://www.opendemocracy.net/en/democraciaabierta/new-york-citys-movement-networks-resilience-reworking-and-resistance-in-a-time-of-distancing-and-brutality/.
47. For discussion of this trend, see Robert Gottlieb, *Care-Centered Politics: From the Home to the Planet* (MIT Press, 2022); Dipali Anumol, Sinduja Raja, and Q. Manivannan, "Politics of Care," in *The Contemporary Reader of Feminist International Relations*, ed. Catherine Goetze and Khushi Singh Rathore (Routledge, 2025); Matthew J. Wolf-Meyer, ed., *Proposals for a Caring Economy* (University of Minnesota Press, 2025).

48. Right to Counsel NYC Coalition and Housing Justice for All, *Going on Rent Strike in New York During COVID-19: Guide & Resources* (Right to Counsel NYC Coalition and Housing Justice for All, 2021), https://d3n8a8pro7vhmx.cloudfront.net/righttocounselnyc/pages/100/attachments/original/1585739362/RTCNYC.
49. Bhargava and Luce, *Practical Radicals*, 220–223.
50. Kurt Schock and Celina Demetriou, "Nonviolent and Violent Trajectories in Social Movements," in *The Wiley Blackwell Companion to Social Movements* (Wiley-Blackwell, 2018).
51. Hannah Allam, "Trump's Pardons and Purges Revive Old Question: Who Counts as a Terrorist?," *ProPublica*, February 10, 2025, https://www.propublica.org/article/jan-6-pardons-trump-purges-domestic-terrorism-focus.
52. Fernández, *The Young Lords*, 148–149 and 271–272.
53. Bruce Lambert, "Drug Group to Offer Free Needles to Combat AIDS in New York City," *New York Times*, January 8, 1988, A1.
54. Daliah Heller and Denise Paone, "Access to Sterile Syringes for Injecting Drug Users in New York City: Politics and Perception (1984–2010)," *Substance Use & Misuse* 46, nos. 2–3 (2011): 140–149.
55. "Looting and Violence Continues in New York City Despite Unprecedented Curfew," *Guardian*, June 20, 2020, https://www.theguardian.com/us-news/2020/jun/02/new-york-city-looting-despite-curfew.
56. Goria Oladipo, "New York to Pay $13.7m to George Floyd Protesters Arrested or Beaten by Police," *Guardian*, July 20, 2023, https://www.theguardian.com/us-news/2023/jul/20/new-york-nypd-george-floyd-protests-2020.
57. Jennifer Agiesta, "CNN Poll: Trump Losing Ground to Biden Amid Chaotic Week," *CNN*, June 8, 2020, https://www.cnn.com/2020/06/08/politics/cnn-poll-trump-biden-chaotic-week/index.html?.
58. Juliana Menasce Horowitz, Katrin Hurst, and Dana Braga, "Support for the Black Lives Matter Movement Has Dropped Considerably from Its Peak in 2020," Pew Research Center, June 14, 2023, https://www.pewresearch.org/social-trends/2023/06/14/support-for-the-black-lives-matter-movement-has-dropped-considerably-from-its-peak-in-2020/.
59. Donatella della Porta, "Repertoires of Contention," in *The Wiley-Blackwell Encyclopedia of Social and Political Movements*, ed. David A. Snow, Donatella della Porta, Bert Klandermans, and Doug McAdam (John Wiley & Sons, 2013).
60. Brian Mann, "More Than a Million Americans Have Died from Overdoses During the Opioid Epidemic," National Public Radio, December 30, 2021, https://www.npr.org/2021/12/30/1069062738/more-than-a-million-americans-have-died-from-overdoses-during-the-opioid-epidemi.
61. Sascha Garrey, "Making the Private Public: P.A.I.N.'s Actions to Confront the Overdose Crisis at the Met and the Guggenheim," unpublished paper, 2023, written for a class on health activism taught by the author.

62. Brian Mann and Martha Bebinger, "Purdue Pharma, Sacklers Reach $6 Billion Deal with State Attorneys General," National Public Radio, March 3, 2022, https://www.npr.org/2022/03/03/1084163626/purdue-sacklers-oxycontin-settlement.
63. Patrick Radden Keefe, *Empire of Pain: The Secret History of the Sackler Dynasty* (Anchor Books, 2021).

7. HOW ACTIVISTS FORGE RELATIONSHIPS WITH ALLIES AND OPPONENTS

1. "Restaurant Owners Taking the 'High Road' Report Better Loyalty, Creativity and Productivity," Economic Opportunity Institute, February 2, 2012, https://www.opportunityinstitute.org/blog/post/restaurant-owners-taking-the-high-road-report-better-loyalty-creativity-and-productivity/.
2. Joy Ang, Rob Galbraith, and Alison Wilkey, *Pay to Play: How Big Real Estate Money Is Leaving New York Tenants in the Dust* (Housing Justice for All; Public Accountability Initiative; and Community Voices Heard, April 2022), https://housingjusticeforall.org/resource/pay-to-play-how-real-estate-money-is-leaving-new-york-tenants-in-the-dust/.
3. Clio Chang, "Kingston Becomes the First Upstate City to Adopt Rent Control," *Curbed*, August 2, 2022, https://www.curbed.com/2022/08/kingston-upstate-rent-control.html
4. Jason Corburn, *Street Science: Community Knowledge and Environmental Health Justice* (MIT Press, 2005).
5. Corburn, 8.
6. Nina Wallerstein, Bonnie Duran, John G. Oetzel, and Meredith Minkler, eds., *Community-Based Participatory Research for Health: Advancing Social and Health Equity* (Jossey-Bass, 2017).
7. Abigail Watts, Anna L. Araiza, Cristina R. Fernández, Leslie Rosenthal, Ileana Vargas-Rodriguez, Nathalie Duroseau et al., "The Campaign for Universal Free Lunch in New York City: Lessons Learned," *Pediatrics* 148, no. 4 (2021): e2020049734.
8. Watts et al.
9. John Keane, "Civil Society, Definitions and Approaches," in *International Encyclopedia of Civil Society*, ed. Helmut K. Anheier and Stefan Toepler (Springer, 2010).
10. Jane McAlevy, "Make the Road New York: Success Through 'Love and Agitation,' " *Nation*, May 22, 2013, https://www.thenation.com/article/archive/make-road-new-york-success-through-love-and-agitation/.
11. McAlevy.
12. Acumen Fund and Open Society Foundation, *Make the Road: Developing a Membership Model That Builds the Power of Immigrant and Working Class Communities* (Acumen Fund and Open Society Foundation, 2019), https://worldjusticeproject.org/sites/default/files/documents/Case%20Study_Make%20the%20Road.pdf.

13. Neil Barsky, "Shut Down Rikers Island," *New York Times*, July 19, 2015, SR4.
14. "A Deadly Year in NYC Jails," *Brian Lehrer Show*, WNYC, November 14, 2022, https://www.wnyc.org/story/deadly-year-nyc-jails/.
15. *Rikers: An American Jail*, produced by Marc Levin, Mark Benjamin, and Rolake Bamgbose (WPBS, 2017), https://www.pbs.org/wnet/rikers/.
16. Jarrett Murphy, "It Will Take Tenacity and Guts to Shutter One of the Country's Most Notorious Jails," *Nation*, July 2, 2017, https://www.thenation.com/article/archive/it-will-take-tenacity-and-guts-to-shutter-one-of-the-countrys-most-notorious-jails/.
17. Some examples: Ed Morales, "The Perils and Potential of Closing Rikers Island," *City Limits*, November 25, 2015, https://citylimits.org/2015/11/25/the-perils-and-potential-of-closing-rikers-island/; Andre Ward, "Little Has Changed Since I Was Held on Rikers; It's Time to Shift Resources as We Close the Jail," *Gotham Gazette*, April 26, 2023, https://www.gothamgazette.com/130-opinion/11942-key-steps-close-rikers-island-jails; Sahalie Donaldson, "A Timeline on the Closure of Rikers Island," City and State New York, December 2, 2024, https://www.cityandstateny.com/politics/2024/12/timeline-closure-rikers-island/376662/.
18. "Questioning Solitary Confinement for Adolescents at Rikers Island," *PBS Newshour*, February 21, 2014, https://www.pbs.org/newshour/show/questioning-solitary-confinement-teens-rikers-island.
19. Jan Ransom, Sarah Kerr, Caroline Kim, and Malachy Browne, "Footage of Inmate Suicide Captures Dysfunction on Rikers Island," *New York Times*, July 17, 2025, A10.
20. Michael Winerip, Michael Schwirtz, and Benjamin Weiser, "Report Found Distorted Data on Jail Fights," *New York Times*, September 22, 2014, A1.
21. "Case for the Close Rikers Campaign Grant," Open Philanthropy, accessed March 15, 2023, https://www.openphilanthropy.org/grants/justleadershipusa-campaign-to-close-rikers/#id-case-for-the-grant.
22. "Case for the Close Rikers Campaign Grant."
23. "Case for the Close Rikers Campaign Grant."
24. Lippman Commission, *A More Just New York City* (Independent Commission on New York City Criminal Justice and Incarceration Reform, 2017), https://static1.squarespace.com/static/5b6de4731aef1de914f43628/t/5b96c6f81ae6cf5e9c5f186d/1536607993842/Lippman%2BCommission%2BReport%2BFINAL%2BSingles.pdf.
25. " 'No New Jails': Activists Protest at Ford Foundation," *Art Forum*, September 27, 2019, https://www.artforum.com/news/no-new-jails-activists-protest-at-ford-foundation-244824/.
26. "Ending Cycles of Trauma & Harm: Grantmaking to Close Rikers," New York Community Trust, May 1, 2024, https://thenytrust.org/news/ending-cycles-of-trauma-harm-grantmaking-to-close-rikers/.
27. Jayne Mooney and Jarrod Shanahan, "Rikers Island Jail Complex: The Use of Social History to Inform Current Debates on Incarceration in New York City," *Howard Journal of Crime and Justice* 59, no. 3 (2020): 286–304.

28. Stuart Marques, "The Birth, Life and—Maybe—Death of Rikers Island," NYC Department of Records and Information Services, March 22, 2019, https://www.archives.nyc/blog/2019/3/21/the-birth-life-and-maybe-death-of-rikers-island.
29. Richard Nixon, "Remarks About an Intensified Program for Drug Abuse Prevention and Control, June 17, 1971," American Presidency Project, accessed December 12, 2025, https://www.presidency.ucsb.edu/documents/remarks-about-intensified-program-for-drug-abuse-prevention-and-control.
30. Mason B. Williams, "How the Rockefeller Laws Hit the Streets: Drug Policing and the Politics of State Competence in New York City, 1973–1989," *Modern American History* 4, no. 1 (2021): 67–90.
31. Quoted in Marques, "The Birth, Life and—Maybe—Death of Rikers Island."
32. Marques.
33. Michael Schwirtz and Michael Winerip, "Close Rikers Island? It Will Take Years, Billions and Political Capital," *New York Times*, March 2, 2016, A16.
34. "Speaker Mark Viverito's 2016 State of the City Address, Remarks as Prepared for Delivery," New York City Council, February 11, 2016, https://council.nyc.gov/press/2016/02/11/46/.
35. Luke Scrivener, Shanon Tomascak, Erica Bond Erica, and Preeti Chauhan, *New York City Jail Population in 2019* (Data Collaborative for Justice at John Jay College, July 2021), https://datacollaborativeforjustice.org/wp-content/uploads/2021/07/2021_07_09_DOC_Full_Brief_FINAL.pdf.
36. "Average Daily Population in New York City Jails 1910–2023," Vital City, accessed December 12, 2025, https://www.vitalcitynyc.org/dataviz/average-daily-population-in-new-york-city-jails.
37. Michelle Alexander, *The New Jim Crow: Mass Incarceration in the Age of Colorblindness* (New Press, 2010).
38. "Our Mission," Black Lives Matter, accessed December 12, 2025, https://blacklivesmatter.com/about/#vision.
39. Christopher J. Lebron, *The Making of Black Lives Matter: A Brief History of an Idea* (Oxford University Press, 2023).
40. Jeremy Travis, *But They All Come Back: Facing the Challenges of Prisoner Reentry* (Urban Institute Press, 2005).
41. Jason R. Andrews, Yiran E. Liu, and Julio Croda, "Enduring Injustice: Infectious Disease Outbreaks in Carceral Settings," *Journal of Infectious Diseases* 229, no. 2 (2024): 307–309.
42. Council of State Governments Justice Center, *Improving Outcomes for People with Mental Illnesses Involved with New York City's Criminal Court and Correction Systems* (Council of State Governments Justice Center, 2012), https://csgjusticecenter.org/publications/improving-outcomes-for-people-with-mental-illnesses-involved-with-new-york-citys-criminal-court-and-correction-systems/; Elizabeth B. Ford, Kevin D. Silverman, Angela Solimo, Y. Jude Leung, Allison M. Smith, Connor J. Bell, and Monica Katyal, "Clinical Outcomes of Specialized Treatment Units for Patients with Serious

Mental Illness in the New York City Jail System," *Psychiatric Services* 71, no. 6 (2020): 547–554.

43. Michael Jacobson, Elizabeth DeWolf, Margaret Egan, and David Hafetz, "Beyond the Island: Changing the Culture of New York City jails," *Fordham Urban Law Journal* 45, no. 2 (2017): 373.

44. Daniel Selling, David Lee, Angela Solimo, and Homer Venters, "A Road Not Taken: Substance Abuse Programming in the New York City Jail System," *Journal of Correctional Health Care* 21, no. 1 (2015): 7–11.

45. Cynthia Golembeski, Gabriel Eber, Carolyn Sufrin, Jacqueline Lantsman, and Homer Venters, "Discretionary Ethics and Governing Public Affairs in Jails and Prisons: Upholding Constitutional Rights to Health and Safety," in *Empowering Public Administrators*, ed. Amanda M. Olejarski and Sue M. Neal (Routledge, 2024).

46. Nicholas Freudenberg, "Jails, Prisons, and the Health of Urban Populations: A Review of the Impact of the Correctional System on Community Health," *Journal of Urban Health* 78, no. 2 (2001): 214–235.

47. Meghan A. Novisky, Kathryn M. Nowotny, Dylan B. Jackson, Alexander Testa, and Michael G. Vaughn, "Incarceration as a Fundamental Social Cause of Health Inequalities: Jails, Prisons and Vulnerability to COVID-19," *British Journal of Criminology* 61, no. 6 (2021): 1630–1646.

48. Richard Schiffman, "The Garden Inside Purgatory," *New York Times*, October 6, 2019, MB1.

49. Katal Center for Health, Equity, and Justice, *Reflections and Lessons from the First Two Phases of the #CLOSErikers Campaign: August 2015–August 2017* (Katal Center, 2018), 13.

50. Katal Center for Health, Equity, and Justice, 13.

51. Office of the New York City Mayor, *Smaller, Safer, Fairer: A Roadmap to Closing Rikers Island* (Office of the New York City Mayor, 2018), https://criminaljustice.cityofnewyork.us/wp-content/uploads/2018/04/Smaller-Safer-Fairer.pdf.

52. Matthew Haag, "N.Y.C to Close Rikers for Jail Reform," *New York Times*, October 17, 2019, A1.

53. Katal Center for Health, Equity, and Justice, *Reflections and Lessons from the First Two Phases of the #CLOSErikers Campaign*, 27.

54. Emily Ngo, "Adams Vows Systemic Change If Elected NYC Mayor, Wants 'Balanced Conversation' on Rikers," *Spectrum News*, October 4, 2021, https://ny1.com/nyc/all-boroughs/politics/2021/10/05/inside-city-hall-eric-adams-rikers-island.

55. Gabriel Sayegh, "Op-Ed: Mayor Adams Talks About Closing Rikers While Working to Keep It Open," *Amsterdam News*, June 6, 2024, https://amsterdamnews.com/news/2024/06/06/mayor-adams-talks-about-closing-rikers-while-working-to-keep-it-open/.

56. "Zohran Mamdani Details How He Will Close Rikers Island," posted September 8, 2025, by Forbes Breaking News, YouTube, https://www.youtube.com/watch?v=F2AlzrMMJaM.

57. Jonathan Lippman and Melissa Mark-Viverito, "Closing Rikers Island Is a Moral Imperative," *New York Times*, March 31, 2017, https://www.nytimes.com/2017/03/31/opinion/closing-rikers-island-is-a-moral-imperative.html.
58. Katal Center for Health, Equity, and Justice, *Reflections and Lessons from the First Two Phases of the #CLOSErikers Campaign*, 29–30.
59. Corey Johnson, "Fix the System," Speech at John Jay College, May 16, 2019, via New York City Council, accessed December 12, 2025, https://council.nyc.gov/data/fix-the-system/speaker-speech-on-criminal-justice-reform/.
60. "Statements from NYC Council Speaker Adams and Criminal Justice Chair Rivera on Reappointment of Independent Rikers Commission to Help Advance Closure and Replacement with Borough-Based Jails, as Required by Law," New York City Council, October 23, 2023, https://council.nyc.gov/press/2023/10/23/2484/.
61. "About COBA," Correction Officers' Benevolent Association, accessed December 12, 2025, https://cobanyc.org/learn-about-coba/.
62. Jarrod Shanahan, "Solidarity Behind Bars: NYC's Correction Officers' Benevolent Association," *Brooklyn Rail*, September 2017, https://brooklynrail.org/2017/09/field-notes/Solidarity-Behind-Bars-NYCs-Correction-Officers-Benevolent-Association/
63. Michael Schwirtz and Michael Winerip, "At Rikers, a Roadblock to Reform," *New York Times*, December 14, 2014, A1.
64. Schwirtz and Winerip, A1.
65. Schwirtz and Winerip, A1.
66. Benjamin Weiser, "Former Jail Guard Union Chief Wins Early Release from Bribery Sentence," *New York Times*, February 24, 2003, A16.
67. Katal Center for Health, Equity, and Justice, *Reflections and Lessons from the First Two Phases of the #CLOSErikers Campaign*, 34–35.
68. Katal Center for Health, Equity, and Justice, 17.
69. Nunez et al. v. New York City Department of Correction and the City of New York, 1:11-cv-05845, (S.D.N.Y.), Opinion and Order Regarding Appointment of a Nunez Remediation Manager, May 13, 2025, https://www.documentcloud.org/documents/25940103-nunezruling/.
70. Jack Newfield and Paul Du Brul, *The Permanent Government: Who Really Rules New York?* (Pilgrim Press, 1981).
71. Jiada Valenza, " 'You Come Back a Year Later and Fight for More': Retiring Dick Gottfried Reflects on 52 Years in the State Assembly," *Gotham Gazette*, July 14, 2022, https://www.gothamgazette.com/state/11445-dick-gottfried-retires-state-assembly-reflects.
72. Luis Ferre-Sadurni, "A Champion of Liberal Causes in New York to Retire After 52 Years," *New York Times*, December 13, 2021, A17.
73. Gabriel Sayegh, "Jeffrey Aubry, Champion for Justice in New York, Leaves a Remarkable Legacy," *Queens Daily Eagle*, July 2, 2024, https://queenseagle.com/all/2024/7/2/opinion-jeffrion-aubry-a-champion-for-justice-in-new-york-leaves-a-remarkable-legacy.

74. John W. Kingdon, "How Do Issues Get on Public Policy Agendas?," in *Sociology and the Public Agenda*, ed. William J. Wilson (SAGE Publications, 1993).
75. Vernice D. Miller, "Planning, Power and Politics: A Case Study of the Land Use and Siting History of the North River Water Pollution Control Plant," *Fordham Urban Law Journal* 21, no. 3 (1993): 721.
76. Jennifer Gonnerman, "Before the Law," *New Yorker*, September 29, 2014, https://www.newyorker.com/magazine/2014/10/06/before-the-law.
77. Katal Center for Health, Equity, and Justice, *Reflections and Lessons from the First Two Phases of the #CLOSErikers Campaign*, 11.

8. HOW ACTIVIST CAMPAIGNS INTERACT WITH LOCAL, NATIONAL, AND GLOBAL MOVEMENTS

1. Steven Greenhouse and Jana Kasperkevic, "Fight for $15 Swells Into Largest Protest by Low-Wage Workers in US History," *Guardian*, April 15, 2015. https://www.theguardian.com/us-news/2015/apr/15/fight-for-15-minimum-wageprotests-new-york-los-angeles-atlanta-boston.
2. Yannet Lathrop, T. William Lester, and Matthew D. Wilson, *Quantifying the Impact of the Fight for $15: $150 Billion in Raises for 26 Million Workers, with $76 Billion Going to Workers of Color* (National Employment Law Project, 2021), https://s27147.pcdn.co/wp-content/uploads/Data-Brief-Impact-Fight-for-15-7-22-2021.pdf.
3. This profile is based on several detailed and informative case studies of the Fight for $15 campaign, including Steven Greenhouse, *Beaten Down, Worked Up: The Past, Present and Future of American Labor* (Knopf, 2019), 231–251; Steven Greenhouse, " 'The Success Is Inspirational': The Fight for $15 Movement 10 Years On," *Guardian*, November 23, 2022, https://www.theguardian.com/us-news/2022/nov/23/fight-for-15-movement-10-years-old; Vincent Pasquier, "The 'Fight for 15' Movement: An Experimental Mobilisation at the Crossroads of the 'Old' Labour and 'New' Social Movements," in *Experimenting for Union Renewal: Challenges, Illustrations and Lessons*, ed. Mélanie Laroche and Gregor Murray (European Trade Union Institute, 2024); Jason Spicer, Robert Manduca, and Tamara Kay, "National Living-Wage Movements in a Regional World: The Fight for $15 in the United States," in *Reimagining the Governance of Work and Employment*, ed. Dionne Pohler (Cornell University Press, 2020); Maite Tapia and Tashlin Lakhani, "Organizing Fast Food: Opportunities, Challenges, and the SEIU," in *Purple Power: The History and Global Impact of SEIU*, ed. Luís L. M. Aguiar and Joseph A. McCartin (University of Illinois Press, 2023).
4. Wendi C. Thomas, "How New York's 'Fight for $15' Launched a Nationwide Movement," *American Prospect*, January 4, 2016, https://prospect.org/economy/new-york-s-fight-15-launched-nationwide-movement/.
5. Steven Greenhouse, "With Day of Protests, Fast-Food Workers Seek More Pay," *New York Times*, November 29, 2012, https://www.nytimes.com/2012/11/30/nyregion/fast-food-workers-in-new-york-city-rally-for-higher-wages.html.

6. Greenhouse, *Beaten Down, Worked Up*, 234.
7. Richard Anker, *Estimating a Living Wage: A Methodological Review* (International Labor Organization, 2011).
8. "Minimum Wage Is Not Enough: A True Living Wage Is Necessary to Reduce Poverty and Improve Health," Policy Brief, Drexel University Center for Hunger-Free Communities, December 2021, https://drexel.edu/hunger-free-center/research/briefs-and-reports/minimum-wage-is-not-enough/.
9. Alex Swerdloff, "How a Fast Food Worker Became an Activist," *Civil Eats*, January 2, 2018, https://civileats.com/2018/01/02/inside-the-life-and-struggle-of-a-fast-food-worker-turned-activist/.
10. Restaurant Law Center and National Restaurant Association v. City of New York and Lorelei Salas, 360 F. Supp. 3d 192 (S.D.N.Y. 2019), https://scholar.google.com/scholar_case?case=2435718207277722252&hl=en&as_sdt=6,33
11. Swerdloff, "How a Fast Food Worker Became an Activist."
12. Jared Gans, "Judge Pauses NYC $18-Per-Hour Requirement for Delivery Workers Amid Lawsuits," *Hill*, July 8, 2023, https://thehill.com/regulation/court-battles/4087013-judge-pauses-nyc-18-per-hour-requirement-for-delivery-workers-amid-lawsuits/.
13. Emma Cohn and Jennifer Sherer, "A Review of Key 2024 Ballot Measures: Voters Backed Progressive Policy Measures," Economic Policy Institute, November 7, 2024, https://www.epi.org/blog/a-review-of-key-2024-ballot-measures-voters-backed-progressive-policy-measures/.
14. Lew Blank, "Voters Think It's Time to Raise the Minimum Wage," Data for Progress, April 26, 2024, https://www.dataforprogress.org/blog/2024/4/26/voters-think-its-time-to-raise-the-minimum-wage.
15. "Our Fight," Starbuck Workers United, accessed December 13, 2025, https://sbworkersunited.org/our-fight/.
16. Patrick Whittle, "Chipotle Agrees to Pay After Closing Store That Sought Union," Associated Press, March 27, 2023, https://apnews.com/article/chipotle-union-store-closure-settlement-lawsuit-af89f99249bd805fd714751bae040181.
17. Claudia Irizarry Aponte, "Staten Island's Amazon Labor Union Joins Forces with the Teamsters," *City*, June 10, 2024, https://www.thecity.nyc/2024/06/10/amazon-union-teamsters-staten-island/.
18. Mariya Strauss, "The Fight for $15 Goes to College," *New Labor Forum*, 25, no. 3 (2016): 107–111.
19. Ruth Milkman, "New Forms of Struggle: The 'Alt-Labor' Movement in New York City," in *City of Workers, City of Struggle: How Labor Movements Changed New York*, ed. Joshua B. Freeman (Columbia University Press, 2019).
20. Janice Fine, "Worker Centers: Entering a New Stage of Growth and Development," *New Labor Forum* 20, no. 3 (2011): 45–53.
21. Kent Wong, "A New Labor Movement for a New Working Class: Unions, Worker Centers, and Immigrants," *Berkeley Journal of Employment and Labor Law* 36, no. 1 (2015): 205–213.

22. William Finnegan, "Dignity Fast food Workers and a New Form of Labor Activism," *New Yorker*, September 8, 2014, https://www.newyorker.com/magazine/2014/09/15/dignity-william-finnegan.
23. Greenhouse, " 'The Success Is Inspirational.' "
24. Associated Press, "Fight for $15, Black Lives Matter Groups Join Forces," *Voice of America*, March 24, 2017, https://www.voanews.com/a/fight-for-15-black-lives-matter-groups-join-forces/3780009.html.
25. Ruth Milkman, Stephanie Luce, and Penny Lewis, "Occupy Wall Street," in *The Social Movements Reader*, 3rd ed., ed. James M. Jasper and Jeff Goodwin (Wiley, 2015).
26. Agence France Presse, " 'Indignant' Protests to Go Global on Saturday," *France 24*, October 15, 2011, http://www.france24.com/en/20111015-indignant-protests-go-global-saturday.
27. James Anderson, "Some Say Occupy Wall Street Did Nothing. It Changed Us More Than We Think," *Time*, November 15, 2021, https://time.com/6117696/occupy-wall-street-10-years-later/.
28. Tapia and Lakhani, "Organizing Fast Food."
29. Stephane Fortado, "Workplace Sexual Abuse, Labor and the #MeToo Movement," *Labor Studies Journal* 43, no. 4 (2018): 241–244.
30. "Survey Shows Two in Five Women in Fast-Food Industry Face Sexual Harassment on the Job," National Partnership for Women and Families, accessed December 13, 2025, https://nationalpartnership.org/news_post/women-in-fast-food-industry-face-sexual-harassment-html/.
31. Kathy Durkin, "Workers strike at McDonald's," *Workers World*, September 25, 2018, https://www.workers.org/2018/09/39157/.
32. Jonathan Rosenblum, *Beyond $15: Immigrant Workers, Faith Activists, and the Revival of the Labor Movement* (Beacon Press, 2017); Nevin Cohen, Janet Poppendieck, and Nicholas Freudenberg, "Food Justice in the Trump Age: Priorities for Urban Food Advocates," *Journal of Food Law and Policy* 13 (2017): 43.
33. Cardinal Timothy Dolan, "Our Moral Duty to Raise the Wage: New York's Archbishop Backs Boosting Minimum Pay to a Level That Enables Families to Support Themselves," *New York Daily News*, February 24, 2016, https://www.nydailynews.com/2016/02/24/our-moral-duty-to-raise-the-wage-new-yorks-archbishop-backs-boosting-minimum-pay-to-a-level-that-enables-families-to-support-themselves/.
34. Saru Jayaraman, " 'ROCing' the Industry: Organizing Restaurant Workers in New York," in *The New Urban Immigrant Workforce*, ed. Sarumathi Jayaraman and Immanuel Ness (Routledge, 2015).
35. José Oliva, "The Restaurant Opportunities Center," in *Food Movements Unite!* ed. Eric Holt Giménez (Food First Books, 2011).
36. Marcy Goldstein-Gelb and Luz S. Marin, "Winning Rights: The Role of Worker Centers in Protecting the Most Vulnerable Workers," *American Journal of Public Health* 113 (2023): 832–833.

37. Stephanie Ross, "Varieties Of Social Unionism: Towards a Framework for Comparison," *Just Labour* 11 (2007): 16–34.
38. Swerdloff, "How a Fast Food Worker Became an Activist."
39. Sarah Jaffe, "This Group Pioneered the Fight for $15," *Nation*, July 5, 2016, https://www.thenation.com/article/archive/this-group-pioneered-the-fight-for-15-can-they-transform-the-fight-for-affordable-housing-too/.
40. Finnegan, "Dignity Fast food Workers and a New Form of Labor Activism."
41. Finnegan.
42. Finnegan.
43. Ava Martinez, "21 U.S. States Are Raising the Minimum Wage in 2025—Here's What We Know," *HR Digest*, January 2, 2025, https://www.thehrdigest.com/21-u-s-states-are-raising-the-minimum-wage-in-2025-heres-what-we-know/.
44. Aurelia Glass, "Trump Just Cut the Minimum Wage for Hundreds of Thousands of Private Sector Workers," Center for American Progress, April 11, 2025, https://www.americanprogress.org/article/trump-just-cut-the-minimum-wage-for-hundreds-of-thousands-of-private-sector-workers/.
45. John Madison, *Project 2025: The Blueprint and Mandate for Leadership* (A. W. Publishing, 2024), 605.
46. Eyal Press, "No Tax on Tips," New Yorker, July 28, 2025, https://www.newyorker.com/magazine/2025/08/04/no-tax-on-tips-is-an-industry-plant?
47. Madison, *Project 2025*.
48 Gwynne Hogan, "Fast Food Chains Could Lose Right to Do Business in NYC, Under New Bill to Protect Workers," *Gothamist*, September 19, 2022, https://gothamist.com/news/council-ramps-up-pressure-on-nyc-fast-food-restaurants-to-protect-workers-rights.
49. David A. Fahrenthold and Talmon J. Smith, "How Restaurant Workers Help Pay for Lobbying to Keep Their Wages Low," *New York Times*, January 17, 2023, https://www.nytimes.com/2023/01/17/us/politics/restaurant-workers-wages-lobbying.html.
50. Theda Skocpol, "The Rise and Resounding Demise of the Clinton Plan," *Health Affairs* 14, no. 1 (1995): 66–85.
51. "Mark Hannay (2012)," Roosevelt House Public Policy Institute at Hunter College, June 20, 2012, https://www.roosevelthouse.hunter.cuny.edu/?conference-speaker=mark-hannay.
52. "Mark Hannay, Metro New York Health Care for All," Everybody In: Racial Equity & Medicare for All Conference, April 17, 2023, https://medicareforall23.sched.com/metrohealth.
53. Judy Gonzalez, "A Brief History of Single Payer," *NYSNA Single Payer Newsletter*, Fall 2023, https://cf-simple-s3-origin-cloudfrontfors3-146697677730.s3.amazonaws.com/pco/campaigns/singlePayer/2023-11SinglePayerNewsletter.pdf.
54. Make the Road New York (@MaketheRoadNY), "Coverage for All Coalition Campaign Condemns Assembly Leaders for Failing to Expand Health Coverage for All

8. HOW ACTIVIST CAMPAIGNS INTERACT WITH MOVEMENTS

Low-Income Immigrant New Yorkers," Twitter (now X), June 21, 2023, accessed May 15, 2024, https://twitter.com/MaketheRoadNY/status/1671881490643439616.

55. John M. Glen, *Highlander: No Ordinary School, 1932–1962* (University Press of Kentucky, 2014).
56. David Moberg, "Back to Its Roots: The Industrial Areas Foundation and United Power for Action and Justice," in *The New Chicago: A Social and Cultural Analysis*, ed. John B. Koval, Larry Bennett, Michael Bennett, Fassil Demissie, Roberta Garner, and Kil-joong Kim (Temple University Press, 2006).
57. "About Us," Midwest Academy, accessed December 13, 2025, https://midwestacademy.com/about-us/.
58. Health Policy Advisory Center, John Ehrenreich, and Barbare Ehrenreich, *The American Health Empire: Power, Profits and Politics* (Vintage Books, 1970); David Kotelchuck, ed., *Prognosis Negative: Crisis in the Health Care System* (Vintage Books, 1976).
59. Merlin Chowkwanyun, "The New Left and Public Health the Health Policy Advisory Center, Community Organizing, and the Big Business of Health, 1967–1975," *American Journal of Public Health* 101, no. 2 (2011): 238–249.
60. "About Us," Popular Democracy, accessed December 13, 2025, https://populardemocracy.org/about/.
61. "The New York City Food Policy Alliance," Equity Advocates, accessed December 13, 2025, https://www.nyequityadvocates.org/community-organizing.

9. HOW ACTIVISTS EVALUATE THEIR WORK

1. For background on the sexual and reproductive health justice movement, see Kelli Stidham Hall, Goleen Samari, Samantha Garbers, Sara E. Casey, Dazon Dixon Diallo, Miriam Orcutt et al., "Centring Sexual and Reproductive Health and Justice in the Global COVID-19 Response," *Lancet* 395, no. 10231 (2020): 1175–1177; Zakiya Luna and Kristin Luker, "Reproductive Justice," *Annual Review of Law and Social Science* 9, no. 1 (2013): 327–352; Kimala Price, "What Is Reproductive Justice? How Women of Color Activists Are Redefining the Pro-Choice Paradigm," *Meridians* 19, no. S1 (2020): 340–362; Loretta Ross, "Understanding Reproductive Justice," in *Feminist Theory Reader*, ed. Carole Ruth McCann, Seung-Kyung Kim, and Emek Ergun (Routledge, 2020); Loretta J. Ross, "Reproductive Justice as Intersectional Feminist Activism," *Souls* 19, no. 3 (2017): 286–314; Loretta Ross and Rickie Solinger, *Reproductive Justice: An Introduction* (University of California Press, 2017).
2. "Black Women on Universal Health Care Reform," ad placed by Women of African Descent for Reproductive Justice, *Washington Post*, August 16, 1994, https://www.fordfoundation.org/wp-content/uploads/2020/02/black-women-health-care-reform.jpg.
3. "Sexual and Reproductive Justice," New York City Department of Health, accessed December 13, 2025, https://www.nyc.gov/site/doh/health/health-topics/sexual-reproductive-justice-nyc.page#.

4. Joy Press, "How the First Abortion Speak-Out Revolutionized Activism," *Vanity Fair*, October 19, 2022, https://www.vanityfair.com/news/2022/10/abortion-stories-speakout.
5. Edith Evans Asbury, "Women Break Up Abortion Hearing," *New York Times*, February 14, 1969, 42.
6. Susan Brownmiller, "Everywoman's Abortions: 'The Oppressor Is Man,'" *Village Voice*, March 27, 1969.
7. Press, "How the First Abortion Speak-Out Revolutionized Activism."
8. Bill Kovach, "Rockefeller, Signing Abortion Bill, Credits Women's Groups," *New York Times*, April 12, 1970, 47.
9. Geoff Watts, "Jean Pakter," *Lancet* 380, no. 9837 (2012): 104.
10. James Colgrove, *Epidemic City: The Politics of Public Health in New York* (Russell Sage Foundation, 2011), 69–71.
11. Jean Pakter and Frieda Nelson, "Abortion in New York City: The First Nine Months," *Family Planning Perspectives* 3, no. 3 (1971): 5–12.
12. Jean Pakter, Donna O'Hare, Frieda Nelson, and Martin Svigir, "Two Years Experience in New York City with the Liberalized Abortion Law—Progress and Problems," *American Journal of Public Health* 63, no. 6 (1973): 524–535.
13. Roe v. Wade, 410 U.S. 113 (1973).
14. "Douglas v. Holloman: Historic Case," Center for Constitutional Rights, last modified October 9, 2007, https://ccrjustice.org/home/what-we-do/our-cases/douglas-v-holloman.
15. Jennifer Nelson, *Women of Color and the Reproductive Rights Movement* (NYU Press, 2003), 140–142.
16. Felicia Kornbluh, *A Women's Life Is a Human Life* (Grove Press, 2023), 243–249.
17. Kornbluh, 236–237.
18. Kornbluh, 261.
19. Judy Klemesrud, "Complacency on Abortion: A Warning to Women," *New York Times*, January 23, 1978, A18.
20. Joyce Wilcox, "The Face of Women's Health: Helen Rodriguez-Trias," *American Journal of Public Health* 92, no. 4 (2002): 566–569.
21. Kornbluh, *A Women's Life Is a Human Life*, 306.
22. Kornbluh, 280.
23. Kornbluh, 251.
24. CARASA News, "Principles of Unity," *CARASA News*, January 1980, Sophia Smith Collection, Smith College, https://compass.fivecolleges.edu/object/smith:1356807.
25. CARASA News.
26. Ros Petchesky and Rayna Rapp, *Women Under Attack: Abortion, Sterilization, and Reproductive Freedom* (Committee for Abortion Rights and Against Sterilization Abuse, 1979), 11.
27. Kornbluh, *A Women's Life Is a Human Life*, 264–266.
28. Kornbluh, 263.
29. Kornbluh, 237.

30. Petchesky and Rapp, *Women Under Attack*, ix.
31. Petchesky and Rapp, 61–62.
32. Ashley Fetters, "Everybody Cares About Pregnancy Discrimination," *Atlantic*, August 3, 2018, https://www.theatlantic.com/family/archive/2018/08/everyone-cares-about-pregnancy-discrimination/566717/.
33. Dina Bakst and Sarah Brafman, "Testimony Before the New York City Commission on Human Rights, January 30, 2019," A Better Balance, accessed December 13, 2025, https://www.abetterbalance.org/wp-content/uploads/2019/03/Testimony_PregnancyCaregiver_FINAL.pdf.
34. Cited in Fetters, "Everybody Cares About Pregnancy Discrimination."
35. Mark Evan Edwards, "Pregnancy Discrimination Litigation: Legal Erosion of Capitalist Ideology Under Equal Employment Opportunity Law," *Social Forces* 75, no. 1 (1996): 247–268.
36. Bakst and Brafman, "Testimony Before the New York City Commission on Human Rights."
37. "Why We Need the Pregnant Workers Fairness Act: Stories of Real Women (2012)," A Better Balance, January 29, 2019, https://www.abetterbalance.org/resources/why-we-need-the-pregnant-workers-fairness-act-stories-of-real-women-2014/.
38. "It Shouldn't Be a Heavy Lift," A Better Balance, January 1, 2013, https://www.abetterbalance.org/resources/it-shouldnt-be-a-heavy-lift/.
39. "Dr. Wendy Chavkin, Letter to Council Member James Vacca," A Better Balance, November 29, 2012, https://www.abetterbalance.org/resources/chavkin-letter/.
40. Bakst and Brafman, "Testimony Before the New York City Commission on Human Rights, January 30, 2019."
41. Bakst and Brafman.
42. Grace Segers, "Ocasio-Cortez's Victory Is Already Reshaping New York Politics," City and State New York, June 28, 2018, https://www.cityandstateny.com/politics/2018/06/ocasio-cortezs-victory-is-already-reshaping-new-york-politics/178319/.
43. Sophie Gardner, "The Decade-Long Journey to End Pregnancy Discrimination," *Politico*, July 7, 2023, https://www.politico.com/newsletters/women-rule/2023/07/07/the-decade-long-journey-to-pregnancy-accommodations-00105167.
44. Dina Bakst, "Pregnant, and Pushed Out of a Job," *New York Times*, January 30, 2012, https://www.nytimes.com/2012/01/31/opinion/pregnant-and-pushed-out-of-a-job.html.
45. Gardner, "The Decade-Long Journey to End Pregnancy Discrimination."
46. In the last few years, activists and scholars have debated what words to use to describe those who are pregnant. Some advocate the use of "pregnant people" to acknowledge the fact that sex doesn't always align with gender identity and that transgender women who identify as men can become pregnant. Others use the term "pregnant women," among others. Some feminists make the case that since the vast majority of pregnancies occur in women, and society has historically discriminated against pregnant women, dropping the term "women" risks erasing that history. I recognize the value of open

discussion of what language to use and the strong feelings on all sides. I choose to use "pregnant women and others" as the generic term and "pregnant women" in other cases. For more on this topic, see Jessica Clarke, "Pregnant People?." *Columbia Law Review* 119, no. 6 (2019): 173–199; Marisa Gates, "Transgender Pregnancies and the PDA," *Tulane Journal of Law and Sexuality* 31 (2022): 75; and Kinnon R. MacKinnon, Ariel Lefkowitz, Gianni R. Lorello, Brett Schrewe, Sophie Soklaridis, and Ayelet Kuper, "Recognizing and Renaming in Obstetrics: How Do We Take Better Care with Language?," *Obstetric Medicine* 14, no. 4 (2021): 201–203.

47. Joseph Goldstein, "Why New York Faltered in Making Childbirth Safer for Black Mothers," *New York Times*, January 7, 2024, A1.
48. "Four in 5 Pregnancy-Related Deaths in the U.S. Are Preventable," United States Centers for Disease Control, September 19, 2022, https://www.cdc.gov/media/releases/2022/p0919-pregnancy-related-deaths.html#.
49. "President's Corner: NYHealth Testimony on Maternal Mortality and Morbidity in New York City," New York Heath Foundation, December 7, 2020, https://nyhealthfoundation.org/2020/12/09/nyhealth-testimony-on-maternal-mortality-and-morbidity-in-new-york-city/.
50. Heather H. Burris, Molly Passarella, Sara C. Handley, Sindhu K. Srinivas, and Scott A. Lorch, "Black-White Disparities in Maternal In-Hospital Mortality According to Teaching and Black-Serving Hospital Status," *American Journal of Obstetrics and Gynecology* 225, no. 1 (2021): 83.e1–83.e9; Elizabeth A. Howell, Natalia N. Egorova, Amy Balbierz, Jennifer Zeitlin, and Paul L. Hebert, "Site of Delivery Contribution to Black-White Severe Maternal Morbidity Disparity," *American Journal of Obstetrics and Gynecology* 215, no. 2 (2016): 143–152.
51. Dána-Ain Davis, "Obstetric Racism: The Racial Politics of Pregnancy, Labor, and Birthing," *Medical Anthropology* 38, no. 7 (2019): 560–573.
52. Diksha Sundrival, "How Did Cordielle Street and Sha-Asia Semple Die?," *Cinemaholic*, July 20, 2022, https://thecinemaholic.com/how-did-cordielle-street-and-sha-asia-semple-die/.
53. Claudia Irizarry Aponte, " 'Every Day I Wake Up Fighting For Her': A Year After the Childbirth Death of Amber Rose Isaac, What's Changed?," *City*, April 20, 2021, https://www.thecity.nyc/2021/04/20/year-after-childbirth-death-of-amber-rose-isaac-whats-changed/.
54. Jessica Madris, "Why Did This Black Woman Die During Treatment for Postpartum Depression?," *Daily Beast*, November 8, 2021, https://www.thedailybeast.com/why-did-denise-williams-a-black-woman-die-during-treatment-for-postpartum-depression.
55. See, for example, Linda Villarosa, "Why America's Black Mothers and Babies Are in a Life-or-Death Crisis," *New York Times Magazine*, April 11, 2018, https://www.nytimes.com/2018/04/11/magazine/black-mothers-babies-death-maternal-mortality.html; Duaa Eldeib, "She Says Doctors Ignored Her Concerns About Her Pregnancy. For Many Black Women, It's a Familiar Story," *Pro Publica*, December 27, 2022,

https://www.propublica.org/article/stillbirths-pregnancy-mothers-parents-racial-disparities#:.

56. April M. Falconi, Samantha G. Bromfield, Trúc Tang, Demetria Malloy, Denae Blanco, Susan Disciglio, et al., "Doula Care Across the Maternity Care Continuum and Impact on Maternal Health: Evaluation of Doula Programs Across Three States Using Propensity Score Matching," *EClinicalMedicine* 50 (2022), https://www.thelancet.com/journals/eclinm/article/PIIS2589-5370(22)00261-9/fulltext.
57. Michelle Zambrano, "Testimony Before Joint—Senate Standing Committee on Health, Mental Health, and Medicaid Reimbursement on Integration of Doula Services in NY State, March 7, 2023," New York Coalition for Doula Access, https://www.nysenate.gov/sites/default/files/ny_coalition_for_doula_access_n.pdf.
58. Andrea J. Wang, "Gutierrez Touts New Doula Program," *Bushwick Daily*, September 26, 2022, https://bushwickdaily.com/news/gutierrez-new-city-doula-program/?utm_sour.
59. Olga Segura, "Bx (Re)Birth and Progress—the Black Birth Workers Caring for Bronx Mothers," *Bronx Frontlines*, March 31, 2023, https://bronxfrontlines.substack.com/p/bx-rebirth-and-progressthe-black.
60. Marie Runyon interview with Katy Cecen, transcript, "Professionalism, Activism, & Politics in Birth Care," *Your Birth Partner Podcast*, December 14, 2020, https://yourbirthpartners.org/transcripts/#027.
61. Julia Chinyere Oparah, "Introduction: Beyond Coercion and Malign Neglect: Black Women and the Struggle for Birth Justice," in *Birthing Justice*, ed. Alicia D. Bonaparte and Julia Chinyere Oparah (Routledge, 2023).
62. "Council Passes Historic Maternal Health Package to Help Address Racial Disparities, Most Severely Affecting Black Women and Birthing People," New York City Council, August 11, 2022, https://council.nyc.gov/press/2022/08/11/2240/.
63. Paige Bellenbaum, testimony, Committees on Women and Gender Equity and on Mental Health, Disabilities and Addiction, New York City Council, June 25,2024, https://legistar.council.nyc.gov/View.ashx?M=F&ID=13184045&GUID=0D2FA824-273A-438A-9114-9EC30D403412.
64. Lorena Kurousias, testimony, Committees on Women and Gender Equity and on Mental Health, Disabilities and Addiction, New York City Council, June 25,2024, https://legistar.council.nyc.gov/View.ashx?M=F&ID=13184045&GUID=0D2FA824-273A-438A-9114-9EC30D403412=.
65. "Black Women on Universal Health Care Reform," ad placed by Women of African Descent for Reproductive Justice, *Washington Post*, August 16, 1994, https://www.fordfoundation.org/wp-content/uploads/2020/02/black-women-health-care-reform.jpg.
66. Suzanne Staggenborg, "Movement and Countermovement Mobilization in the US Abortion Conflict," *PS: Political Science & Politics* 58, no. 1 (2025): 65–68.
67. Barbara Klugman, " 'Effective Social Justice Advocacy: A Theory of Change Framework for Assessing Progress': Reflections on the Terrain Since Its Publication in 2011," *Sexual and Reproductive Health Matters* 31, no. 3 (2023): 2267199.

68. Barbara Klugman, "Effective Social Justice Advocacy: A Theory-of-Change Framework for Assessing Progress," *Reproductive Health Matters* 19, no. 38 (2011): 146–162.
69. Klugman.
70. Susana Otálvaro, Juan Miguel Gallego, and Paul Rodríguez-Lesmes, "De-Normalizing Smoking in Urban Areas: Public Smoking Bans and Smoking Prevalence," *Economics & Human Biology* 48 (2023): 101202.
71. Sanjay Basu, Ankita Meghani, and Arjumand Siddiqi, "Evaluating the Health Impact of Large-Scale Public Policy Changes: Classical and Novel Approaches," *Annual Review of Public Health* 38, no. 1 (2017): 351–370.
72. Abigail Watts, Anna L. Araiza, Cristina R. Fernández, Leslie Rosenthal, Ileana Vargas-Rodriguez, Nathalie Duroseau et al., "The Campaign for Universal Free Lunch in New York City: Lessons Learned," *Pediatrics* 148, no. 4 (2021): e2020049734.
73. Amy Ellen Schwartz and Michah W. Rothbart, "Let Them Eat Lunch: The Impact of Universal Free Meals on Student Performance," *Journal of Policy Analysis and Management* 39, no. 2 (2020): 376–410.
74. Some useful sources on evaluating activism include Michael C. Fagen, Ehren Reed, Jackie Williams Kaye, and Leonard Jack Jr., "Advocacy Evaluation: What It Is and Where to Find Out More About It," *Health Promotion Practice* 10, no. 4 (2009): 482–484; Juniper Glass, " 'Advocates Change the World; Evaluation Can Help': A Literature Review and Key Insights from the Practice of Advocacy Evaluation," *Canadian Journal of Program Evaluation* 32, no. 1 (2017): 46–64; Alissa Marchant, Cory Georgopoulos, and Shelli Golson-Mickens, *Collective Power Framework and Indicators: Measuring the Redistribution of Power in Coalitions* (Innovation Network, 2024), https://www.innonet.org/media/Collective-Power-Framework-and-Indicators_Final.pdf; Manuel Pastor, Jennifer Ito, and Rachel Rosner, *Metrics That Matter for Building, Scaling, and Funding Social Movements* (USC Dornsife Program for Environmental and Regional Equity, 2011), https://search.issuelab.org/resource/transactions-transformations-translations-metrics-that-matter-for-building-scaling-and-funding-social-movements.html; and Sonia Taddy-Sandino, Anna Saltzman, and Shayla Spilker, "The Art and Science of Developmental and Advocacy Evaluation," *New Directions for Evaluation* 2021, no. 171 (2021): 19–29.
75. Some useful references on community-based participatory research and participatory action research include Jason Corburn, *Street Science: Community Knowledge and Environmental Health Justice* (MIT Press, 2005); Flora Cornish, Nancy Breton, Ulises Moreno-Tabarez, Jenna Delgado, Mohi Rua, Ama de-Graft Aikins et al. "Participatory Action Research," *Nature Reviews Methods Primers* 3, no. 1 (2023): 34; Meredith Minkler and Nicholas Freudenberg, "From Community-Based Participatory Research to Policy Change," *Handbook of Engaged Scholarship: Contemporary Landscapes, Future Directions* 2 (2010): 275–294; Amy J. Schulz, Barbara A. Israel, Angela G. Reyes, Donele Wilkins, and Stuart Batterman, "Promoting Health Equity with Community-Based Participatory Research: The Community Action to Promote Healthy Environments (CAPHE) Partnership," in *Global Handbook of Health Promotion Research*, vol. 3, *Doing*

Health Promotion Research, ed. Didier Jourdan and Louise Potvin (Springer International Publishing, 2023); Nina Wallerstein, Bonnie Duran, John G. Oetzel, and Meredith Minkler, eds., *Community-Based Participatory Research for Health: Advancing Social and Health Equity* (John Wiley and Sons, 2017).

76. Ava Kikut-Stein, Kathleen Givan, Paulette Branson, Jeffrey Fishman, Kavon Bailey, Michelle Paolicelli et al., "Youth Participatory Action Communication Research: A Model for Developing Youth-Driven Health Campaigns," *Health Communication* 40, no. 6 (2025): 1062–1077; Abby C. King, Feyisayo A. Odunitan-Wayas, Moushumi Chaudhury, Maria Alejandra Rubio, Michael Baiocchi, Tracy Kolbe-Alexander et al., "Community-Based Approaches to Reducing Health Inequities and Fostering Environmental Justice Through Global Youth-Engaged Citizen Science," *International Journal of Environmental Research and Public Health* 18, no. 3 (2021): 892; Peggy M. Shepard, "Advancing Environmental Justice Through Community-Based Participatory Research," *Environmental Health Perspectives* 110, no. S2 (2002): 139–140.

77. David Michaels, *The Triumph of Doubt: Dark Money and the Science of Deception* (Oxford University Press, 2020).

78. See Karen M. Douglas, Joseph E. Uscinski, Robbie M. Sutton, Aleksandra Cichocka, Turkay Nefes, Chee Siang Ang et al., "Understanding Conspiracy Theories," *Political Psychology* 40 (2019): 3–35; Porismita Borah, "Politicization of Health Issues: Misinformation and Social Media," in *Communication and Misinformation: Crisis Events in the Age of Social Media*, ed. Kevin B. Wright (Wiley-Blackwell, 2025); Marie-Jeanne Leonard and Frederick L. Philippe, "Conspiracy Theories: A Public Health Concern and How to Address It," *Frontiers in Psychology* 12 (2021): 682931.

79. Kyrah Berthiaume, "Protecting Public Health Amid Misinformation and Scientific Illiteracy: Federal Actions Necessitating State Interventions," Social Science Research Network, April 13, 2025, https://ssrn.com/abstract=5326000.

80. Petchesky and Rapp, *Women Under Attack*, 11.

10. WHAT NEXT? TRANSLATING LESSONS INTO PRACTICE

1. New York City Comptroller Brad Lander, *Spotlight Minimum Wage* (Bureau of Budget, February 2023), https://comptroller.nyc.gov/wp-content/uploads/documents/Spotlight-Minimum-Wage.pdf.

2. New York City Comptroller Brad Lander, *Evictions Up, Representation Down: How New York City Is Undermining the Right to Counsel* (Bureau of Policy and Organizing, May 2025), https://comptroller.nyc.gov/reports/evictions-up-representation-down/.

3. New York State Comptroller Thomas DiNapoli, *New Yorkers in Need: Homelessness in New York State* (Office of the New York State Comptroller, January 2025), https://www.osc.ny.gov/files/reports/pdf/new-yorkers-in-need-homelessness-nys.pdf.

4. Lindsey Smith Tallie and Barry Popkin, "The Promise and Pitfalls of 'Make America Healthy Again,'" *Lancet Diabetes & Endocrinology* 13, no. 4 (2025): 274–275; Lawrence O.

Gostin, Sarah A. Wetter, and Peter Lurie, "Can a New Commission Make America Healthy Again?," *JAMA Health Forum* 6, no. 3 (2025): e251304–e251304.

5. Centers for Disease Control and Prevention, "Ten Great Public Health Achievements—United States, 1900–1999," *MMWR: Morbidity and Mortality Weekly Report* 48, no. 12 (1999): 241–243; Barbara Starfield, "Is US Health Really the Best in the World?," *JAMA* 284, no. 4 (2000): 483–485; Laudan Aron and Steven H. Woolf, eds., *US Health in International Perspective: Shorter Lives, Poorer Health* (National Academies Press, 2013); "Personal Health Issues (2001–2024)," Gallup, accessed December 18, 2025, https://news.gallup.com/poll/1648/personal-health-issues.aspx#.
6. Donatella Della Porta, "Conceptualising Backlash Movements: A (Patch-Worked) Perspective from Social Movement Studies," *British Journal of Politics and International Relations* 22, no. 4 (2020): 585–597.
7. Sara E. Gorman, *The Anatomy of Deception: Conspiracy Theories, Distrust, and Public Health in America* (Oxford University Press, 2024); Michael E. Mann and Tom Toles, *The Madhouse Effect: How Climate Change Denial Is Threatening Our Planet, Destroying Our Politics, and Driving Us Crazy* (Columbia University Press, 2016).
8. M. Anthony Mills and Price St. Clair, "The Strange New Politics of Science," *Issues in Science & Technology* 41, no. 3 (2025); *The MAHA Report: Make Our Children Healthy Again* (White House, 2025), https://www.whitehouse.gov/wp-content/uploads/2025/05/MAHA-Report-The-White-House.pdf.
9. Alfred Sköld, "Hope in the Time of Hopelessness," *Nordic Psychology*, March 30, 2025, 1–14.
10. See, for example, Josh Bivens and Asha Banerjee, "Inequality's Drag on Aggregate Demand," Economic Policy Institute, May 24, 2022, https://www.epi.org/publication/inequalitys-drag-on-aggregate-demand/; Fahd Ahmed, Tom Angotti, Jennifer Jones Austin, Shawn Blumberg, and Robin Steinberg, "The Long Crisis: Economic Inequality in New York City," *CUNY Law Review* 18, no. 1 (2014): 153; Anastasia Koutavas, Sophie Collyer, Yajun Jia, and Christopher Wimer, *Spotlight on the Racial Wealth Gap in New York City* (Center on Poverty and Social Policy at Columbia University; Regional Plan Association, January 2025), https://robinhood.org/wp-content/uploads/2025/02/PT_Racial_Wealth-Gap_1.21_rev_FINAL.pdf.
11. "$1.3 Million for New York City's Grassroots Movements," North Star Fund, March 20, 2025, https://northstarfund.org/2025/03/nyc-grants/.
12. "New Statewide Survey Highlights New Yorkers' Concerns About Healthcare Affordability," Community Service Society, March 10, 2022, https://www.cssny.org/news/entry/new-statewide-survey-highlights-new-yorkers-concerns-about-healthcare-affor#.
13. Jeffrey M. Jones, "More in U.S. See Health Coverage as Government Responsibility," Gallup, December 9, 2024, https://news.gallup.com/poll/654101/health-coverage-government-responsibility.aspx.
14. Alliance for Safety and Justice and the Independent Rikers Commission, *New York City Crime Survivors Speak: A Citywide Survey of Victims' Views on Safety and Justice* (Alliance

for Safety and Justice; Independent Rikers Commission, May 2024), https://static1.squarespace.com/static/5b6de4731aef1de914f43628/t/671133ff8d73f94748bca0d6/1729180672733/NYC+Crime+Survivors+Speak+Report+-+October+2024.pdf.

15. Samuel J. Abrams, "Capitalism Isn't the Enemy—What Young Voters Really Want," Deseret News, July 11, 2025, https://www.aei.org/op-eds/capitalism-isnt-the-enemy-what-young-voters-really-want/.
16. Travis N. Taylor, "American Voters Overwhelmingly Back MAHA Policies, Support Spans Party Lines," Center for Excellence in Polling, May 16, 2025, https://excellenceinpolling.com/poll/american-voters-overwhelmingly-back-maha-policies-support-spans-party-lines/.
17. "Surprising New Research Finds Americans Oppose Technology That Kills Us, Support Technology That Saves Lives," Tavern Research, August 21,2025, https://www.tavernresearch.com/research-and-writings/voters-split-on-rfk-jr-health-agenda.
18. Erin McAleer, "Op-Ed: We Can't 'Make America Healthy Again' Without SNAP and Medicaid," Foodtank, July 2025, https://foodtank.com/news/2025/07/op-ed-we-cant-make-america-healthy-again-without-snap-and-medicaid/.
19. Ezra Klein, "MAHA Is a Bad Answer to a Good Question," *New York Times*, August 22, 2025, https://www.nytimes.com/2025/08/22/opinion/ezra-klein-podcast-rachael-bedard-david-wallace-wells.html.
20. This name is not to be confused with the existing New York Alliance for Healthcare Justice, a coalition of health-care workers, faith leaders, community health advocates, and patients fighting for all New Yorkers to have access to affordable, quality care. This worthy new organization (see https://www.nyhjustice.org/aboutfocuses) on health care rather than the full range of health and social justice issues I suggest.
21. World Health Organization, *Primary Health Care: Report of the International Conference on Primary Health Care, Alma-Ata, USSR, 6–12 September 1978* (World Health Organization, 1978).
22. Ravi Narayan and Claudio Schuftan, "People's Health Movement," in *International Encyclopedia of Public Health*, vol. 5, ed. Kristian Heggenhougen and Stella Quah (San Diego Academic Press, 2008).
23. "People's Health Movement at 25: the Struggle for Health for All continues," People's Health Dispatch, December 19, 2025, https://phmovement.org/peoples-health-movement-25-struggle-health-all-continues.
24. See the People's Movement for Health website at https://phmovement.org/.
25. See People's Health Movement, *Global Health Watch 6* (Bloomsbury Academic, 2022); People's Health Movement, *Mobilizing for Health Justice: Global Health Watch 7* (Daraja Press, 2025), https://darajapress.com/publication/mobilizing-for-health-justice-en/.
26. See Chiara Bodini, Martina Consoloni, Valerio D'Avanzo, Delia Da Mosto, Sara Gerotto, Silvia Giaimo et al., "Community Development and Health Promotion in Contemporary Policy: Results from an Action-Research Project in Bologna (Italy)," *Community Development Journal* 58, no. 4 (2023): 614–633; Myrna van Pinxteren, Christopher J. Colvin, and Sara Cooper, "Using Health Information for Community

Activism: A Case Study of the Movement for Change and Social Justice in South Africa," *PLOS Global Public Health* 2, no. 9 (2022): e0000664; Anuj Kapilashrami, Katherine E. Smith, Suzanne Fustukian, Mor Kandlik Eltanani, Sue Laughlin, Tony Robertson et al., "Social Movements and Public Health Advocacy in Action: The UK People's Health Movement," *Journal of Public Health* 38, no. 3 (2016): 413–416.

27. World Health Organization, *Healthy Cities: Effective Approach to a Rapidly Changing World* (World Health Organization, 2020), https://iris.who.int/bitstream/handle/10665/331946/9789240004825-eng.pdf.
28. Shuan Danielli, Hutan Ashrafian, and Ara Darzi, "Healthy City: Global Systematic Scoping Review of City Initiatives to Improve Health with Policy Recommendations," *BMC Public Health* 23, no. 1 (2023): 1277.
29. David Rosner, ed., *Hives of Sickness: Public Health and Epidemics in New York City* (Rutgers University Press, 1995); Richard H. Shryock, "The Origins and Significance of the Public Health Movement in the United States," *Annals of Medical History* 1, no. 6 (1929): 645; Sandra Opdycke, *No One Was Turned Away: The Role of Public Hospitals in New York City Since 1900* (Oxford University Press, 2000); John Duffy, *The Sanitarians: A History of American Public Health* (University of Illinois Press, 1992).
30. David A. Ansell, *County: Life, Death and Politics at Chicago's Public Hospital* (Chicago Review Press, 2003); Jason Corburn, *Cities for life: How Communities Can Recover from Trauma and Rebuild for Health* (Island Press, 2021); Jenna M. Loyd, *Health Rights Are Civil Rights: Peace and Justice Activism in Los Angeles, 1963–1978* (University of Minnesota Press, 2014); Randy Shilts, *And the Band Played On: Politics, People, and the AIDS Epidemic* (Souvenir Press, 2011).
31. See, for example, Hillel W. Cohen and Mary E. Northridge, "Getting Political: Racism and Urban Health," *American Journal of Public Health* 98, no. S1 (2008): S17–S19; Sharon Friel, Marco Akerman, Trevor Hancock, Jacob Kumaresan, Michael Marmot, Thomas Melin et al., "Addressing the Social and Environmental Determinants of Urban Health Equity: Evidence for Action and a Research Agenda," *Journal of Urban Health* 88, no. 5 (2011): 860–874; Suhas Gondi and Dave A. Chokshi, "Cities as Platforms for Population Health: Past, Present, and Future," *Milbank Quarterly* 101, no. S1 (2023): 242; Margit Mayer, "The 'Right to the City' in Urban Social Movements," in *Cities for People, not for Profit*, ed. Neil Brenner, Peter Marcuse, and Margit Mayer (Routledge, 2012); Timothy Milewa and Evelyne de Leeuw, "Reason and Protest in the New Urban Public Health Movement: An Observation on the Sociological Analysis of Political Discourse in the 'Healthy City,'" *British Journal of Sociology* 47, no. 4 (1996): 657–670.
32. Benjamin H. Bradlow, "Urban Social Movements and Local State Capacity," *World Development* 173 (2024): 106415.
33. Bradlow, 106415.
34. Sidney Tarrow, *Movements and Parties: Critical Connections in American Political Development* (Cambridge University Press, 2021).
35. Frederick Douglass, "If There Is No Struggle, There Is No Progress," West India emancipation speech, Canandaigua, New York, August 3, 1857, via Black Past,

January 25, 2007, https://www.blackpast.org/african-american-history/1857-frederick-douglass-if-there-no-struggle-there-no-progress/.

36. Quoted in Maisha-Maureen Auma, "Kimberlé Crenshaw's Influence on My Thinking with Regard to Transformative Justice, in *"Reach Everyone on the Planet . . . ": Kimberlé Crenshaw and Intersectionality*, ed. Gunda Werner Institut in the Heinrich Böll Foundation (Heinrich-Böll-Stiftung, 2019), 28.
37. Jane McAlevey, *No Shortcuts: Organizing for Power in the New Gilded Age* (Oxford University Press, 2016), 10.
38. McAlevey, 179–198.
39. Ashley Dager, "Calls for Healthcare Coverage for Everyone Regardless of Immigration Status," CBS6 News WRGB Albany, March 1, 2023, https://cbs6albany.com/news/local/calls-for-healthcare-coverage-for-everyone-regardless-of-immigration-status.
40. Mark Hannay, "Metro New York Health Care for All," Everybody In: Racial Equity & Medicare for All Conference, April 17, 2023, https://medicareforall23.sched.com/metrohealth.
41. First defined by women of color in 1994 to inform the development of the Clinton health plan, Women of African Descent for Reproductive Justice published a statement signed by more than eight hundred women insisting that any national health-care plan must address the unmet reproductive health needs of Black women.
42. "About Us," Sister Song, accessed December 18, 2025, https://www.sistersong.net/about-x2.
43. Frances Fox Piven and Richard Cloward, *Poor People's Movements: Why They Succeed, How They Fail* (Vintage, 1977), 36.
44. "Political Activism and Advocacy: Driving Policy Change," Everything Policy, July 10, 2024, https://www.everythingpolicy.org/post/political-activism-and-advocacy-driving-policy-change.
45. Joshua B. Freeman, *Working Class New York Life and Labor Since World War II* (New Press, 2000), 125–142.
46. Paul Burstein, "Social Movements and Public Policy," in *How Social Movements Matter*, ed. Marco Giugni, Doug McAdam, and Charles Tilly (University of Minnesota Press, 1999).
47. Nancy MacLean, *Democracy in Chains: The Deep History of the Radical Right's Stealth Plan for America*, 2nd ed. (Penguin, 2023).
48. "Who We Are," Atlas Network, accessed December 18, 2025, https://www.atlasnetwork.org/who-we-are.
49. Sebastian Haunss and Darcy K. Leach, "Social Movement Scenes: Infrastructures of Opposition in Civil Society," in *Civil Societies and Social Movements*, ed. Derrick Purdue (Routledge, 2007).
50. Janet M. Conway, *Edges of Global Justice: The World Social Forum And Its "Others"* (Routledge, 2012).
51. Louisa Chafee, "Total Cost of Three Selected Categories of Unpaid Fines and Charges in New York City," New York City Independent Budget Office, April 5, 2023, https://www.ibo.nyc.ny.us/iboreports/unpaid-fees-fines-letter-april-2023.pdf.

52. Emily A. Benfer, "Contaminated Childhood: How the United States Failed to Prevent the Chronic Lead Poisoning of Low-Income Children and Communities of Color," *Harvard Environmental Law Review* 41 (2017): 493.
53. Kim Phillips-Fein, *Fear City: New York's Fiscal Crisis and the Rise of Austerity Politics* (Metropolitan Books, 2017).
54. Michael Barbaro, "Behind N.Y. Gay Marriage, an Unlikely Mix of Forces," *New York Times*, June 26, 2011, A1.

INDEX

Page numbers in *italics* refer to illustrations.

INDEX